COLONIAL PA

COLONIAL PATHOLOGIES

American Tropical Medicine, Race,

and Hygiene in the Philippines

Warwick Anderson

DUKE UNIVERSITY PRESS   DURHAM AND LONDON   2006

© 2006 Duke University Press

All rights reserved

Printed in the United States of America
on acid-free paper ∞

Designed by Heather Hensley

Typeset in Sabon by Keystone Typesetting, Inc.

Library of Congress Cataloging-in-
Publication Data appear on the last printed
page of this book.

Contents

Acknowledgments

As my interest in the entwined histories of American tropical medicine and racial thought has endured now for most of my career, the intellectual debts that have accumulated are countless. Only the most pressing can be acknowledged here. Charles Rosenberg and Rosemary Stevens guided my first studies of colonial public health at the University of Pennsylvania. At Harvard, Allan Brandt, Arthur Kleinman, Evelynn Hammonds, and Mary Steedly helped me to reshape and develop many of my arguments. Colleagues in the Department of Anthropology, History and Social Medicine at UCSF, and in the History Department at Berkeley—in particular, Adele Clarke, James Vernon, Philippe Bourgois, Vincanne Adams, Tom Laqueur, Sharon Kaufman, and Dorothy Porter—encouraged me to return to the book manuscript and provided inspiration and support. At Madison, I benefited greatly from the advice of colleagues in the Department of Medical History and Bioethics and at the Center for Southeast Asian Studies. Conversations with Judy Leavitt, Rick Keller, Mike Cullinane, Al McCoy, Courtney Johnson, Victor Bascara, and Maria Lepowsky proved especially valuable. Jean von Allmen, with characteristic efficiency, ensured I had time for writing.

Bob Joy, Dan Doeppers, and Barbara Rosenkrantz read earlier versions of the book manuscript and peppered me with their questions, challenges, and doubts. I may not have responded adequately to all of their queries, but without their engagement the book would be the poorer. I was fortunate to have such generous and careful readers.

It was the enthusiasm and support of Vince Rafael that enabled me to complete this book. He and many other scholars of the Philippines, especially Michael Salman and Paul Kramer, have guided me through new territory and provided intellectual sustenance.

I would also like to thank Michelle Murphy, Jono Wearne, Matt Klugman, Martin Gibbs, Chris Shepherd, Peter Phipps, Dan Hamlin, and Kiko Benitez for research assistance. Kiko, too, read much of the manuscript and gave me helpful advice. Gabriela Soto Laveaga assisted with translation of some of the Spanish material and pointed me to Latin American analogies.

Without the enthusiasm and persistence of Ken Wissoker at Duke University Press, it is unlikely that I would ever have completed this book. Ken and Anitra Grisales have smoothed the path to publication and allayed most of the author's anxieties along the way.

This project was supported financially through a fellowship from the Social Science Research Council and the American Council of Learned Societies. I received travel grants from the Rockefeller Archive Center, the University of Pennsylvania, Harvard University, the Pacific Rim Research Program of the University of California, and the University of Wisconsin-Madison.

I am grateful for the assistance of archivists and librarians at the University of Pennsylvania, the College of Physicians of Philadelphia, the American Philosophical Society, the Countway Medical Library and other Harvard libraries, the U.S. National Archives and Records Administration, the Library of Congress, the History of Medicine Division of the National Library of Medicine, the Bentley Library at the University of Michigan, the Bancroft Library at the University of California-Berkeley, the Kalmanowitz Library at UCSF, the Hagley Museum and Library, the Alan Mason Chesney Archives at Johns Hopkins University, the Wisconsin Historical Society Library, the Ebling Library of the University of Wisconsin-Madison, the Rockefeller Archive Center, the U.S. Army Military History Institute at Carlisle Barracks, the Massachusetts Archives, the Philippine National Archives, and the Rizal Library at Ateneo de Manila.

I have presented portions of this work at numerous institutions over the past fifteen years: through comment and discussion on these occasions, the book has emerged much improved. Sections of it have also benefited from the remarks of editors and anonymous reviewers for the following journals: *Critical Inquiry*, the *Bulletin of the History of Medicine*, the *American Historical Review*, *Positions*, and *American Literary History*.

Above all, I want to thank family and friends for gracefully putting up with my peculiar preoccupation with the history of colonial medicine — my own family, of course, but also the family of Ken and Rochelle Goldstein, who looked after me in Philadelphia. It is to the memory of Kenneth S. Goldstein that this book is dedicated.

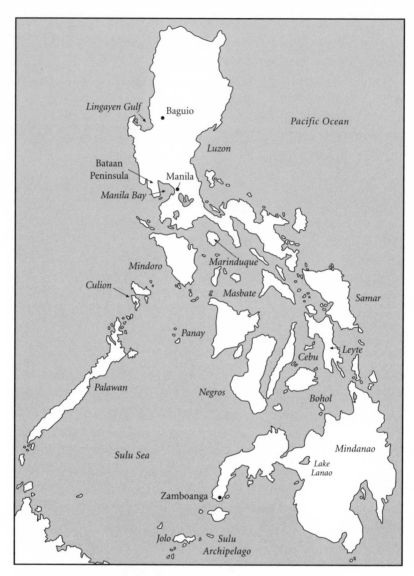

MAP I. Philippine archipelago.

INTRODUCTION

"The only things that matter in this fallen world," Rudyard Kipling advised his friend W. Cameron Forbes in 1913, "are transportation and sanitation."[1] Forbes, the governor-general of the Philippines and a fastidious Harvard man, believed that the greater of these was sanitation. Indeed, since the defeat of Spanish forces in the archipelago in 1898, the American colonial authorities had eagerly taken up the burden of cleansing their newly acquired part of the Orient, attempting to purify not only its public spaces, water, and food, but also the bodies and conduct of the inhabitants. According to Victor G. Heiser, who was director of health in the Philippines from 1905 to 1915, it had to be understood that "the health of these people is the vital question of the Islands. To transform them from the weak and feeble race we have found them into the strong, healthy and enduring people that they may yet become is to lay the foundations for the successful future of the country."[2] American military and civil health officers thus dedicated themselves to registering and refashioning Filipino bodies and social life, to forging an improved sanitary race out of the raw material found in the Philippine *barrio*. Hygiene reform in this particular fallen world was intrinsic to a "civilizing process," which was also an uneven and shallow process of Americanization.

I want in this book to recapture the civic vision of medicine and science in a specific colonial setting. That is, I would like to describe how the political rationality of American colonialism became manifest in a technical discourse on bodily practice, mundane contact, and the banalities of custom and habit. I am suggesting, in particular, that in framing disease potential, medical officers might also assemble a flexible, and sometimes unstable, framework for constituting racial capacities and colonial bodies.[3] Experiencing hygiene thus could also be a means of experiencing empire and race. Indeed, racialized agency was constructed and contested in the colonial Philippines more through the projects of hygiene and bodily reform than any other means — certainly more so than through esoteric anthropological debate.[4]

In the Philippines during the first years of the twentieth century, military medical officers developed a novel, and at first distinctively American, understanding of the tropics and the bodies inhabiting the region. The exigencies of guerilla combat in the archipelago had reshaped the American medical officer's knowledge of risk and containment, of stress and fit, suggesting new methods of tropical disease control and population management. Fears of contagion, of the pathological consequences of contact with native races, largely supplanted older assumptions of environmental danger, of the hazards of geographical displacement. The mismatch of race and place — which once had suggested the inevitable degeneration of Europeans in conditions of moist heat — soon seemed less threatening to invading whites than contact with diseased or meretriciously "healthy" natives. Disease prevention, in these circumstances, required behavioral and bodily reform of local inhabitants, the sort of discipline and surveillance that could turn raw army recruits into obedient and hygienic soldiers. Segregation, with the construction of hygienic enclaves for whites, generally seemed impractical in the Philippines. In order to contain microbial *insurrectos*, the Philippine *barrio* would instead come to resemble a well-ordered American army camp.[5] New germ theories informed emerging techniques of population management; microbiologists provided the intelligence and monitored the progress of hygiene reform, following a colonial military logic.

When military medical officers later marched confidently into the civil health service, the rules of sanitary engagement changed little. As Reynaldo C. Ileto puts it, "The image of the conquering soldier soon became transformed into that of the crusading sanitary inspector."[6] Bodily and behavioral reforms came to be promoted less as techniques of pacification than as part of a civilizing project, as the development of "republican" virtue and self-restraint among Filipinos, or simply as progress and modernization.[7] By 1902, the well-ordered laboratory, more than the army camp, appeared to represent the exemplary site for modern Filipino bodies and culture: the archipelago was frequently characterized as a laboratory of hygienic modernity. American medical officers linked the attainment of Filipino self-government to corporeal and cultural transformation, to the establishment of hygienic identities in the colonial laboratory, but most of them expected the process would take generations. They triaged Filipinos as infantile, immature subjects, unready yet for self-government of body or polity — as *formes frustes* stalled on the trajectory from native to citizen.[8] In the colonial setting, the racializing of liberal governmentality implied the conditions of its deferral.[9] Accordingly, American administration of disease control and medico-moral uplift, the civilizing project, would have to continue indefinitely. Many Filipinos, however, thought otherwise, and by the 1920s they had secured control of the health service, changing its patterns of deployment. American medical officers dispersed, some back to the army, others to colonize the emerging international health services and the urban public health departments of the United States, adapting Philippine techniques as they went.

This book charts the colonial development and deferral of what might be called "biomedical citizenship."[10] Feminist scholars have argued that citizenship in Europe and North America has in practice been differentiated by gender; they point to attempts (always partial and flawed) to construct a masculine public sphere of abstract rights and a feminine private sphere of affect, desire, and embodiment.[11] The apparently disembodied individual citizen of modernity conventionally was predicated on a white, male norm. Nancy Stepan has therefore suggested that in the colonial setting "the history of embodiment must be seen as part of the story of citizenship and its limits."[12] In the Philippines, this means tracking the development of civic bacteriology — following medical bureaucrats as they quickly moved from mapping biological difference onto a "tropical" territory to mapping human difference and civilizational potential in the new American possessions. Microbiology rapidly became civic destiny, organized into a typology that positioned immature native germ-carriers (and distributors) against responsible, clean, yet especially vulnerable whites.[13] But on this occasion the taxonomy was not fixed: some Filipinos might eventually be trained to behave hygienically; they could, so it seemed, metamorphose into recovering natives and therefore embark on the career of the probationary citizen-subject, on becoming modern. Progressive American medicos imagined themselves eventually, many generations hence, producing germ-free Filipino citizens: it is in this sense that colonial hygiene became a liberal strategy of deferral, not exclusion.[14]

Racial hygiene in the Philippines was a harbinger of development regimes elsewhere. By the 1920s, other colonial states were not just policing the boundaries of civility but extending them, canalizing and mobilizing the bodies and cultures of the colonized along with those of the colonizers. A perfunctory and still largely typological social evolutionism was suggesting new, though faint and fraught, trajectories for native subjectivity, fresh possibilities for the technologies of self-government. Frequently, American activities in the Philippines seemed to offer models for such scientific and progressive intervention. But historians of colonial medicine who focus on the nineteenth century or perhaps on less liberal regimes generally have not analyzed this distinctive late-colonial mode of population management and identity formation. Ann Laura Stoler, for example, has argued that in the Dutch East Indies during this period, "native and mixed-blood 'character' was viewed as fixed in a way that European 'character' was not"—even though she recognizes that in other ways the "social geography of empire underwent profound restructuring in the early-twentieth century."[15] Toward the end of *Colonizing the Body*, David Arnold observes that after 1914 biomedical ideas and practices began to exert more influence over the identities and relationships of the Western-educated Indian middle class as well as "to infiltrate and inform public debate and political language to a quite remarkable degree."[16] But he does not elaborate on this concluding insight. If many historians of colonial medicine appear thus to stop prematurely, historians of international health services and developmental states may start their narrative too late. For example, Frederick Cooper, like most other African historians, assumes that the developmentalist, or "modernizing," colonial state dates only from the 1940s (as it may well in sub-Saharan Africa, though not elsewhere).[17] What I want to do here, then, is to suggest continuities between the late-colonial civilizing process and international development projects—that is, I want to trace the genealogy of development back to the medical mobilization of civic potential in the Philippines in the early twentieth century.[18]

American hygienists were, in effect, bringing the adult Filipino into the colonial public sphere as both menace and mimic—"half devil and half child," as Kipling put it in his verse "The White Man's Burden." In framing a Filipino social body, medical officers claimed authority over the most private of daily activities; personal and domestic life became constituents of the public performance of personal and domestic hygiene.[19] The Filipino emerged in this medico-moral vision as an immature, contaminating type, but also as a potentially reformable one if subject to the right techniques of the body. Thus the construction of colonial boundaries, which were always too porous anyhow, was often less compelling than the fabrication and management of colonial trajectories.[20] The sense of menace — "a difference that is almost total but not quite" — could shade into an obsession with mimicry, "a difference that is almost nothing but not quite."[21] In Philippine public health programs during this period, such figures of paranoia and narcissism, expressed in terms of potential for contamination or as gradations of civic virtue, are held in tension with each other.

The examination of the corporeal contingencies of civic status represents the lower stratum of an emerging body of literature on identity formation in the Philippines under the Spanish and American regimes. Reynaldo C. Ileto has reconstructed Philippine revolutionary mentality and traced the invention of "the Filipino" in the late nineteenth century. In *White Love*, Vicente L. Rafael described the American colonial interest in racializing Filipinos and their history.[22] During the past few years, Michael Salman has identified the Philippine prison as a site for creating self-governing subjects, for the production of citizens, laborers, and commodities. Paul Kramer implicates anthropology and exhibitions in the construction of a new colonial order in the archipelago.[23] Of course the historian of medicine has to work with the markings of bodies, Filipino and American, and especially their orifices and excretions, the more private and intimate parts of colonial power. It seems to me that what we all do, in our various ways, high and low, is reveal the construction of a "sensationalized racial contrast" in the Philippines and explain how colonial subjects, thus rendered visible and accessible, would then be trained or prepared for conversion or assimilation, an end indefinitely delayed.[24] As Michael Taussig, in a different context, once put it, "The frontier provides the setting within which the problem of discipline magnifies the savagery that has to be repressed and canalized by the civilizing process."[25] Or one might say that in the colonial laboratory of the Philippines, American health officers were licensed to express a fascination with that which the native cannot be allowed fully to repress.

In imagining their new colony as a laboratory of hygiene and modernity, American medical officers were indulging in a form of magical thinking, creating sympathetic associations in the hope of changing the world. For most colonial bureaucrats, the laboratory not only was an appealing representational space, but also seemed to allow a manipulation of the scale of things, so that macro may become micro and then be magnified again.[26] This scalar technology proved especially alluring in a colonial setting, where so much seemed macroscopically complex or otherwise uncontrollable until translated into docile specimens. But conditions in the archipelago could never become thoroughly laboratory-like. Most Filipinos failed to feel the attraction of a laboratory, and not even the more fastidious of Americans really wanted to spend all their lives in one. The rhetoric of the "colonial laboratory" lingered, but the sense of control it expressed was often belied in the turmoil of the Philippine public sphere, where the laboratory might either be unknown or deemed irrelevant or mistaken.[27] Rather than a site of absolute control, the real laboratory was, for Filipinos, more likely a site of contestation, negotiation, or apathy. But the laboratory did, nonetheless, exert some influence on local conditions; eventually it helped to shape the way Filipinos thought about their bodies and their society; and it adjusted and regulated spatial practice, even if it was never completely hegemonic.

In the colonial arena of public health work, the brashness and bluster of white American males as well as their moments of diffidence and self-distrust are revealed with startling clarity. American medical officers in the Philippines were all white men, whereas in the United States during this period some women had begun to infiltrate public health departments. A few American women served as medical missionaries, but they remained marginal to the clubs and offices of Manila. Filipino women increasingly resorted to nursing, and some others graduated from the local medical schools, but their presence was not felt in high-status public health activities until the early 1920s. The Bureau of Health was thus predominantly a distant theater for the rehearsal and performance of white American male virtue.

Begun as a study of the colonial inculcation of hygiene and civic decorum in Filipinos, the book has become, perhaps more penetratingly, an examination of the distressed and assertive colonial culture of bourgeois white males — which was always more than simply a vessel for paranoia and narcissism, though it was that too.[28] As they investigated, treated, and attempted to discipline allegedly errant Filipinos, American medicos were revealing previously hidden aspects of their own characters and disclosing their fears and anxieties in alien circumstances. Most of the colonial health officers had graduated from the reformed, scientific medical schools of major eastern universities; many had transferred directly into the civil health services from the army medical department; some moved up through the ranks of the expanding U.S. Public Health Service. They tended to see themselves as progressive and pragmatic representatives of modern American science—a laboratory science they hoped to substitute for politics. They clung to Protestant rectitude, affirmed the manly ideals of self-mastery and restraint, and expressed contempt for softness. They extolled relentless industry and strenuous physical activity in circumstances that seemed inimical to such virtues. Obsessed with systematic documentation and the marshalling of fact, they demonstrated confidence in the power of bureaucratic intervention and technology to transform Philippine environment and society.[29] The American tropics presented special opportunities for progressive bureaucratic activities, but also their testing ground. Many American scientists and physicians— some of them unmarried or socially isolated—found the conditions extremely trying, and a few of these "prosthetic Gods" broke down, lost their nerve, and became unmanned.[30] In the tropics, then, American scientists and physicians felt compelled to reinvent their whiteness and harden their masculinity. Alongside the science of native pathology, health officers developed a positive and perhaps sadly overassertive science of white physiology and mentality. White male bodies and white male minds were repeatedly differentiated from those of Filipinos and insulated from apparently hostile and degenerative surroundings, especially from moist heat, germs, and Filipino social life. Physicians sought to construct a white corporeal armature—a hard, sporty indifference—to their multiply challenging milieu. But often their whiteness and manliness proved disappointingly fragile or corruptible.[31]

In order to appreciate the scope of this book, it is important to consider the "colonial" as a process and category in the history of medicine and public health more generally. By this I mean more than the mere accumulation of homologies or family resemblances, the notion that if it looks like something else it must somehow be related—that all medicine, for example, is somehow colonial in its relation to the body of the patient.[32] Rather, I am suggesting that one can put together a specific genealogy of metaphors, practices, and careers that links the colony with the metropole and with other colonies, that one might follow people, technologies, and ideas as they move from one site to another. The medical doctors and bureaucrats I write about were itinerants, with a global view of things that historians, so preoccupied with the local and constrained by nation or region, are only now coming to appreciate. In a generally uncritical, unreflective way, these colonial technicians were prepared to find the modern in the colony, the colonial in the metropole. In this case, the traffic between the United States and the Philippines, the Pacific crossing, enables us to recognize that colonial technologies of rule could also be used to develop the "nation" and its various disciplines in both locations.[33] The experience of empire allowed American scientists and physicians to bring many colonial bureaucratic practices — and even a new sense of themselves — back to urban health departments in the United States and elsewhere between 1910 and 1920. José David Saldívar, among others, has urged us to look at the borderlands between the United States and Mexico as "the spaces where the nation begins and ends."[34] But we should remember that the colonial laboratories of the Philippines, Puerto Rico, and Hawaii also were borderlands, where many "experts" were experimenting with various national bodies, including their own.[35]

In the first part of the book, I describe the engagement of American military medicine with the tropics during the Philippine-American War. The whiteness and the manliness of most American troops seemed both more visible and more vulnerable in a torrid struggle against Filipinos; the task of the military medical officer was to prevent and treat disease and degeneration in these conditions. Many of the medical practices examined in chapter 1, especially those focusing on care of the body and disposal of excrement, anticipated later colonial preoccupations. In chapter 2, I suggest that the strategies and tactics of colonial warfare against guerilla forces favored a rapid extension of military hygiene into Philippine social life. The administrative logic of pacification, or crowd control, implied the laying down across the tropical terrain of sedimentary strata of disciplinary structures, including military hygiene. It is within this new bureaucratic matrix that bacteriology and parasitology began to acquire political and civic significance.

Focusing on research under the emerging civil regime, chapter 3 explains the gradual medical exoneration of the tropical environment as a directly pathogenic agent (for the white physical body if not for mentality) and the growing racialization of germ carriage and distribution. Both research programs had begun during the war, but they were augmented during civil government in the laboratories of the Manila Bureau of Science and the Army Board for the Study of Tropical Diseases. It appeared that so long as they followed military stipulations of hygiene, whites had little to fear from the climate; rather, the Filipino was now figured in colonial science as a dangerous and promiscuously contaminating racial type and the major threat to white health. The following chapter continues to explore the biopolitical implications of this racialized tropical pathology. Chapter 4 considers in particular the colonial health officer's obsession with native excrement — how the image of the "promiscuous defecator" was used to mark racial and social boundaries as well as to indicate just how porous and imperiled these distinctions could be. I describe here the mapping of purity and danger onto white American and Filipino bodies, with a concomitant differentiation of colonial space and social life into the laboratory and the unsanitary market, the toilet and the field, Clean-Up Week and the disorderly fiesta.

When white American medicos set out to reshape public space and private activities in the Philippines, they did so with an assertiveness that often proved delusory and poignant. To amplify a theme running through the first half of *Colonial Pathologies*, chapter 5 returns to the anxieties and insecurities of the white American bureaucrats who were attempting to discipline Filipino bodies and promote civic virtue in the tropics. Even as they disparaged Filipinos and demanded that this "inferior" race try ineptly to become more like them, white males found themselves enfeebled, baffled, and thwarted. Colonial nerves repeatedly undermined colonial assertion. Conventionally, American males attributed their own mental and moral deterioration to the strain of conducting civilized brain-work in a humid climate; but by the 1920s, some psychological experts had begun to discount devitalization as a cause and instead found evidence of an internal personality disorder, an individual maladaptation to civilized social life, a return of the repressed. Just as a few "natives" supposedly were to acquire a relatively spineless superego, the destabilizing tropics had become lodged deep within the minds of civilized white men.

Enfeebled or not, public health officers remained capable of changing the lives of many Filipinos. Chapter 6 considers the Culion leper colony, an exemplary combination of army camp, laboratory, and small American town and a site for the biological and civic transformation of those considered most unclean and least socialized. Deemed marginal to Philippine society, lepers appeared ironically to be the most eligible for modern biomedical citizenship. Through hygiene and treatment protocols linked to civic performance, lepers in the exemplary microcolony were expected to achieve "emancipation" in advance of the nonlepers of the macrocolony. Of course, the model lepers at best were only in remission and thus merely incipient or probationary citizens; they were deemed unsatisfactory mimics of white practices, mere dressed natives. Culion, like the rest of the archipelago, was in practice an island where cure and self-government remained asymptotic projections, not validated attainments.

The remainder of the book describes, in various ways, the disintegration, repair, and persistence of the white American grid of racial intelligibility in the colonial Philippines. Racial typologies became increasingly unstable and unsatisfying through the 1920s and 1930s, and the texture of ideas about race, culture, and environment proved ever more friable. White males became unnerved, Filipino "mimicry" made them uneasy, and enthusiasm for technological solutions came to displace confidence in race management. Internal contradictions, deficiencies, and discomfort exercised the most corrosive influences on racial frameworks during this period, not explicit local resistance and refusal or liberal reaction to North American eugenics or, later, to Nazi race policies.

These last two chapters examine the Rockefeller Foundation hookworm and malaria programs in the Philippines during the 1920s and 1930s. The leaders of the hookworm project regarded it as a means of medically recolonizing the archipelago after the Filipinization of the health department. In chapter 7, I examine their medical effort—beyond Culion—to reiterate hybrid, imitative subject positions for Filipinos. Most strikingly, Rockefeller emissaries regarded the Filipino bureaucrats who had supplanted Americans as flawed or profane copies of white experts: Filipinos were still seductively attesting to their developmental delay, their unreadiness for self-government. Therefore only Americans were eligible to lead programs of hygiene reform, to undertake the task, as Ruth Rogaski puts it, of "connecting the privy to the nation."[36] And yet, an awareness of supposed Filipino mimicry, an uncanny sense of the copy, could also subvert Americans' self-confidence, revealing again the brittleness of their own masterful identity. In contrast, the leaders of the malaria program—described in chapter 8—eventually tried to circumvent, rather than openly disparage and reform, local culture. This final chapter suggests that in the emerging international health services ideas of race were not so much abandoned as pragmatically nudged aside in favor of the exploration of regional ecologies and an emphasis on technical intervention. Indeed, when it seemed necessary to bring the "human factor" back into the equation, a rackety version of the older racial hygiene often reemerged in international health and development programs, at least until the invention of medical anthropology in the 1960s.

It may seem at first that I am writing in opposition to science, hygiene, and civic virtue. In order to avoid such misunderstanding, I feel obliged to express my enthusiastic personal and professional affiliation with all three enterprises. But I remain interested in how estimates of hygiene have framed racial and civic identities, how hygiene reform has mobilized people, made them more tractable, and enabled them to think differently about their bodies, social life, and place in the world. In this case, I am especially interested in the typological construction of hygiene and civic potential for white Americans and Filipinos, that is, in the way hygiene once took specific racial form, and how this convenient racial biology came for a time to represent human destiny.

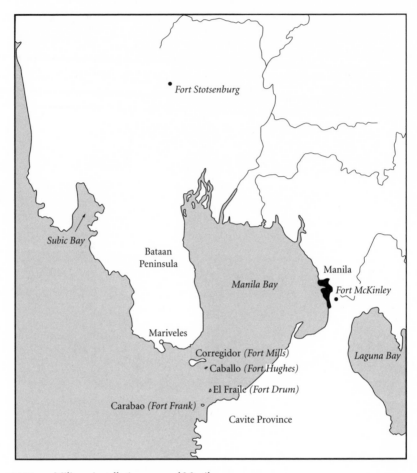

MAP 2. Military installations around Manila.

Chapter One

AMERICAN MILITARY MEDICINE FACES WEST

On June 13, 1900, Captain S. Chase de Krafft, M.D., a volunteer assistant surgeon with the American forces in the Philippines, reported from his post at Balayan the death from "hemoglobinuric fever" of Private Glenn V. Parke of the 28th Regiment. In January, Parke had fallen out of a march "from physical exhaustion" and was sent to the hospital in Manila. When he rejoined his company a few months later he appeared to be well but soon succumbed to "malarial fever intermittent." On the long, hot march to Balayan, Parke had fallen out again and was admitted to the post hospital with an acute attack of diarrhea. After daily doses of quinine and thrice-daily strychnine, the soldier soon returned to duty. But his malarial fever recurred: back in hospital he was "seized with a severe attack of bilious vomiting," and later his urine was red and scanty. The bilious vomiting, diarrhea, and fever persisted, along with pain over the liver; his entire body was soon "saffron-colored." His urine became darker and more concentrated. Within a few hours, the patient sank into delirium and then coma, dying early in the morning. Parke had told the surgeon he was twenty-three years old, though most suspected he was no more than twenty-one; in any case, his body was quickly buried in the north side of the cemetery at Balayan.

De Krafft then turned his attention to ensuring the well-being of the remaining troops.[1]

Tropical disease would take the lives of many U.S. soldiers during the Philippine-American War. From General Wesley Merritt's assault on Manila on July 31, 1898, until the war gradually eased in 1900, more than six hundred soldiers were killed or died from wounds received in battle, and another seven hundred died of disease.[2] The record of Parke's clinical course presents in unusual detail an example of diagnosis and treatment in the medical corps of the U.S. Army during the first year of the campaign. The army surgeon in the field was still likely to attribute illness to exhaustion or reckless behavior and to favor explanations that implied a mismatch between bodily constitution and circumstance. In his extensive case notes, de Krafft nowhere mentions germs, even though the microbial causes of diarrhea and malaria had been established for many years. Parke's feces were not cultured for bacteria; his blood was not examined for the malaria parasite. Instead, the surgeon carefully described the vitality and appearance of the patient, the strength of his pulse, the qualities of his dejecta, and the hourly variations in body temperature. The diagnosis was expressed not in terms of any causative organism but as a type of fever, a bodily response not identified with any inciting agent. In a tropical environment, in conditions that supposedly depleted white constitutions, the surgeon turned naturally to stimulants — strychnine, quinine, mustard plasters, and eggnog — to rally Parke's resisting powers.[3] There was no suggestion that a medication might attack directly a microbe or other specific cause. The surgeon hoped to restore his patient's balance and vitality and thus combat the nonspecific challenges of overwork or feckless behavior in trying foreign circumstances.

The surgeon's meticulous attention to this individual case reveals more than just the expediency and deftness required in clinical engagement under such grueling conditions. It also indicates medical priorities in the U.S. military at the outset of the war. In an elaborate epidemiological reconstruction of the effects of the Philippine-American War on the local population, Ken de Bevoise has estimated that the annual death rate in the archipelago, previously a high thirty per thousand, soared to more than sixty per thousand between 1898 and 1902, and that more than seven hundred thousand Filipinos died in the fighting or in concomitant epidemics of cholera, typhoid, smallpox, tuberculosis, beriberi, and plague.[4] Displaced and destitute, sometimes crowded into reconcentration camps, ordinary Filipinos were especially vulnerable to disease. Endemic infection, previously contained, flared into epidemics; new diseases, some perhaps carried by invading troops, soon became rife. But the spread of disease among local communities was not, in the early stages of war at least, the main concern of the medical corps of an attacking army.

The job of a military surgeon, recently codified in the U.S. Army, was clearly delimited.[5] During battle, the care and evacuation of sick and wounded soldiers would inevitably preoccupy the military surgeon; at other times, in the respite from the demands of surgical treatment of acute cases, the surgeon worked to ensure the sanitation of camps and the hygiene of troops. "A military surgeon who believes he is appointed for the sole purpose of extracting bullets and prescribing pills," according to Captain Charles E. Woodruff, M.D., was "a hundred years behind the times."[6] The medical officer was also a sanitary inspector, responsible for the scrutiny of food, provision of adequate clothing, ventilation of tents, disposal of wastes, and the general layout and "salubrity" of camps. In the past, according to Woodruff, the military surgeon might have restricted himself to preventing and eradicating "hospital contagion" — gangrene among the wounded and fever (usually typhus) among long-term inmates — but now, in the "modern era," he had a duty to provide for the well-being of troops. Thus de Krafft, after hastening the disposal of Parke's body, had gone about trying to prevent other cases. "The army medical officer," noted a contemporary observer, "ceased to be primarily a general practitioner in becoming the administrative officer of a sanitary bureau, with certain clinical duties when accident or the failure of prevention placed the individual soldier for special care in a hospital ward."[7]

In seeking to protect white soldiers, the military surgeon in the Philippine-American War repeatedly assayed the nature of the territory and climate and the character and behavior of troops and local inhabitants. Like medicine more generally, army sanitary science was heedful of environment, social life, and morality; always conservative, it tried to guard against any radical departure from the body's accustomed locale and mode of existence. Alterations in living conditions, in patterns of human contact, and in exposure to different climates might exert a direct impact on the soldier's body and temperament, or they might imply some perilous modification of his microbial circumstances. For troops like Parke, going to the tropics to fight a war meant encountering a peculiar new physical environment and exotic disease ecology. The conditions would be incongruent with those that whites experienced in most of the United States, and therefore potentially harmful in ways as yet undetermined. To predict and stave off disease, the medical officer had

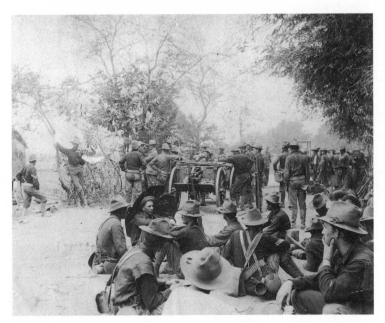

FIGURE I. U.S. troops on the road to Malalos, 1899 (RG 165-PW-81608, NARA).

to understand the effect of an alteration in circumstances or habits on his charges and learn how to mitigate or combat the pathological concomitants of change and mobility. To stay healthy the soldier must either reassert his previous pattern of life or establish a different means of coping with the novel environment and deployment. Military medicine in the Philippines thus was predicated on appraisal of territory, climate, and behavior; it sought constantly to protect the vulnerable alien race from strange circumstances and dangerous habits and to teach presumably transgressive soldiers how they might inhabit a new place with propriety and in safety.

Most of the troops in the Philippines would describe themselves as white — the term crops up repeatedly in letters and reports — so it is tempting to regard military medicine, at least in part, as an effort to gauge white vulnerability and to strengthen white masculinity in trying foreign circumstances.[8] Indeed, it often proves difficult to extricate concerns about the character of whiteness from fears of disease in the tropics. Would the white race degenerate and die off in a climate unnatural to it? Would the discord of race and place produce a deterioration of white physique and mentality that shaded into disease? Were the tropics inimical to the white man? Such questions still puzzled medical officers and soldiers alike. Most of the time, of course, military surgeons like de Krafft were preoccupied with alleviating disease and treating injuries. But sanitary duties ensured that medical officers would also strive to restructure and secure the boundaries of white masculinity in the colonial tropics, to determine how to preserve Anglo-Saxon virility and morality in a hostile region, a place bristling with physical, microbial, and native foes. As so often in the past century, the U.S. Army provided a model, an ideal space, for working out political and social problems that also beset the unruly public sphere — whether in the metropole or the colony. Thus the care and disciplining of white troops would come to serve as a test case for how to manage white American colonial emissaries and later as a guide to how natives might be reformed into self-disciplined "nationals."[9] In order to understand these subsequent transfers and substitutions it is necessary to take a closer look at the fighting white man and his tropical burden.

TO THE PHILIPPINES

Admiral George Dewey's victory over the Spanish fleet in Manila Bay on May 1, 1898 — one of the early engagements of the Spanish-American War — signaled the entry of a new colonial power into Southeast Asia. President William McKinley hurriedly arranged to send a military expedition, assembled mostly in the western states, to take possession of the Philippines. But by the time the U.S. Army arrived later in 1898, Spanish authority had collapsed, and Emilio Aguinaldo's rebel forces had taken control of most of the provinces. The commander of the Spanish garrison in Manila surrendered to the expeditionary forces, and so Filipino troops, spurned as allies, decided to entrench themselves around the city. In the Treaty of Paris, signed on December 10, 1898, Spain disregarded Filipino nationalist aspirations and formally awarded the United States sovereignty of the archipelago. During the next four years, American forces engaged in a bitter and brutal campaign against the Philippine *insurrectos* in order to secure the new possessions.[10] The logic of westward expansion was to leave the United States with a Southeast Asian empire, one that would last another forty or so years. In supplanting Spain, America thus unexpectedly took its place in the region alongside the Dutch in the East Indies, the British in Malaya and Hong Kong, and the French in Indochina. But for U.S. colonialists, these older European imperial entanglements would more commonly constitute object lessons than models worth emulating.

The troops had arrived in an archipelago of over seven thousand islands, supporting a population of close to seven million people, most on the island of Luzon. With a mean annual temperature of eighty degrees Fahrenheit, an average humidity of 79 percent, and distinct wet and dry seasons, the climate of Manila assuredly is tropical, however one might imagine that indefinite quality. The rainy season lasts from June through November, after which the weather can be quite pleasant, tempered by sea breezes. Although Manila's average temperature may be a little higher and its humidity a little less, it seemed to many Americans that the weather there might be similar to conditions prevailing in Rangoon, Bombay, and Calcutta.[11] It was in any case a climate few Americans had experienced.

As Benedict Anderson has remarked, "Few countries give the observer a deeper feeling of historical vertigo than the Philippines."[12] In the late sixteenth century, the Spanish had occupied Luzon and made Manila their capital. After three hundred years of Spanish clerical colonialism, fewer than 10 percent of the local inhabitants were literate in Spanish, yet some of the Catholic religious orders — the Jesuits and Dominicans especially — had supported pioneering natural history and astronomical research, and from the seventeenth century had even sponsored universities in the archipelago. Thus José Rizal, novelist, physician, and nationalist, in the 1880s reflected that "the Jesuits, who are backward in Europe, viewed from here, represent Progress; the Philippines owes to them their nascent education, and to them the Natural Sciences, the soul of the nineteenth century." Various religious orders had established hospitals for the poor, and colleges for the small *mestizo* and *criollo* elite. The San Francisco Corporation founded the San Lazaro Hospital in 1578, initially for the poor in general but after 1631 reserved for the increasing number of lepers. In Manila, the Hospital de San Juan de Dios, for the care of poor Spaniards, opened in 1596; and the Hospital de San José was established in Cavite in 1641. The University of Santo Tomás, which the Dominicans founded in 1611, belatedly allowed the organization of faculties of medicine and pharmacy in 1871. Scientific and medical journals soon proliferated: the *Boletín de medicina de Manila* (1886), the *Revista farmacéutica de Filipinas* (1893), the *Crónicas de ciencias médicas* (1895), and others. Provincial medical officers, the *médicos titulares*, were first appointed in 1876; and the Board of Health and Charity, equivalent to a public health department, was established in 1883 and expanded in 1886. Sanitary conditions in the capital were changing during this period. The government put sewers underground in Manila during the 1850s; in 1884, the Carriedo waterworks opened, giving the city the purest water in Southeast Asia.[13] The central board of vaccination had been producing and distributing lymph since 1806; by 1898 there were 122 regular vaccinators — notoriously inept and

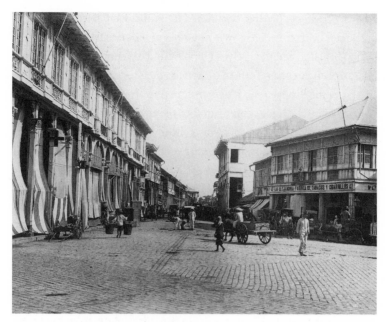

FIGURE 2. Manila street scene, Binondo 1899 (RG 165-PW-35-9, NARA).

lazy — passing the time in Manila and the major towns.[14] In 1887, the Spanish colonial authorities set up the Laboratorio Municipal de Manila to examine food, water, and clinical samples — but evidently it was rarely used.[15] Nonetheless, it is clear that recognizably modern structures of public health and medical care were taking shape in Manila and its immediate hinterland.

The 1870s had witnessed vast improvements in communication with Europe and an expansion of traffic between metropole and colony. From 1868, vessels could use the Suez Canal, reducing the journey between Europe and the Philippines from four months to one month by steamer. In 1880, cable linked Manila more closely to Europe than ever before. Better connections with Spain reduced the influence of foreign traders in Manila and encouraged Spaniards to move to the islands. In 1810, there had been fewer than four thousand *peninsulares* and Spanish *mestizos* in the archipelago, mostly clustered in Manila (compared to several million *indios* throughout the archipelago); in 1876, four thousand *peninsulares* and more than ten thousand *mestizos* and *criollos* lived in the Philippines; by 1898 the numbers had swelled to more than thirty-four thousand Spaniards, including six thousand government officials, four thousand army and navy personnel, and seventeen hundred clerics.[16]

As they increasingly became committed to nationalism, science, anticlericalism, and political reform, a growing number of *mestizos* and *criollos* in the archipelago began to call themselves Filipinos and to represent themselves as *ilustrados*, or enlightened reformers.[17] In part, the progressive sentiment, expressed first in the Propaganda movement, derived from Spanish liberal and secular agitation, which had culminated in the revolution of 1868 — just as the conservative reaction in Spain was echoed in the Philippines after the 1872 Cavite rebellion. But local factors also contributed. The school reforms of 1863 had established a framework, still grossly inadequate, for a state system of primary education. Improved commercial opportunities allowed the expansion of the middle class; ambitious and progressive Filipinos began sending their sons to France and Spain for higher education; talented local candidates resented the *peninsulares*, who took most of the top government posts; and more efficient communication helped to break down regional separatism and conflict in the islands. Furthermore, racial distinctions became especially marked toward the end of the century, and there emerged "a tendency to thrust the native aristocracy into a secondary place, to compel them to recognize 'white superiority,' to a degree not so noticeable in the earlier years of Spanish rule."[18] Initially, local ambitions and resentments found expression in moderate groups such as Rizal's Liga Filipina. But in 1892, Andrés Bonifacio organized the Katipunan, an anticlerical and anti-Spanish brotherhood that in 1896 led an insurrection against Spanish control. The friars attributed disaffection to "*Franc-Masonería*," for them the epitome of everything pernicious in modern life; and the Spanish army attempted to suppress the rebellion, employing such brutality that even moderates turned against Spanish rule.[19] But by the time Aguinaldo was able to declare the Philippine Republic in 1899, the United States had claimed the archipelago.

José Rizal, the so-called First Filipino, was one of the leaders of the rising generation of nationalists. From the Jesuits at the Ateneo de Manila Rizal had received a solid grounding in the sciences, even if he subsequently argued that Jesuit education had seemed progressive only because the rest of the Philippines was mired in medievalism. But at Santo Tomás, studying science, he found that the walls "were entirely bare; not a sketch, nor an engraving, nor even a diagram of an instrument of physics." A mysterious cabinet contained some modern equipment, but the Dominicans made sure that Filipinos admired it from afar. The friars would point to this cabinet, according to Rizal, to exonerate themselves and to claim that it was really "on account of the apathy, laziness, limited capacity of the natives, or some other ethnological or

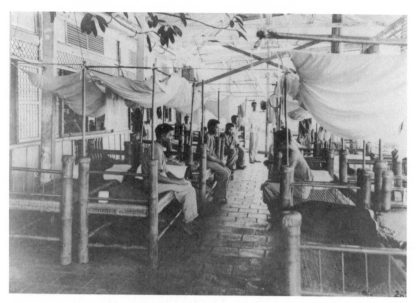

FIGURE 3. Interior of the Spanish Bilibid Hospital. Courtesy of the Rockefeller Archive Center.

supernatural cause [that] until now no Lavoisier, Secchi, nor Tyndall has appeared, even in miniature, in this Malay-Filipino race!"[20] (Still, it should be recalled that nowhere else in Southeast Asia was education available at such an advanced level.)[21] In 1882, Rizal traveled to Spain to study medicine, and he later visited France and Germany. He was astonished and embarrassed by the political and scientific backwardness of the imperial power. In Europe, medicine, political activism, and the writing of his brilliantly sardonic novels occupied most of his time, but after Rizal returned to the Philippines and was confined at Dapitan, he also began collecting plants and animals and discovered new species of shells.[22] During this period, Rizal engaged in a copious, self-consciously enlightened correspondence with Ferdinand Blumentritt, the Austrian ethnologist, and translated into Spanish many of his works on the Philippines.[23] For Rizal, a commitment to science and reason informed patriotism, and patriotism implied a scientific orientation to the world. Unimpressed, the clerical-colonial authorities executed the First Filipino in 1896.

Rizal did not live to see the United States completing the work of Spain and crushing the nationalist forces. The Philippine-American War would directly and indirectly cause widespread sickness, injury, and suffering as well as destroy much of the recently constructed apparatus of education and public health in the archipelago. The nascent, weak public health system broke down completely, the Filipino sick and wounded overwhelmed local hospitals, vaccination ceased altogether, and colleges and universities either closed or struggled to graduate students. Thus as Americans assumed control they found little evidence of previous scientific and medical endeavor and felt justified in representing the Spanish period as a time of unrelieved apathy, ignorance, and superstition, in contrast to their own self-proclaimed modernity, progressivism, and scientific zeal.

THE ARMY MEDICAL DEPARTMENT

When John Shaw Billings addressed the graduating class of the Army Medical School in 1903, he celebrated the great progress in military medicine he had observed over the past fifty years. Billings recollected that the president of the Army Medical Board who examined him in 1861 had been inclined to reminisce along the same lines, praising the recent introduction of anesthesia and the new operations for excision of joints. The examining surgeon in those days had heard of the clinical thermometer and the hypodermic syringe but doubted that either would prove useful. The young physician, soon to join the Army of the Potomac, was asked to describe "laudable pus" and the best means of securing healing by second intention. He was questioned on the means of preventing malaria and typhoid fever among troops. "If I had referred to bacilli, hematozoa, flies and mosquitoes, as you would probably do, I don't think I should have passed." Just as the symbol of the old military surgeon was the scalpel, his new emblem ought to be the microscope. "Forty years ago the microscope was mainly used by physicians as a plaything, a source of occasional amusement," Billings recalled. "Today the microscope is one of our most important tools."[24] Although the bookish sanitarian was perhaps overestimating the bacteriological grasp of most military surgeons and ignoring the difficulties of using the new techniques in the field, it was true that during the previous forty years the role of the army medical officer had changed beyond recognition.

The intellectual and professional transformation of military medicine encompassed both its therapeutic and its prophylactic aspects. The new medical officer combined clinical duties with administrative tasks designed to prevent disease outbreaks, or at least to provide early warning of them. Of course, in times of war it was still the care of the sick and wounded that took most of the time and energy of the military surgeon. Since the Civil War, changes in the combat zone and in medical technology had transformed the scope and character of these clinical duties. By the 1890s, antiseptic methods prevailed in the operating room, primary union could be secured in gunshot wounds, depressed skull fractures were operable, and wounds of the intestine, once considered beyond surgical relief, on occasion were sutured in risky laparotomies. The military surgeon was more confident and optimistic than ever before in his ability to intervene clinically. General George M. Sternberg, M.D., the surgeon general of the army and the president of the Association of Military Surgeons, in 1895 observed that his colleagues, as a consequence of these advances, would have "to devote much more time to individual cases than was thought necessary during our last war."[25] The army needed more medical staff, with better training, and it needed more ambulance officers and sanitary assistants to take on the first-aid work. The trained surgeon could then move from the firing line, where staunching hemorrhage was the most that could be done, to the new field hospital, where he now might operate.[26]

If all had gone well, by the time the wounded soldier arrived at a distant field hospital, an elastic bandage (or, more likely, the old-fashioned tourniquet) would have been applied on the firing line to stop any hemorrhage, and at the dressing stations bleeding vessels tied with ligatures of catgut or silk and wounds plugged with gauze.[27] In the field hospital, the patient might receive opium to relieve pain and to prevent the "depression of shock," though some medical officers preferred to administer alcohol by mouth, enema, or hypodermic injection, on occasion combining it with nitroglycerine. At the hospital, surgeons took special care to remove any foreign bodies, any contaminants, and they would enlarge the wound if necessary. "One speck of filth, one shred of clothing, one strip of filthy integument left in ever so small a wound will do more harm, more seriously endanger life, and much longer invalid the patient, than a wound half a yard long in the soft parts, when it is kept aseptic," warned one military sugeon.[28] If the campaign had been long and severe, with the soldiers hard-pressed and huddled together without bathing facilities or changes of clothing, "they are quite apt to get into a horrible condition of filth and the presumption will be in favor of every wound being infected and apt to do badly."[29] In such conditions, conservative treatment was often fatal, and any attempt at asepsis would be better than none.

Of course strict asepsis was usually impossible in the field. And even when antiseptics were available, it was sometimes hard to find the large quantities of pure water required to dilute them. "You can imagine our horror," a surgeon recalled, "to find ourselves in the midst of a dozen or two operations with dirty, bloody hands and instruments, blood, vomited matter and other filth strewn on the ground, and no water to clean up."[30] Nor was it easy to keep boiling water clean on an open campfire: the smoke would rise and spread dirt and soot on it. Operations in the open and even in tents would quickly be covered in dust if the wind rose, often making even "the antiseptic lotions look like mud."[31] The exigencies of battle left no time for microscopic examinations or bacteriological cultures: the surgeon depended still on his senses and acted in response to his disgust with obvious filth and foreign matter. For surgeons, even those trained in microbiology, dirt simply implied the presence of germs of infection. And on the firing line and in the field hospital, dirt was everywhere.

Increasingly, between battles and skirmishes, the military surgeon performed sanitary duties too. "The progress and popularization of sanitary science were such that commanding officers did not dare to pass unnoticed the suggestions of their medical officers," noted a contemporary observer (and an inveterate optimist).[32] The sanitary science of the military officer was still, in practice, largely predicated on knowledge of the geographical landmarks of disease, although empirical suspicions of unhealthiness could in theory be tested bacteriologically. Most physicians at the end of the nineteenth century expected to find a specific microbial pathogen for each disease, but these etiological agents, even the more cosmopolitan bacteria, might still have a distinctive geographical distribution. Captain Edward L. Munson, M.D., in his massive *Theory and Practice of Military Hygiene*, conceded that mosquitoes might transmit malaria, but still he wondered if drinking water from marshes or swamps would also give rise to the disease.[33] Professor J. Lane Notter, an international expert on military hygiene, advised an audience of medical officers that, while each disease is "due to a specific microorganism," all diseases "like plants and animals, can only flourish within certain geographical limits."[34] Qualities of soil, water, and climate gave some pathogens sustenance and not others: the sanitary officer therefore continued to monitor the situation and ventilation of the camp. For the moment, bacteriology might adjust or extend the preexisting framework of geographical pathology; it would take another decade or more to dismantle the old conceptual edifice altogether.

Medical geographers during the nineteenth century had suggested a great many landmarks to identify pathological agency. For most of the century scholars had assumed that the environment might exert a direct noxious effect on the human constitution, with the exact outcome depending ultimately on hereditary and behavioral factors.[35] But since the 1870s, it seemed that indirect mechanisms—microbiological mediators of physical and social circumstances—would incite most diseases.[36] This presented a practical problem for the military surgeon in the field since conditions were not stable enough for a detailed, painstaking search for microbial nuisances. Medical officers rarely had easy access to a laboratory, and microscopes and culture media were scarce; nor was there time to wait for bacteriological confirmation of pathogenic organisms. In order to act expeditiously, the military physician often fell back on the old, timeworn geographical settings and correlates of pathology.[37]

In practice, then, bacteriology had touched little more than the margins of the military surgeon's spatial imagination. Munson advised that the location of the camp was "a matter of the greatest importance in maintaining the health and efficiency of troops," but this precept was rarely put to bacteriological test. Thus Munson drew on commonplace empirical knowledge when remarking that "newly ploughed ground should never be employed for camping purposes, although a site which has long been under cultivation is usually healthful." He generally recommended a pure, dry, sandy soil: "Exhalations from damp ground are powerfully depressing to the vitality of the human organism, and favor the occurrence of rheumatism and neuralgia as well as the invasion of the system by infectious germs, certain of which best retain their vitality and perpetuate their kind amid such environment."[38] More fastidiously still, Colonel C. M. Woodward advised his fellow surgeons that the ground for camp should be elevated, bordering on a rapidly running stream, and away from any swamps. Every tent must be raised during the day to permit free circulation of air. "Company quarters," he advised, "should always be kept thoroughly policed and freed from all appearance of evil—that is, all scraps of paper and refuse of any kind should not be allowed to collect on or about quarters or in camp, for although they may not be positively unsanitary in their presence, they look so."[39] Professor Notter urged medical officers to avoid valleys so narrow that the air stagnates, ground immediately above marshes, and fresh clearings. "Dampness of soil adds immeasurably to camp diseases"; but he argued that sandy soils also "act prejudiciously both by not disinfecting these organic matters and by their drying power, so that when clouds of sand are raised by the wind, these clouds carry particles of organic matter." Men should never be allowed to sleep below the level of the ground, in excavated tents, "exposed to ground-air emanations."[40] The decaying of organic material in the soil suggested the presence of pathogenic germs—but on few occasions were these suppositions tested.

Colonel Dallas Bache, M.D., expected that "certain sanitary interrogatories will be put to any important situation, and the replies carefully considered," before a place was chosen for camp: "manifestly a very great range of questions upon climate, soil, water, and waste disposal must be met."[41] Evidence pointed, for instance, to a "malady of the wind" — as of the sea — requiring the hygienist to consider carefully the lay of the land and its ventilation. The attributes of the soil, including its texture, temperature, and water and mineral content, also had "well-established or highly probable relations to health," contributing to the origin or spread of many diseases.[42] "We cannot afford to neglect the evidence," Bache warned his colleagues in 1895, "that makes a close ally of the soil with malaria, and proclaims it the nursery of neuralgia, catarrhs, rheumatism, and consumption; more constant and insidious foes to the military community than the Indian." He suggested that the new science of bacteriology had simply indicated that the soil "offers itself as a culture medium or refuge in general terms" for the agents of cholera, typhoid fever, diarrhea, and dysentery.[43] These diseases might lurk in the environment, ready to subvert the soldier's health.

Conditions of military life also drew attention to the health threats of overcrowding and the need for meticulous group discipline and personal hygiene. Thus concern with the management of populations would often accompany territorial appraisal on the march. Just as the new bacteriology might be superimposed on old landmarks of geographical pathology, so too might it give further pathological depth to old fears of bad behavior and unregulated social contact. The danger of contracting venereal disease, especially from prostitutes of another race, was well recognized, but increasingly it was suspected that even nonvenereal social contact with one's peers might prove risky.[44] Therefore the bodies and habits of soldiers, as much as the territories they passed over, needed constant surveillance and care. It was important, from the beginning, to ensure that recruits derived from sturdy and reliable stock. Since the 1880s, all recruits went through a physical examination and a cursory assessment of mentality and character before enlistment. The advantage of this procedure, according to Bache, was that it rejected "material that would swell the death and discharge rates."[45] "A man who is incapable of sustaining the fatigue of a four-mile march," noted Colonel Herbert Burrill, M.D., "would be an incubus on the rapid movement of troops."[46] Worse, he was also more susceptible to disease, whatever its cause, and perhaps more likely to pass it on. Munson observed that "recruits must be of trustworthy physique and sound constitution before the military character can be developed, and the physically, mentally and morally defective are hence to be uniformly rejected as unfit for service." The army would take sober men from the "lower walks of life and the laboring classes" and train their character and body.[47] Those resistant to military discipline must be excluded. In his revision of *Tripler's Manual*, Colonel Charles R. Greenleaf, M.D., an assistant surgeon general of the army, insisted that no recruits be drawn from the "vagrant and criminal classes."[48] Munson, too, advised against admitting "men whose physical faults render them unfit for duty and susceptible to disease, whose undetected affections may be transmitted to others or whose moral obliquities induce malingering and desertion."[49]

Military surgeons knew from experience that physical training and discipline could transform eligible raw material into good soldiers. As Munson wrote, "Strength, activity, endurance and discipline, combined with sound bodily health, are the first requisites of the soldier." These qualities, he argued, were "the foundation upon which the whole structure of military efficiency rests." But mental and moral training must always accompany physical development; otherwise the recruit would become just "sluggish muscle piled on the back of a listless and indifferent mind and an irresolute and halting will." Instead, the ideal citizen-soldier should be "of manly character, willing, brave, steadfast, zealous, enthusiastic, of good humor, and possessed of initiative." Munson wanted thus to make "the man in the ranks a part of an intelligent machine to act at the voice of a commander."[50] This efficient performance demanded an education in temperance and self-restraint. In accordance with the emphasis on a simple mode of life, the soldier was advised against dietary indiscretion and alcohol abuse. It was important more generally to regulate intake and excretion to achieve a balance of the bodily system. The soldier's clothing, for example, ought to ensure that he maintained a stable temperature and evaded heatstroke, fatigue, and any diseases brought on by chill. The army ration would deliver a balanced diet of protein, starch, fat, and salts.[51]

The well-trained soldier was expected to recognize and avoid sanitary hazards, especially those related to disposal of excreta. Munson, throughout his career in the army, and later as advisor to the Bureau of Health in the Philippines, would warn of the dangers of promiscuous defecation, a failing that at least seemed readily disciplined in white soldiers. Experience had convinced him that "the care of latrines is a most important factor in the preservation of the health of the command." Indeed, "raw troops living like savages in their disregard of sanitary principles, without moving camp as often as do these savages, cannot fail to be scourged by epidemic disease as a result of their ignorance and neglect." Education and camp inspection were unremitting; "camp police" would discipline those who refused to find the distant latrines.[52] In the military service, the removal of excreta and the maintenance of personal cleanliness would normally receive more emphasis than in white civilian life, in recognition of the special health risks of shared and often crowded living conditions. The personal hygiene of soldiers in the line was regulated as never before. Since the 1880s, far in advance of the British army, all military posts in the United States had provided bathing facilities for troops. Each American soldier was now required "to wash the face, head, neck and feet once daily, cleanse the hands prior to each meal and bathe his entire body at least as often as once in five days." His personal cleanliness and propriety had become "a constant object of solicitude on the part of his superiors."[53]

When epidemics broke out among troops, as they often did despite even the best policing, the military hygienist set about to inquire into their history and predisposing causes and then recommend measures of control. In the 1890s, the sanitary officer could draw on a large repertoire of interventions. These included isolation of the diseased, prevention of crowding, purifying of food and water, avoidance of unripe or decomposing vegetables, eradication of "soil pollution," whitewashing or burning of infected localities. destruction of infected articles. disinfection of privies, urinals, sinks, and drains, checking of ventilating appliances, protection from dampness, the daily airing of bedding, healthy amusements and exercise, prevention of intemperance and promiscuity, and, in the case of smallpox, vaccination.[54] It was gradually becoming more likely that the surgeon would seek to identify a microbial cause of the epidemic and, if successful, attune his response accordingly. In the summer of 1898, when typhoid, or camp fever, spread among the troops assembling in the United States to fight the war with Spain, General Sternberg appointed a board of investigation that included Major Walter Reed, M.D., to show what could be done with new scientific techniques.[55] The board visited all the large camps in the United States, studying the water supply, the quality and quantity of food, the nature of the soil, the arrangement and size of tents, the location of sinks, and the disposal of human waste. "Scientific investigations of the blood," including application of the Widal test for the typhoid organism, indicated that most of what had passed for "malarial fever of a protracted variety" should have been diagnosed as typhoid. Frequently, the presence of typhoid was deliberately hidden: "in one command the death-rate from indigestion was put down as fifteen percent."[56] The board carefully assessed the various proposed explanations for the epidemic. They concluded it derived not from sending northern men into a southern climate or from the locality or simply the massing of so many men in one place. Rather, the cause was "camp pollution," that is, the improper disposal of excreta. On hearing of this conclusion, Sternberg recommended to the adjutant general that subordinates clean up the camps, discourage flies, and sterilize the excreta of typhoid cases.[57] But by then the disease had mostly run its course.

At the end of the nineteenth century, an education in the principles of modern hygiene was supposed to inform the military surgeon's sanitary work. When a candidate passed the medical department's competitive examinations, he had to attend a four-month (later eight-month) course at the Army Medical School in Washington, D.C. Sternberg had established the school in 1893 to teach army regulations, customs of service, examination of recruits, care and transportation of the wounded, and field hospital management. Special emphasis was placed on military hygiene and sanitation and on "clinical and biological microscopy, particularly as bearing on disinfection and prevention of disease."[58] Billings taught military hygiene, Reed instructed students in bacteriology, Major Charles Smart, M.D., was in charge of sanitary chemistry, and Professor C. W. Stiles lectured on parasites in man. According to Dr. Charles H. Alden, the school's director, the courses provided for "a study of Hygiene in all its various branches, of air and water and their impurities, clothing, food, exercise, barrack and hospital construction, sewerage and drainage, sanitary chemistry and practical bacteriology." Laboratory work was a prominent feature of the course, supposedly "consuming most of the students' time."[59]

In 1898, at the beginning of a long tropical war in the Philippines, the army medical service appeared to exercise more influence over the care of troops than ever before. Even if the medical department's grasp on bacteriology was still weak at times, its organizational structure was stronger than ever. At the outbreak of the Spanish-American War the department consisted of 177 commissioned officers and 750 enlisted men. A permanent sanitary organization was attached to each regiment. For every 1,000 of strength, there were now 3 medical officers, 1 hospital steward, 2 acting hospital stewards, 1 nurse, 1 cook, and 3 orderlies; 2 company bearers were detailed for every 100 men on the line. Each division, 10,000 men strong, was provided with a field hospital, including 9 medical officers and 27 privates, members of the hospital corps, male nurses or "sanitary soldiers," who cared for the sick and wounded.[60] In the recent past, line and staff were inclined to scorn medical officers for their attempts to "coddle" soldiers. But this attitude was changing. The military surgeon possessed the authority accorded to his rank, the growing dignity of his profession, and now the freshly minted currency of laboratory science. Woodruff found that he rarely needed to compel ordinary soldiers "to get well," for they would "readily submit to all reasonable restrictions and methods of treatment, and many unreasonable ones too."[61] The military surgeon toward the end of the nineteenth century was gaining confidence in his new expertise, grappling with bacteriology, and attempting to incorporate novel pathogens into familiar patterns of environmental and social etiology. But his skills would be severely tested abroad, among the foreign disease ecology of the tropics.

AMERICAN MILITARY MEDICINE IN THE TROPICS

The warfare around Manila at first was mostly of a continental type, with the deployment of columns and the entrenchment of positions. The medical department was hard-pressed with the care of wounded and the establishment of divisional or general hospitals, though some public health work did begin soon after the occupation of Manila. During the first year of the war, the medical service concentrated on surgery and devising an easily movable front line, a more or less constant means of supply and evacuation, and well-determined depots for the sick in the general hospitals. The volunteer surgeons and those from the National Guard generally proved unprepared for war conditions. According to Lieutenant Colonel John van Rensselaer Hoff, M.D., the leading administrative reformer in the sanitary bureau, there was, among regimental medical officers and hospital stewards, "scarcely an officer or man who possessed the slightest knowledge of medico-military matters." Indeed, the medical department was "quite as much in need of training in the theory of the special military work of the sanitary corps, as were the troops of the line in their routine of 'fours right and fours left.' "[62] Lieutenant Colonel Jefferson D. Griffiths, M.D., the medical director of the Missouri National Guard, found his new circumstances particularly challenging. "As surgeons," he recalled, "we thought we could amputate a limb. We were familiar with laparotomies, and had an idea that we were fully competent to deal with the necessities of the occasion. Many of us even thought we knew something about the proper sanitation of camps, and disinfection." But after a few weeks in the military, "we found our ignorance was sublime."[63]

Most of the surgeons streaming into military service found themselves in

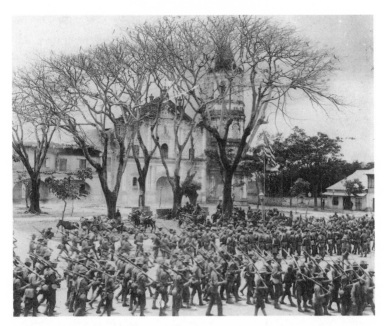

FIGURE 4. Square at Malalos, March 1899 (RG 165-PW-3H, NARA).

Griffith's predicament. In particular, the contract surgeons had no special training in military hygiene and knew nothing of army administrative procedures. So pressing was the need for surgeons that the rigorous physical and professional examinations for entry into the medical department had been suspended. Few volunteers possessed Henry F. Hoyt's experience of frontier medical practice and knowledge of modern hygiene. The "red-haired Indian-fighter," as he called himself, had set up a practice in New Mexico and tended railway workers there, before becoming commissioner of health for St. Paul, Minnesota, where he vaccinated widely and opened a bacteriology laboratory. Assigned as chief surgeon in the Second Division, Eighth Army Corps, Hoyt arrived in Manila in December 1898. The general advance of the army on Aguinaldo's trenches around the city was his first experience under fire. Wearing a white cork East India helmet, "being fearful of sunstroke in the tropics under a campaign hat," the medical officer gave first aid to the wounded and then sent some back for "aseptic surgery."[64] Regulations called for two men of the hospital corps to carry each litter, but Hoyt soon saw that "even six white men" could not manage it "in that hot, humid tropical climate," and he recommended that "Chinese coolies" be substituted.[65] The army continued to advance through "rough country and impenetrable jungle," all the while dodging brisk sniper fire, leaving transportation for the wounded far in the rear. The retreating army had destroyed the bridges, and ambulances could not cross the streams. Although the railway track was quickly repaired, Aguinaldo had kept most of the rolling stock. But using "a bunch of Igarote [sic] prisoners as motive power," Hoyt was able to improvise boxcars as ambulances for the wounded. When a fierce battle outside Malalos left four Americans dead, thirty wounded, and eleven with "heat exhaustion," he even tried ferrying the casualties by canoe.[66]

In May 1899, Hoyt established the first field hospital in the islands. He selected five "commodious houses" and connected them with a bamboo porch, an expedient that won praise from Senator Albert Beveridge when he visited. Soon afterwards, an ambulance brought Simon Flexner and Lewellys Barker, a pathologist and a physician from the Johns Hopkins University, keen to study tropical disease. According to Hoyt, they were like most young American men, "wild to get a taste of real war at the front."[67] But they did not linger. Hoyt himself had by then tasted rather too much of the Philippines. During the advance from Malalos he was "seized with a severe attack of amebic dysentery" and "fainted away." Sent to the new convalescent hospital on Corregidor Island, he grew worse and was ordered home. "The change and sea air did wonders," and, as he neared his homeland, he began to gain strength.[68]

Lieutenant Franklin M. Kemp, M.D., also remembered clearly his first time under fire, as the army attacked Aguinaldo's trenches. Kemp, like Hoyt an experienced hygienist, had arrived in Manila in August 1898 and spent the next few months in "the teaching of men to save their lives, or those of their comrades when wounded." During his daily drill and lecture, Kemp gave the men practical instruction in minor surgery, first aid, and transportation of the wounded. "They were taught to regard the first aid packet as their most precious possession, after their rifle."[69] On the night of February 4, 1899, as the American forces moved out of Manila, Kemp stationed the hospital corps with litters along the Singalong Road and was soon busy dressing the wounded who staggered out from the brushwood. As they retreated, Filipinos kept up a "constant and severe cross-fire," yet "the hospital corps men seemed to be ubiquitous, going from one pit to another, across open spaces, apparently bearing charmed lives."[70]

By April, when the army was advancing on Santa Cruz, Laguna, Kemp had learned to put the hospital corps five or ten paces in the rear of each company, with Chinese bearers a further hundred yards behind. The Chinese were proving themselves better able to withstand the intense heat than American litter-bearers, and with "the usual Oriental stoicism" they often worked "apparently beyond the limits of human endurance." They were under the charge of a private in the hospital corps "who could swear volubly in Chinese and was further assisted by a huge navy revolver and a big stick."[71] For two weeks the troops moved through country that had never carried wheeled transportation before: they were compelled to make roads, build bridges, and ford rivers, with little to guide them. But Kemp and his corps were by then prepared for such conditions: "My coolies would have the locality all cleaned up before the train arrived, the carts containing the medical, the surgical and the sterilizing chests coming next. In a few minutes the division field hospital would be established and in thorough running order, rounds made, operating table improvised and all dressings and operations performed. Ambulances would be parked and cleaned and made ready for instant use."[72]

And before long, they would pack up and move on again. After crossing the Pasig River, the troops endured the hardest day's march that Kemp could remember. All day, under fire from the enemy, they trudged across rolling land, "destitute of water," covered with "rank weeds and grass to one's waist," intersected with deep ravines, with absolutely no shade and a temperature of 110 degrees Fahrenheit. "Water gave out early in the morning," Kemp wrote; "tongues were so swollen that one could not speak; men dropped down in simple heat exhaustion or in convulsions, not one at a time, but in squads of five or six." Even in the seasoned 14th Infantry, almost 40 percent of the complement succumbed that day.[73] Kemp was kept busy in his improvised hospital till late at night.

Lieutenant Colonel Henry Lippincott, M.D., the chief surgeon for the Division of the Pacific and Eighth Army Corps, recalled that the wounded and sick generally did well during the early stages of the Philippines campaign, and the medical department performed its duties "cheerfully and efficiently."[74] "Of course we had excellent surgeons on the firing line" — men like Hoyt and Kemp — who "saw the wounded were well cared for before transportation, whether by ambulance, rail, or water, to the First Reserve [Hospital], and the men arrived in as good condition as could be expected."[75] Lippincott had converted the Spanish military hospital into the First Reserve Hospital in August 1898, a few days after the fall of Manila. Erected just twelve years earlier, the hospital accommodated between eight hundred and a thousand patients. The wards seemed well constructed "and very large and roomy, but the location [was] bad owing to the swampy surroundings." Not surprisingly,

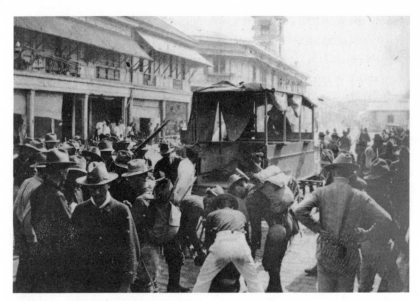

FIGURE 5. Wounded arriving in Manila, c. 1899 (RG 200-PI-46A, NARA).

the "sewer and closet arrangements, like everything of the kind in Manila, were unsanitary," but they were soon altered to resemble "the good features of the hospitals in America." Initially, all the sick and seriously wounded came to this large hospital, but less than a month later Lippincott established the Second Reserve in an abandoned convent, for the overflow from the First Reserve. In November 1898, the Corregidor Hospital opened on a site that Lippincott described as "a model spot for a large hospital."[76] The environmental conditions of the island seemed to revitalize most American soldiers: the temperature was ten degrees below Manila's, there was no malaria, shade trees abounded, and the saltwater bathing was excellent.

Yet medical conditions were not as satisfactory as Lippincott implied. Lieutenant Colonel Alfred A. Woodhull, M.D., Lippincott's successor as chief surgeon in Manila, reported that the two reserve hospitals were "swollen out of all proportions," and barracks had to be used for the overflow.[77] He was disturbed above all by the condition of the First Reserve Hospital: "The hospital grounds have been in a wretched state of police; the Hospital Corps seems to have neither system nor order for its control; there is no dining room, no proper facilities for the preparation of food or its distribution . . . the wards that I have incidentally passed through have been dirty and in poor order, they are horribly overcrowded and insufficiently manned."[78] He had found a "large and foul bathroom and privy" next to the main kitchen; many of the wards were "polluted with the remains of food."[79] During the wet season, the tent wards were awash with water, "literally an ankle deep."[80] Lieutenant Conrad Lanza, confined to the hospital in June 1899, complained that the army ration he received was "uneatable" and members of the hospital corps were "habitually disrespectful and inattentive."[81] Nurse Mary E. Sloper alleged that the sputum of tuberculosis patients overflowed receptacles onto the floor; and the two large jugs in the center of the ward, filled daily with fresh drinking water, contained bugs and worms in the slime at the bottom. According to Nurse Sloper, patients slept in dirty linen, discarded by previous inmates, and their bodies were never washed.[82] Conditions in hospitals outside Manila were scarcely better. The hospital at Corregidor remained under canvas six months after its establishment. The field hospitals proved woefully inadequate too. "There are innumerable regimental hospitals that in my judgment are pernicious," Woodhull lamented, "but which are authorized and supported. These are rendezvous of idlers and malingerers made possible merely because efficient medical officers, or in fact any at all, cannot be assigned to them."[83]

Others echoed Woodhull's complaints of inadequate medical staffing. Hoyt repeatedly pointed out the deficiencies in personnel, ambulances, and transportation at the front. He could count on only two surgeons on duty with each regiment when, for "service in the tropics," there should be at least three. Kenneth Fleming, in the hospital corps, wrote to his "dear ones at home" to tell them that "the Stuerd is sick and the Dr. is in Bunate and that leaves me in a pretty tight place but their is nothing much to do hear but hold sick call and I can atend to one company . . . I havent killed any body yet and I don't intend to do that."[84] Major General H. W. Lawton criticized the scarcity of medical attendants in his division: "At present one surgeon is forced to travel a line of mud and water . . . a distance of some four miles by road in performance of his duties, and he is far from being well himself." To send someone to his assistance would leave another command entirely without medical services.[85] In response to these and other complaints, Sternberg dispatched more contract surgeons and hospital corps. But soon after arriving, many of them would fall ill. Of the medical officers "actually on duty in Luzon, seven are disqualified on account of sickness," Woodhull reported, and many others had been "placed upon selected duty on account of their health." The chief surgeon found himself constantly shifting the remaining healthy medical officers from one battalion to another. It was difficult to keep up. Woodhull's first knowledge of an expedition was often "an announce-

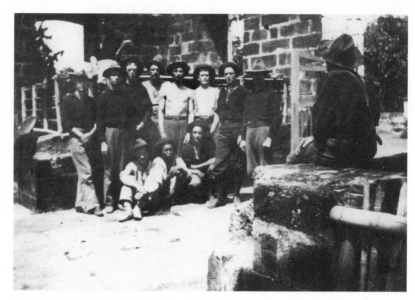

FIGURE 6. U.S. Ambulance Corps, c. 1899 (RG 200-PI-11C, NARA).

ment from [the regiment] that it was moving off with an inadequate medical force."[86] Sternberg sent out even more contract surgeons, but within months Woodhull was listing another twenty-five vacancies, each case a result of "sickness," "gastro-enteritis," "dysentery," "repeatedly breaking down," or just "weakened health."[87]

The duties of those medical officers who remained fit were long and arduous. During the wet season the roads they traveled became quagmires, and on crossing the rice fields "not infrequently the officers are wet up to their waists even when it is not raining." The daily sick call often took several hours when companies were scattered across many miles of defenses. "The weather is always warm," Woodhull reported, "and the atmosphere is generally humid, so that when the sun is unobstructed its direct rays are distressing and it is always oppressive in the field."[88] Woodhull found many of his contract surgeons lacking in aptitude and industry under these conditions. Among them was a man who had worked well in the field but had "no more judgment than to turn over sick call to his wife" and therefore marked himself as "certainly not the sort of person from whom the best service can be obtained." Indeed, Woodhull constantly expected "to hear of his breaking down." Another was "notoriously frail physically" and "exceedingly slow and over-cautious." Others appeared to be malingering or else just "dead wood." "It is very trying," Woodhull wrote, "to be credited with such as these

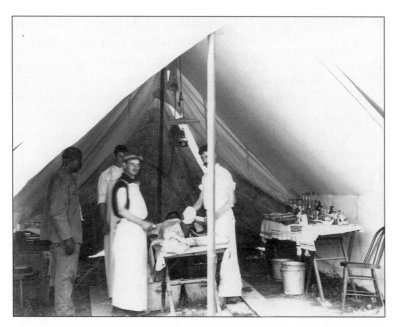

FIGURE 7.   Operating station, c. 1899 (RG 165-PW-G, NARA).

and expected to get good work out of them."[89] Most of the contract surgeons were merely "young men of small personal experience," and very few had made "a special study of the diseases of this climate."[90]

THE RACIAL ECONOMY OF THE TROPICS

In January 1900, Lieutenant P. C. Fauntleroy, M.D., proudly described his Second Division field hospital at Angeles, which then consisted of nine adjoining dwellings, all connected by bamboo and nipa covered ways. The water from the well seemed pure enough, but even so Fauntleroy made sure it was always filtered and boiled. The hospital bedding was regularly disinfected and boiled to prevent the spread of tinea, measles, and other skin irritations. Fauntleroy suspected that the origin of the many cases of malaria and intestinal disease he encountered was "to be found in the constant exposure while on the march and especially on outpost duty at night, to the prevailing conditions natural to this section, and to the flooding of the land for agricultural purposes," which had made the ground damp. "Irregular and often hasty eating of food" may have added to the level of morbidity.[91] These environmental and behavioral explanations did not mean that the medical officer discounted germs as the causes of disease; it was just that germs seemed to possess older geographical and moral correlates. In perplexing cases of fever, Fauntleroy would look for malaria parasites in the blood, but generally he could discern clear clinical signs — often a distinctive rash or fever pattern — indicating a specific disease and excusing him from deploying the microscope.

Lippincott reported that most of the "diseases incidental to the tropics" could be encountered in the Philippines. Dysentery was always present; leprosy was common, and enteric fever, or typhoid, "long ago became fastened to the coast line." The "inordinate activity of the skin" made severe "dermatic affections" nearly universal among white soldiers. "Slight injuries often result in long unhealed ulceration," the chief surgeon noted, "and this is due to excessive perspiration with its attending debility."[92] Vaccination and revaccination of the troops against smallpox "of a type especially severe to the white"[93] and endemic among Filipinos went on "as systematically as the drills at a well-regulated post."[94] "Malarial poisoning" was widespread, though not nearly as malignant as first feared; all the same, many regiments, beset with sporadic outbreaks, had required quinine prophylaxis. Not surprisingly, the wet season was the harbinger of death and disease, since "the camps were not only quagmires, but the soldiers were often drenched for days together." The results of this miserable predicament were dysentery, persistent diarrhea, rheumatism, enteric fever, and more malaria. During 1899, the worst year of the campaign, 36 officers and 439 soldiers were killed or died from wounds received in action, 8 officers and 131 soldiers died from "other forms of violence," and 16 officers and 693 men fell to disease, principally diarrhea and dysentery, smallpox and typhoid. Additionally, more than 1,900 soldiers were transferred back to the United States on account of sickness. The American army in the Philippines therefore lost through death, discharge, or transfer almost 14 percent of the average mean strength present (which was a little under 28,000 men). The sick rate — a more accurate measure of the incapacity of an army — was of course much higher.[95]

Although it was now generally accepted that "climate cannot generate fever no more than it can generate plants and animals," most physicians and their patients continued to believe that tropical conditions would reduce an alien race's general resistance to disease and present it with novel microbial pathogens for which it was unprepared.[96] Malaria had become prevalent among white troops because "the depressing influence of the tropical climate lessens the individual's normal resisting powers and thereby prepares a favorable soil for the invasion of parasites."[97] Even familiar, cosmopolitan diseases exerted a more deleterious effect in the devitalizing tropics. Smallpox "in this latitude and longitude," according to Hoyt, was "very fatal, especially to the white man."[98] The experience of Major Charles F. Mason, M.D., in treating typhoid among American soldiers in the Philippines convinced him that "the disease is more severe than in the temperate zone, and more fatal in its results."[99] Sternberg warned, "The spread of diarrhea and dysentery is indirectly promoted and their danger aggravated by the alternate heat and rains of a tropical climate and by the lowering of vital powers consequent on heat exhaustion."[100] Notter, too, had observed that "the mortality from enteric fever in hot climates is always more than in temperate zones," owing no doubt to "the diminished resistant power of the individual." The more potent "undermining factors" appeared to be youth and recent arrival in the foreign environment. Yet he had also noticed how "prolonged residence in a hot climate doubtless deteriorates the system" and led to the diminution of Anglo-Saxon "energy" — though he hastened to assure his readers that "the influence of 'climate' as a direct etiological factor of cholera or enteric fever . . . is baseless in fact."[101]

The encounters of military surgeons in the Philippines seemed to confirm that the white race was likely to degenerate and sicken in the tropics. According to Greenleaf, "the principal medical feature" of the San Isidro campaign in April 1899 was the "severe physical hardship" white troops endured: "The very bullock trains had to be helped by hand, under intense heat and atmospheric humidity." As a result, many soldiers succumbed to exhaustion, and 530 of them, almost 15 percent of the command, were admitted to the field hospital. Such incidents reinforced the conviction, held by physicians and ordinary soldiers alike, that "the Anglo-Saxon cannot work hard physically in the tropics without suffering physical harm from the sun and climate."[102] This meant in practice that only Filipinos and Chinese should perform heavy manual labor, such as lugging ambulance litters. But what was fighting a war if not a form of hard labor? Few medical officers doubted that the typical white soldier, marching and fighting "under very exhausting conditions of country and climate," could not "endure the same amount of nerve tension and physical strain that he can in a temperate zone." "Recuperation and convalescence in this climate are slow," reflected Greenleaf, and "were an epidemic of any character to occur among men in that condition, its effects would probably be very disastrous."[103] In Mason's opinion, "the great majority of white men in the tropics suffer a gradual deterioration of health and year by year become less and less fit for active service."[104] American sojourners might watch as "the sun cast long fingers of light" through the banana palms; they might gaze on "a blue sky, a gray beach, besprinkled with beautifully tinted shells" — but they were never allowed to forget the "generally accepted fact that [whites] cannot permanently adapt to the climatic conditions of this zone."[105]

The mental and moral qualities of the white race, finely attuned to a more stimulating environment, seemed especially likely to jangle and twang in tropical circumstances. The common enervation might on occasion slide into serious mental disorder. In the opinion of Surgeon Joseph A. Guthrie, "The Philippine sun seems to have a powerful influence upon the body, an overstimulating effect, like unto the surcharged x-ray, penetrating the skin along the nerve fibers and exerting its influence upon the entire nervous system."[106] Munson, in contrast, was convinced that tropical service inevitably caused "a depression of vital and nervous energy" and bred "nostalgia, ennui and discontent" among nonnative troops. Soon they became "wearied, fagged, and unable to concentrate their ordinary amount of brain power on any one subject."[107] Episodes of the "depressing condition known as nostalgia," brought on by fighting far from home in a foreign climate, occurred regularly, especially among the less worldly rural recruits. "In individual cases of illness," Greenleaf reported, "nostalgia became a complication that aggravated original disease and could not be removed while the patient remained in the islands."[108] "The sudden transfer to a foreign land," recalled Major Louis Mervin Maus, M.D., "separation from sweethearts, wives and family, the constant influence of conversation regarding the horrors of tropical diseases and climate, mental forebodings as to evil happenings, produced in a large number of the men, unaccustomed to absence from home, nostalgia which gradually merged into mental depression, apathy, loss of vitality, neurasthenia, melancholia and insanity."[109] Reeling between overstimulation and depression, the common soldier was struggling to maintain his usual equable temperament. At home, many came to believe the heat had driven men mad. In February 1900, the *Evening Star* in Washington, D.C., warned that "during the last three months nearly 250 demented soldiers have been sent across the continent [to Washington] and it is said that 250 more will arrive soon from Manila. In nearly all cases the men are violently insane."[110]

In 1902, reviewing the lessons of recent tropical service, Munson concluded that there was "ample proof that tropical heat and humidity produce marked changes in body-function which exert an effect adverse to the health and existence of all but the native-born." Heat and humidity increased European body temperature and perspiration while reducing pulse rate, blood pressure, and urine production. The number and function of "red blood corpuscles" diminished in whites transplanted to the tropics. Therefore, even if they avoided specific disease, "residence in hot climates, under circumstances of ordinary life, has an adverse effect on the white race." Speaking from experience, Munson could not doubt that "the Anglo-Saxon branch of the Teutonic stock is severely handicapped by nature in the struggle to colonize the tropics."[111] It mattered little whether Providence or evolutionary mechanism had matched race to climate: whatever the explanation, whites in the tropics were out of place, and degeneration and disease would be the natural rewards of environmental transgression.

The apprehensions and anxieties of American medical officers were hardly novel. Most medical authorities and social theorists in the nineteenth century held that the boundaries within which an individual could stay healthy and comfortable coincided with the region in which his race had long been situated. To venture beyond this natural realm in any circumstances seemed hazardous; to go abroad and fight a war on treacherous ground was to court disaster. For the past century, medical geographers had discussed whether Europeans might adapt themselves, or acclimatize, to a tropical environment — and the answer was still, even in the 1890s, unsettled. A general sense of climatic anxiety and pessimism pervaded the medical and colonial literature. Thus E. A. Birch, in Andrew Davidson's *Hygiene and Diseases of Warm Climates*, explained to his readers that a tropical climate would always be "inimical to the European constitution." A continued high temperature seemed to produce in the white body "an excessive cutaneous action, alternating with internal congestions." Although "the effort of nature is to accommodate the constitution to the newly established physiological requirements," there would be an inherent racial limit to this functional adjustment.[112] It comes as no surprise that the conventional concern about racial displacement was applied to the Philippines. Benjamin Kidd, an English social Darwinist, believed that "the attempt to acclimatize the white man in the tropics must be recognized as a blunder of the first magnitude. All experiments based on the idea are foredoomed to failure." On the eve of the U.S. Army's invasion of the Philippines, Kidd pointed out that "in climatic conditions that are a burden to him, in the midst of races in a different and lower stage of development; divorced from the influences that have produced him, from the moral and political environment from which he sprang, the white man . . . tends to sink slowly to the level around him." For in the tropics, "the white man lives and works only as a diver lives and works under water."[113]

But not all was lost on diving into the tropics. Medical officers in the Philippines gradually became more confident that proper attention to personal hygiene at least slowed the decay of the white racial constitution in a foreign environment. Thus the care of the body and the tempering of behavior might preserve and supplement the white soldier's powers of resistance and so mitigate the presumed transgression against nature. In other words, personal hygiene would perhaps allow alien Americans to function as if in sealed hermetic microenvironments, to equip themselves with a sanitary armature against the climate. Evidently, if a white American soldier was to withstand his depleting circumstances, his "habits, his work, his food, his clothing, must be rationally adjusted to his habitat" — not to make him like the locals but to protect him from going native. The basic precepts of tropical hygiene were simple enough: avoid the sun, stay cool, eat lightly, drink alcohol in moderation or not at all. In Mason's experience, "errors of diet, abuse of alcoholics, chilling after over-heating, especially at night, excessive fatigue, and the use of the heavy cartridge belt" had all been "powerful disposing factors" to invaliding and death in the tropics.[114]

The proper attire, diet, and conduct of American troops in the Philippines excited much expert commentary. Captain Matthew F. Stelle, M.D., in discussing the appropriate dress for a soldier in the tropics, admitted he had scarcely heard of khaki before 1898, but since then it had rapidly replaced blue as the distinctive coloration of the U.S. soldier. The lighter color, which deflected the sun, certainly seemed better adapted to the tropics. But he remained convinced that the old campaign hat used in the Philippines absorbed and concentrated the sun's rays and was "the most certain, rapid and permanent hair-eradicator that was ever invented."[115] Mason confirmed the hat's evil effects. He reported that a thermometer placed under a felt campaign hat registered 100.2 degrees, but under a khaki hat, left out in the sun, it never exceeded 92 degrees. His conclusion was that the campaign hat was "not fit for tropical service."[116]

When Stelle first ventured into the tropics, it seemed he was asked at least forty times a day, "Have you got an abdominal bandage?" "People were daft on the subject," he said. Although he later came to believe that "no greater fake was ever perpetrated" and that it was "a bad habit, a vice, a disease," he had become addicted to it, as had so many others, and "nothing but death can rescue us."[117] Guthrie was equally convinced that the popular flannel abdominal bandage was unnecessary, yet he continued to advise Americans in the tropics to protect their abdomen with a blanket when sleeping, to prevent them "chilling" through evaporation of sweat.[118] Members of the Philippine Commission, the new executive government, also concluded that the "abdominal band is necessary for perhaps fifty percent of Anglo-Saxons. One can try to do without it, but if one develops diarrhea, the best thing to do is wear it."[119] Captain Woodruff, however, expressed his objections to abdominal bands and other warm clothing with characteristic bluntness: "We are less in danger of chills," he declared, "than of being devoured by polar bears." The white man in the tropics could not cool off day or night, no matter how hard he tried. In these circumstances, "as little clothing as possible is the rule, and that clothing should be such as to interfere in no way whatever with getting rid of surplus heat."[120]

The effort to formulate the ideal ration for the white man in the tropics was similarly predicated on the perceived need to prevent the accumulation of excessive heat and thus restore the preexisting balance of the white constitution. Munson wanted more vegetables and less protein and fat in order to avoid "hyper-stimulation of the liver."[121] Surgeon Hamilton Stone argued that in the tropics, "where the excretory organs are always overtaxed," there was a marked tendency "for us to eat too much," especially the bulletproof army hardtack, some of it rumored to be left over from the Civil War.[122] Greenleaf, however, did not see any need to change the quantity of the tropical ration but suggested a decrease in the meat component and an increase in cereals. If the "nitrogenous and fatty elements" were reduced, then the diet would approximate that which sustained the local inhabitants.[123] But Woodruff, not surprisingly, challenged this objective too. "If we eat like natives," he predicted, "we will become as stupid, frail and worthless as they are." The real reason disease seemed so severe in the tropics was, he thought, that "the white man is exhausted by idleness and insufficient food and has no resistance." Experience had shown him that "the tropical heat causes a great expenditure of nervous and muscular force," so to balance this, to "supply the wastes and help to prevent exhaustion," more animal food was required, not less.[124] Such debates over white nutrition, dress, and behavior in the tropics would continue for the next twenty years.

MANLY WHITE TROPICAL SOLDIERS

American whiteness and masculinity were both more readily discerned and more highly valued in the tropics than at home; they appeared at once more vulnerable and more necessary.[125] The figure of "whiteness," whether deficient or overassertive, became a means through which Americans declared their presence in the Philippines. The white troops endured fatigue, fever, and nostalgia, all of which seemed to sap or undermine the race's reserves of energy and character. They often felt out of place, not in sympathy with tropical circumstances. Their medical officers attributed racial deterioration and disease to a mismatch between bodily constitution and environment — sometimes the environment was directly noxious, at other times it was microbiologically mediated. Soldiers felt awry and uncomfortable; their doctors confirmed and further specified the pathological consequences of displacement into a foreign climate and exotic disease ecology.

If whites were proving so vulnerable to tropical conditions, what was to be done? Medical officers sought to limit the troops' contact with microbes, especially the unfamiliar ones that appeared to prevail in the new territory. Moreover, they attempted to manage the selection, conduct, clothing, diet, and personal hygiene of soldiers in order to build up resisting powers and strengthen the constitution. In multiple ways, then, the military sanitarian was delimiting the boundaries of whiteness in the Philippines, counterposing it to an unwholesome and morbific climate and ecology and thus refiguring what it would mean to be a real white man — a vigorous American citizen-soldier — in the tropics. Evidently, remaining or becoming successfully white in the tropics was going to entail continual medical surveillance and discipline.

Facing west from California's shores, some Americans observed their whiteness become more visible again, this time in relation to the multiply threatening tropical milieu. Frederick Jackson Turner claimed that the struggle with savages and wilderness on the continental frontier transformed Europeans into Americans.[126] As that frontier closed, a new one opened on the other side of the Pacific, one markedly more militarized and medical. In the crucible of the Philippines "borderlands," American whiteness and masculinity would again be refashioned: now it was the medical officer who took charge of the process and determined the results.

Chapter Two

THE MILITARY BASIS OF COLONIAL
PUBLIC HEALTH

Carl von Clausewitz once remarked that although politics and warfare follow the same logic they use a different grammar.[1] Colonial public health, as it emerged in the Philippines under the American regime, would come to share both logic and grammar with the military sanitary bureau. That is, the mode of action and disciplinary tactics employed by military surgeons to ensure the hygiene and propriety of white troops were invoked, toward the end of the war, to manage the civilian population of the archipelago. New practices of colonial warfare, which required the attraction and pacification of local communities, fostered a transfer of contemporary military-medical strategies of crowd control. Military surgeons, who once had focused attention on raw American recruits, moved into the civil health authority and began to retrain Filipinos in the discipline of hygiene and to render sanitary their *barrios*, or "encampments." The new tropical medicine that developed in the Philippines was therefore as much a manifestation of military administrative logic as an expression of the rising enthusiasm for germ theories. Military strategy and practices of population management, more than laboratory science, would give distinctive form to modern public health in the Philippines. Indeed, the introduction of laboratory methods was dependent upon, and not responsible for, the administrative reform of crowd control and personal conduct in American colonial medicine.

In this chapter I want to chart a military genealogy of modern tropical hygiene.[2] It is necessary, then, to focus on the development of colonial warfare, with its distinctive and novel tactics and styles of deployment. Doctrines of colonial warfare, devised in the 1890s, differed from those of continental engagement. Colonial wars generally were fought in remote countries over large areas of unknown territory: the aim was not the destruction of the enemy, but, as Jean Gottman suggests, the "organization of the conquered peoples and territory under a particular control." "Instead of bringing death into the theater of operations, the aim [was] to create life within it."[3] In 1900, Hubert Lyautey summarized the new principle of colonial strategy: avoid the column and replace it with "progressive occupation." "Military occupation," he wrote, "consists less in military operations than in an organization on the march." The goal was to cover new territory with a network of disciplinary structures, including a network of hygiene. Colonial warfare at the turn of the century was thus recognized as being inseparable from administration. According to Lyautey, "the occupation deposits the units in the soil like sedimentary strata" — it created a new, more favorable terrain.[4] In this sense, the strategy and tactics of modern tropical public health might repeat and enhance colonial military strategy and tactics.[5] Moreover, in a colonial war, with dispersed and mobile military forces whose goal was reformation of the population, there was a special emphasis on developing intelligence (which after all is nothing more or less than military and medical analysis of foreign bodies) and a pressing need for communication, standardization, and registration. These military and medical requirements gave rise to a characteristic form of administration, and it was within this structure that bacteriology and parasitology eventually would be recognized as useful tools.

Fought initially in a conventional continental style, the Philippine-American War late in 1899 assumed more the character of colonial warfare, as Filipinos began to avoid fixed engagements and turn to skirmishes and other guerilla tactics.[6] In the archipelago, and especially in the main island of Luzon, colonial warfare would, toward the end of the campaign, thus become the major conduit through which the administrative practices of the army sanitary bureau flowed into and recanalized a subject population. The notion that colonialists might keep themselves healthy behind a *cordon sanitaire* — the sense that a sanitary enclave might protect them from environmental and social nuisances — was not completely abandoned, but it gradually gave way to efforts, which still to some appeared quixotic, to reform the presumed morals and behavior of "native races," to recultivate the social terrain.[7] The practice of progressive occupation signaled a shift from disregard of the health of local inhabitants to meticulous attention to their personal and domestic hygiene, from enclavist alienation to disciplinary extension. In creating a new public health in the tropics, American colonialists were commencing a "civilizing" project — a "nation-building" program — that might, in the distant future, transform their new subjects into approximate, if not to their minds authentic, citizens.

FROM MILITARY HYGIENE TO
COLONIAL PUBLIC HEALTH

"After things are more settled there is ample time for the germologist," wrote Surgeon Joseph A. Guthrie: in the meantime, "there are macroscopic topics of more consequence."[8] Guthrie's views were common among medical officers during the first year or so of the Philippines campaign: neither their training nor the exigencies of war permitted extensive microbiological investigation, while attention to the older landmarks of pathology and to sustaining the soldier's resisting powers seemed to work well enough. The surgeon initially concentrated on environmental risk and constitutional vulnerability, on knowing the territory and watching his men, on assaying a soil both literal and metaphoric — rarely did he focus on germs, the new seeds of disease. But by the time Guthrie was writing, military conditions had improved for the Americans, the war was dwindling into skirmishes with guerilla bands, and resort to bacteriology was becoming more frequent. The new military circumstances in which microbes were, in a sense, discovered in the Philippines — or at least finally made salient in a war against disease — would confer a deeper social and political meaning on these agents. Germs were no longer mere concomitants of environmental threat: increasingly they might be located in local fauna, which included Filipinos, and tracked through local biological and social networks. After 1900, medical strategies and military tactics derived from mutually reinforcing renditions of the need to contain and discipline the hostile and increasingly mobile agents in the region, whether germ or *insurrecto*.

With the advance of the army into Luzon, the settled conditions Guthrie and others sought were gradually imposed. As Aguinaldo resorted to guerilla tactics, the strategy of General Arthur MacArthur, the army's field commander, came to resemble more and more Lyautey's doctrine of colonial warfare. Thus MacArthur emphasized research and intelligence, that is, the surveillance of the enemy; the column was divided into small fighting units; and the control of populations became more important than the defeat of opposing forces. Destruction was minimized, and a network of disciplinary institutions was laid down, a new terrain was produced, or settled, in step with the advance. MacArthur was obsessed with drill and discipline, clear channels of authority, explicit record keeping, and neatness of dress in subordinates; he found it hard to deal with civilians unless they conformed to military style. Civilians had to be rendered obedient, not with armed force but through administration. "We have to govern them," he wrote, "and government by force alone cannot be satisfactory to Americans."[9]

After 1900 more than five hundred army posts were scattered over the archipelago in an effort to hold enemy territory. As General George M. Sternberg, M.D., reported, "This change in the character of the service required of the troops had an important bearing on the medical administration."[10] The medical officers who once had concentrated at the general hospitals dispersed with the regiments. There were not enough for each garrison in a district to possess its own physician, so hospital corpsmen were often assigned to smaller detachments and subposts. As the army advanced, MacArthur ordered all towns and villages to conform to stringent health standards. He set up municipal and provincial boards of health to manage sanitary conditions and to enforce stipulations of hygienic behavior. Local military surgeons from a nearby post or on secondment organized and watched over the boards. "The sanitary condition of the garrisoned towns and villages is described as having been execrable," Sternberg noted. "Filth of all kinds underlay and surrounded the houses, and the hogs were not the only scavengers."[11] Major L. Mervin Maus, M.D., writing from northern Luzon, imparted that "owing to the hostile condition of the country and the facilities offered for harboring insurrectos and ladrones, etc., the division commander decided to garrison all the principal pueblos in the limits of the division." Maus too found that "the sanitation of the towns was extremely bad when our troops entered them. The habitations of the natives as a rule were surrounded by filth of all kinds — slops, garbage, fecal accumulations, rubbish, and other débris. Weeds and rank vegetation were allowed to grow along the fences, in the yards, and in the streets." But post commanders spoke severely with local officials and soon "a great reformation was accomplished."[12] Similarly, Major Franklin A. Meacham, M.D., reported from Tarlac that "the policing of the grounds around the barracks and buildings occupied by troops is excellent and is regularly done." This had set a good example for the local inhabitants, who were exhorted to follow it. "Where troops are stationed such policing is done by the presidente of the town and by the cabezas of the barrios, under instructions from the commanding officers." As a result, "countless unsanitary evils among the natives have been remedied."[13]

As Lieutenant Colonel Alfred A. Woodhull, M.D., had advised in the many editions of his *Notes on Military Hygiene*, it was "the direct duty of officers of the line in whose hands is the machinery of control, to maintain the whole territory of occupation as unpolluted as a parade ground."[14] Major Edward L. Munson, M.D., recommended that "a complete new sanitary machine, applicable to the special conditions encountered, must be established without delay," even though in colonial settings this apparatus frequently met with disfavor or passive opposition. Such resistance required the military medical officer with civil ambitions to demonstrate "high capacity for organization and administration, combined with good judgment, discretion, force of character and tact."[15] Munson himself attempted to display these qualities as a medical officer in Manila (1902–04), instructor in military hygiene at Fort Leavenworth, acting director of health in the Philippines (1914), editor of *Military Surgeon*, health advisor to governor-general Leonard Wood in the archipelago (1922–25), and finally as commandant of the Medical Field Service School at Carlisle Barracks, Pennsylvania.[16] His career thus sutured together military and colonial hygiene, and he found no impediment to the transfer of military practices into the colonial civil regime. In particular, he liked to make analogies between "military efficiency" and "industrial morale" — military drill and discipline therefore were applicable "with little or no modification to the industrial problems of civil life." Munson believed military and civil "morale work" was fundamentally a "science of human engineering." Reform of customs and habits and improvement in morale could make good soldiers and better citizens. But experience showed him that for some races, including African-Americans and Filipinos, "it takes time to abandon old standards and establish new, even with the assistance of the cohesion under pressure of the military environment."[17] Just as well, then, so it seemed to Munson and his colleagues, American tutelage had some time yet to exert its impact in the archipelago.

From the earliest days of their occupation of Manila, the army set about cleaning up the capital. The interim military Board of Health for Manila, organized by Major Frank Bourns, M.D., in September 1898, had developed the basic arrangements for sanitation and health care delivery in the city. It divided the city into ten districts and appointed a municipal physician to each — again, usually detailed from the military. Lieutenant Harry Gilchrist conducted a census of the city in 1899, providing a demographic inventory that informed later medical activities. During this period, separate hospitals for smallpox, leprosy, and venereal diseases were established, and a veterinary corps organized. A municipal dispensary opened in late 1899.[18] Colonel Charles R. Greenleaf, M.D., reported that the Manila Board of Health, dominated by army officers, had

> made great progress in cleaning the streets of the city, in removing filth that has been accumulating for years, and in regulating, to a certain extent, the purity of the food supply; it has practically stamped out smallpox by forcible vaccination and revaccination, where it was necessary, and held in check the progress of bubonic plague, that, after lodgment in other tropical cities, has speedily become epidemic and caused a frightful mortality; but its work has of necessity been superficial, and the good results can only be maintained by a vigorous support from the military authorities, and by a liberal supply of funds.[19]

Dean C. Worcester, a notoriously rancorous member of the Philippine Commission and later the secretary of the interior in the civil government, went out of his way to praise the efforts of Bourns, an old friend, in "waging war upon the more serious ailments that threatened the health of the soldiers and the public."[20]

An extensive system of sanitary inspectors checked for violations of the regulations. Each of the ten Manila sanitary districts now boasted an American medical officer and subordinate Filipino inspectors, a sanitary corps, responsible for each division. Since the 1870s, the army medical department had performed sanitary inspections of the troops, and now these procedures were transferred over to the civil sphere so as to enable surveillance of the local inhabitants. Munson, referring to military hygiene, remarked that "the skilled sanitary officer should be of methodical and industrious habits, competent in observation, impartial in judgment and conscientious in action." Civil sanitary inspectors required the same qualities. According to the colonial military hygienist, "men, manners, mind, diet, dress and discipline all fall legitimately within the province of the sanitary inspector."[21] As it was in military life, so it would be in civil affairs.

The new civil Board of Health for the whole of the Philippine Islands, established in 1901, included the commissioner of public health and the chief health inspector, with the chief surgeon of the U.S. Army in the Philippines

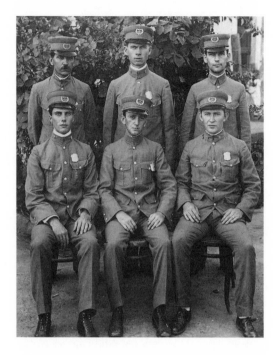

FIGURE 8.
U.S. sanitary inspectors
(RG 350-P-E41.3, NARA).

and the chief quarantine officer of the U.S. Public Health and Marine Hospital Service as honorary members. This body drafted legislation to control the
practice of medicine, dentistry, pharmacy, and veterinary science and supervised the new provincial and municipal boards of health.[22] Policy came from
above, but the demands of routine work and personal contact often led to
considerable flexibility in the actual administration of public health. The local
health boards — over three hundred of them by then — were responsible for
the prosecution of any violations of the sanitary laws and enforced the regulations of the national board. The Filipino elite took charge of these boards,
mediating between the government and local society, although there was
usually an army post surgeon nearby to supervise them.[23] After 1903, the
Filipino doctors who headed the boards were sent to Manila to undergo a
training program to fit them for their responsibilities. Through these off-
shoots the national Board of Health extended its operations to every municipality in the archipelago.[24]

Maus, detailed from the army's medical department, became the first "civil"
commissioner of public health.[25] Just one of a cavalcade of military medical
officers passing confidently into the civil service, Maus found that his new
appointment entailed few changes in the scope and character of his work.

According to Greenleaf, Maus during the war had "established an efficient working system, restored order, replenished supplies, established hospitals, and procured reports that had long been neglected."[26] As health commissioner, he worked eighteen hours a day combating new epidemics of bubonic plague and cholera, writing new health ordinances, attempting to isolate lepers and control venereal disease.[27] But soon after taking up his new post, he fell out with Worcester, who accused him of insubordination and dishonesty. Maus claimed Worcester was annoyed merely because the desk of his brother-in-law, Paul Freer, had been removed from the health commissioner's office.[28] Eventually Maus was forced out: "I submitted my resignation," he recalled, "feeling I could no longer occupy a position which was subjected to such unpleasant surveillance and criticism."[29] But Worcester's attempt to assert control over the Board of Health was short-lived.

In late 1902, Major Bourns was recalled to take temporary charge of the board until Major E. C. Carter, M.D., could take over as commissioner of public health.[30] Soon after taking up his duties, and believing that the Board of Health had by then established "a reasonable control of sanitary affairs in Manila," Carter set out to obtain accurate information on the sanitary conditions of the provinces and to secure a public health service in these outlying regions. He realized that "specially trained men" were required in order to collect "reliable data."[31] To this end, a number of physicians were selected and trained as sanitary inspectors. The board piled up detailed reports on the condition of markets and stores, disposal of garbage, the "situation" of the villages and the character of the "terrain," water supply, prevalent diseases, local ordinances and laws on sanitary matters, the "customs and habits" of the people as they affected health and sanitation, and the diseases found among cattle and other domestic animals. Scarcely a village evaded this rigorous scrutiny. "As each township was visited and inspected," Carter recalled, "a sanitary map of the Philippines" was gradually compiled — a topography both medical and military.[32]

"WHAT ALCHEMY WILL CHANGE THE ORIENTAL QUALITY OF THEIR BLOOD?"

Reporting to President Theodore Roosevelt, Elihu Root, the secretary of war, observed that the army, "utilizing the lessons of the Indian wars, . . . has relentlessly followed the guerilla bands to their fastnesses in mountain and jungle and crushed them." The American military was displaying "splendid virile energy" in difficult tropical conditions; "individual liberty, protection of

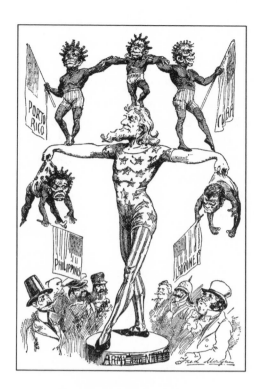

FIGURE 9. "Uncle Sam's new-caught anthropoids" (*Literary Digest*, August 20, 1898). Courtesy of the University of Wisconsin Library.

personal rights, civil order, public instruction, and religious freedom have followed its footsteps."[33] According to Root, the military thus became a liberal reformist force, attracting and pacifying Filipinos and rendering them more docile and amenable to American control. Roosevelt happily endorsed the message. He had already boasted that the army in the Philippines was proving itself "a great constructive force, a most potent implement for the up-building of a peaceful civilization."[34] In 1902, Roosevelt would insist that the aim of the war in the Philippines was "the triumph of civilization over forces which stand for the black chaos of savagery and barbarism." "Our armies do more than bring peace, do more than bring order," he continued. "They bring freedom."[35] Later that year, Roosevelt returned to this theme. In the Philippines, he declared, "the soldier's work as a soldier was not the larger part of what he did. When once the outbreak was over in any place, then began the work of establishing civil administration."[36] On another occasion he noted that "too much praise can not be given to the army for what it has done in the Philippines both in warfare and from an administrative standpoint in preparing the way for civil government."[37]

The republican language of civic virtue infused the rhetoric of imperialists and anti-imperialists alike.[38] Roosevelt saw annexation of the Philippines as the latest installment of the westward expansion that had forestalled corruption in the American republic and renewed independent virtues such as self-reliance, industry, and temperance.[39] Even as imperialism thus benefited the United States, there was a dim prospect of it also promoting civic virtue, with eventual citizen competence and self-government, among Filipinos. But many anti-imperialists regarded empire as a threat to the republic because it might permit the incorporation of races utterly incapable of self-determination. They feared that Filipinos, who seemed permanently unable to maintain orderly governments in the Anglo-Saxon fashion, might join the union. William Jennings Bryan, among others, warned that Filipinos could not become citizens without endangering the republic. He saw no reason to exercise sovereignty over an alien race in a forlorn attempt to elevate it: "Does history justify us in believing that we can improve the condition of the Filipinos and advance them in civilization by governing them without their consent and taxing them without representation?"[40] Imperialism was at variance with constitutional government. The islands should be abandoned and Filipinos left to their own primitive devices.

Regardless of anti-imperialist warnings, the goals of American colonial government would be frankly reformist. With the development of modern legal, medical, and commercial infrastructures and the instilling of bourgeois and democratic values, traditional patterns of social organization were expected to dissolve, and Filipinos to become reconciled to U.S. control.[41] Of course, neither soldier-administrators nor their nonmilitary successors expected Filipinos would soon achieve the civic objectives they had been set. Thus Roosevelt reflected that "it is a very difficult matter, practically, to apply the principles of an orderly free government to an Oriental people struggling upward out of barbarism and subjection."[42] The president was "extremely anxious that the natives shall show the power of governing themselves" — but he expected that such accomplishment would take several generations of tutelage. "The only fear is lest in our over-anxiety we give them a degree of independence for which they are unfit, thereby inviting reaction and disaster."[43] It was, he mused, "a task requiring infinite firmness, patience, tact, broadmindedness."[44]

William H. Taft, the first civil governor of the Philippines, heartily agreed with the president, though he warned that Filipinos were a "sensitive people" who rankled at the label of "savage."[45] All the same, "lacking the American initiative, lacking the American knowledge of how to carry on a government,

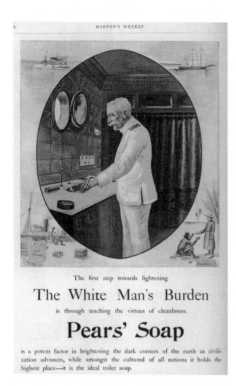

The first step towards lightening

The White Man's Burden

is through teaching the virtues of cleanliness.

Pears' Soap

is a potent factor in brightening the dark corners of the earth as civilization advances, while amongst the cultured of all nations it holds the highest place—it is the ideal toilet soap.

FIGURE 10. "The white man's burden" (*Harper's Weekly*, September 20, 1899). Courtesy of the Wisconsin Historical Society.

any government there must be a complete failure until by actual observation and practice, under the guidance of a people who know how to carry on a government, who understand the institutions of civil liberty, there may be trained a Filipino element." The Ohio Republican thought he knew how to carry on a government; he had been doing so through the Philippine Commission since the middle of 1900, teaching Filipinos "what individual liberty is and training them to a knowledge of self-government." "We have a hope," he testified, "that with the imitative character of the people, with their real desire for improvement . . . we can carry out an experiment and justify our course."[46] But, like Roosevelt, he felt it would take many generations to lift them up to civilization. Part of this uplift would be hygienic. Thus "the gradual teaching of the people the simple facts of hygiene, unpopular and difficult as the process of education has been, will prove to be one of the great benefits given by Americans to this people." Eventually, then, with American guidance, Filipinos might show themselves to be "capable of exercising the self-restraint and conservatism of action which are essential to political stability."[47] Self-government was evidently as much a personal need as a political goal.

Bernard Moses, a Berkeley professor of political science and member of the Philippine Commission, had shaped Taft's views on native development. An expert on Spanish-American history, Moses frequently reflected on the problem of educating "an alien race, whose thoughts are not our thoughts, and whose motives it is not always easy for us to understand." For Moses, "the facts of race distinction" lay at the foundation of colonial administration. Local customs and habits might take generations to change, but he believed Americans had already managed to "infect" Filipinos "with the fever of progress."[48] Through association with "a higher form of life," the "dependent body is drawn into the current of a superior nation's life, and is carried along by the momentum of its progress."[49] However, after millennia of "barbarism" and subjection to the autocratic control of Spain, Filipinos lacked the "political instinct" of Anglo-Saxons. It would be necessary to eradicate the "inordinate conceit" of the *mestizo* — "his inexperience, his half-knowledge was the basis of his confidence" — and to govern the archipelago for many decades before "habit established by long practice will supplement his knowledge and furnish him certain direction in the conduct of his affairs."[50] Independence, if granted within forty years, would inevitably mean a return to barbarism.

Professional orators such as Senator Albert J. Beveridge, a Republican from Indiana, captured eloquently the case for continued civic tutelage of Filipinos. In 1900, Beveridge declaimed that Filipinos were "a barbarous race, modified by three centuries of contact with a decadent race"; therefore they were not capable of "self-government in the Anglo-Saxon sense." "What alchemy," he asked, "will change the Oriental quality of their blood, in a year, and set the self-governing currents of the American pouring through their Malay veins?"[51] Having just returned from the islands, Beveridge was convinced that many years of example would be required before Filipinos were fully instructed in "American ideas and methods of administration," for "in dealing with Filipinos we are dealing with children." Moreover, he believed that God had marked "the American people as His chosen Nation finally to lead in the regeneration of the world," to rescue it from wilderness and savage men.[52] Accordingly, if puerile natives were as yet incapable of self-government, then they must carefully and gradually be taught how to do it, whether they liked it or not: "We govern Indians without their consent, we govern our territories without their consent, we govern our children without their consent." Invigilation and constant discipline must accompany the inevitable "march of the flag."[53]

As Beveridge implied, there were obvious continental models, or ana-
logues, for insular reformation. Taft, for example, lamented that the "Negroes" freed after the Civil War had never been "trained to self-support or
self-help." He argued that education and "industrial independence" might
promote some progress of the "Negro race" and the "Filipino people": "advancement along that path opens up to both the possibility, indeed, the cer-
tainty of attaining all other ideals, intellectual, political, and moral."[54] Roosevelt was somewhat less confident of African-American capacities, but he was
able to discern parallels between the civilizing of American Indians and of
Filipinos. Indeed, the president believed that the civilizing of Indians might
result in "their ultimate absorption into the body of our people," though "this
absorption must and should be very slow."[55] Eventually, civilized Filipinos
would attain self-government, while civilized Indians might become eligible
for American citizenship. It seemed possible that hygiene, education, and industry would in time uplift both groups of "savages," turning natives into
proletarians. From the 1880s the government had been making an effort to
transform displaced American Indians into docile, property-owning, Christian subjects: citizenship was granted to those who took up allotments on the
reservations, and a few children attended boarding schools, such as the Carlisle Indian Industrial School in Pennsylvania.[56] But Roosevelt and many
others still felt that Indians would continue to represent a challenge to the as-
similative capacities of American society. "Some Indians can hardly be moved
forward at all," he wrote. "Some can be moved both fast and far. . . . A few
Indians may be able to turn themselves into ordinary citizens in a dozen years.
Give to these Indians every chance; but remember that the majority must
change gradually, and that it will take several generations to make change
complete."[57] Organized through the civil Bureau of Indian Affairs, plans for
Indian assimilation remained underfunded, halfhearted, and specious.

After Aguinaldo's resort to guerilla warfare late in 1899, the U.S. army,
including the medical department, also readily recognized the similarity of
Indian and Filipino. Scattered across the archipelago in posts and garrisons,
medical officers often remarked on how fighting in the Philippines now called
to mind the occupation of "Indian country" before the coming of the rail-
roads, in advance of the cultivation and settlement of the West.[58] Indeed,
officers and enlisted men in the Philippines, on occasion, would even refer to
Filipinos as Indians and squaws. But there were limits to such analogies. To
most it was evident that Christian, urban Filipinos were not roaming heathens. When Taft famously claimed "it is possible for us to govern them as we

govern the Indian tribes," he was alluding not to "lowland" Tagalogs, but to the non-Christian Moros in the southern Philippines. He continued, "They are nowhere near so amenable to education, to complete self-government, as are the Christian Filipinos." Moreover, colonial warfare in the Philippines differed significantly from the Indian wars. For example, in the United States the Sioux and Cheyenne had been forced onto reservations, and whites took their land; in the Philippines, such displacement was as undesirable as it was impractical. In America, the alleged civilizing of Indians on the reservations was hardly more than gestural and decorous, a poor excuse for expropriation of land. There, pauperism and dependency prevailed, tuberculosis was rife, and agency physicians were scarce and found little time or enthusiasm for hygiene reform.[59] In the Philippines, though, hygiene and civic discipline emerged as part of a specific military strategy and were enforced with precision and care. The army and the emergent colonial state thus attempted an intensive reform and disciplining of Filipinos *in situ*, to render them more docile and amenable to distant American control. The U.S. government conferred the status of national — not quite colonial subject and not quite citizen — on American Indians and Filipinos, but different colonizing processes meant that the implications of this term, especially its implied potential for development and self-government, would diverge in North American and insular settings.[60]

MICROBIAL *INSURRECTOS*

"However much beclouded by sentiment and humanitarianism they may be," Munson wrote in 1911, "the motives primarily actuating the sanitary service are, after all, tactical and economic." Moreover, sanitary tactics were "always to be regarded as consequent upon and subordinate to general military tactics."[61] It was necessary to obtain good information on the strength, position, and movements of human and microbial enemies, on the character of the terrain, and on where casualties have fallen or are likely to fall. New bacteriological techniques could be used to probe the enigmatic foreign environment and to investigate the purity of water and food; or they might also help to locate pathogenic agency within insect and human populations. In the Philippines, bacteriology emerged as a practical tool just when military tactics began to focus on the organization of the population. The earlier medical concerns about terrain, climate, and bodily constitution persisted, but interest in the threat posed by the local fauna became more intense and soon dominated medical strategy, as it did military tactics. Bacteriology, as it developed in the matrix of colonial warfare, became especially helpful in registering individuals and populations: it could generate a standardized documentary record that provided intelligence on past human behavior and monitored conformity to the rules, or discipline, of modern hygiene—whether the subjects were raw recruits to the army or "savages." In 1899, the little bacteriological investigation that occurred in the Philippines had interrogated the perplexing environment and errant or ailing American troops; by 1905, bacteriology abounded, and it focused mostly on Filipino bodies, generally revealing their defiance of civilized military hygiene or their apparent indifference to such discipline.

The distinctive disease ecology that the microscope was revealing in the tropics incorporated Filipinos—as "natural" hosts and carriers of the microbes with which they had evolved—into a network of pathological causation. Filipinos were thus armed—only to be disarmed—with a weapon more insidious than any rifle. "The Filipinos are never free from contagious diseases of one form or another," warned Lieutenant Colonel Henry Lippincott, M.D., "and we can never be sure that they are not bringing infection into our midst."[62] According to Maus, Americans were campaigning against "a densely ignorant race of people, who had as little knowledge or respect for the abc's of sanitation as the American Indian at home."[63] Medical officers for a time forbade contact with the "natives." No matter how clean Filipinos might look or smell, they were still to be distrusted, still potentially unhygienic *insurrectos*. "The natives do not keep their hands clean, although it is said their bodies are washed daily," wrote Guthrie; "at all events, they are not microscopically clean."[64]

Americans felt they battled invisible foes, whether guerilla or microbe, that could merge with ease into the luxuriant natural realm or into a disorderly social world. "One day we may be fighting with thousands of their people [and] the next day you can't find an enemy, they are all 'amigos,'" Captain Delphey T. E. Casteel complained. "They have hidden their rifles and may be working for you for all you know."[65] In a guerilla war, the army took up the slogan "There are no more amigos."[66] As for Major C. J. Crane, every thicket suggested to him the presence of a treacherous Filipino. Insurgents were "hiding in the mangroves or swamps" or disappearing into "rank vegetation and dense undergrowth." In "this struggle with an unseen yet imminent danger," it appeared that "every Filipino is our enemy," and "even the dogs seemed trained to bark peculiarly at an American."[67] An intelligence officer reported from Biñan that Filipinos "are at this date outwardly friendly to the Ameri-

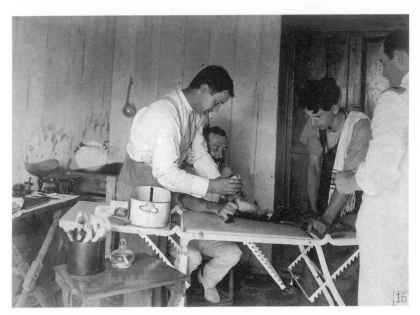

FIGURE 11. Animal necroscopy room, Army Pathological Laboratory, c. 1900 (Johns Hopkins University Commission). Courtesy of the Alan Mason Chesney Archives, Johns Hopkins University.

cans, but secretly aid the insurrection."[68] Indeed, all the fauna in the archipelago, whether human or nonhuman, seemed increasingly duplicitous, ready at any moment to come into focus, to sting, to infect, to shoot. Had not Lippincott warned his fellow surgeons that all Filipinos, like the swamp-dwelling mosquitoes, were potentially carriers of destructive, hidden infection? Guthrie preferred a more explicit analogy. "The glands of the skin are the individuals in a regiment," he explained. "Weaken the individuals and the regiment deteriorates." In the Philippines, he continued, "there is in reserve an array of living things to prey upon the poor alien's depleted cuticle." For example, "insects prevail in vast quantities, their stings and bites add to the enemy's strength, and so we must prepare against many foes."[69]

Most Americans on arriving in the Philippines, according to Surgeon Guthrie, soon became convinced that "the air, water, soil, the whole earth and its sundry encumbrances (living and dead)" were actually "reeking in germs." Thus the visitor "contracted along with his 'Philipinitis,' 'germania.' "[70] While Guthrie treated the ambit claims of the "germologists" with skepticism, many of his colleagues had begun to search for local microbial pathogens and to reveal their passage through human and insect life. From the beginning, the

First Reserve Hospital had possessed a small diagnostic laboratory, but it faltered when its first director contracted typhoid and rapidly succumbed to the disease.[71] The eventual successor, Richard P. Strong, found himself pre-occupied with performing autopsies and making cultures of blood, feces, and urine along with other clinical services — when he was not laid up with Malta fever. But in 1900, Strong, a recent Johns Hopkins graduate afire with en-thusiasm for the new bacteriology, was appointed to an army board to investi-gate the diseases of the archipelago.[72] As hostilities dwindled to skirmishes with bands of partisans, more time and personnel might be spared for re-search. Strong developed his earlier, relatively perfunctory studies of dysen-tery; W. J. Calvert investigated the transmission of plague; and Joseph J. Curry attempted to elucidate the cause of the regional fevers, especially those "un-influenced by quinine administered in large doses."[73] After repeated blood examinations and the use of the Widal test, Curry was able to diagnose many hitherto obscure fevers as typhoid — the rest unfortunately remained obscure. Strong, however, successfully identified an amoeba as the cause of much of the dysentery commonly experienced in the islands. Several other cases that came to autopsy were infected with a microorganism that grew to resemble the standard culture of Shiga's *Bacillus dysenteriae*, which had been sent from Japan. Stirred by these achievements, Strong and his colleagues set out resolu-tely to animate microbiologically the tropical environment and its macro-scopic life forms. He boasted to Sternberg that "the English as yet apparently have no good laboratory in the East, and they have expressed considerable surprise that one has been established and so thoroughly equipped here."[74] From 1900, Manila had a municipal laboratory, derived from the army's hospital laboratory, and before long other bacteriological laboratories were cropping up across the archipelago.

THE COLONIAL POLITICS OF EPIDEMIC DISEASE

The first major test of American bacteriology in the Philippines was an out-break of bubonic plague late in 1899. The disease arrived from Hong Kong and persisted at a low level in the archipelago until 1906. Forty-eight cases occurred in Manila in February 1900; a year later sanitary inspectors re-ported twenty-seven cases.[75] Alexandre Yersin had identified the plague bacil-lus in Hong Kong in 1894, but because the organism, rarely found in the bloodstream, could be extracted only from the obvious buboes, the diagnosis was still made mostly on clinical grounds. Moreover, the discovery of a cause did not, in this case, imply any one mode of transmission. Some physicians still regarded plague as directly contagious; others, like Patrick Manson, believed it derived from contact with clothing, soil, and refuse — the bacillus had recently been found in rats, but Manson regarded them as mere "multipliers of the virus."[76] By 1904, Maximilian Herzog at the Bureau of Science in Manila would wonder if rats and their fleas might actually spread the disease, but he concluded that *Bacillus pestis* most likely gained entry to the body through skin and mucous membranes.[77]

The early sanitary response to plague in Manila involved both control of personal contact and a campaign against rats. All vessels arriving in the islands were inspected for human cases and for rodents, and if they came from an affected port they were quarantined. The Board of Health demanded that those suffering from the disease be isolated; the sickroom was disinfected with corrosive sublimate or carbolic acid, and "all valueless clothing and other effects" were burned. It recommended that the public drink only boiled water, obey "the rules of general hygiene," and regularly remove any trash. "Wearing of shoes and stockings," the board advised, "is an important factor in preventing plague gaining an entrance into the body through wounds."[78] But humans were not the only targets of the public health officers. "In view of the association between plague and rodents," the nascent Board of Health set about waging an "incessant war" against the animals. It told house-owners to replace wooden floors with more sanitary concrete ones, to remove all refuse, and to burn any rat manure. Squads of rat-catchers fanned out over the city, visiting each house and setting traps or laying out bane. They concentrated on areas that had produced the heaviest caseload and examined the associated disease ecology, attempting to confirm etiological suspicions in the bacteriology laboratory. The presence of plague bacilli in some of the local rats seemed to corroborate their suspected role in the transmission of the disease. In February 1902 alone, the squads delivered more than twenty thousand rats to the government laboratory, which examined almost ten thousand microscopically for bacilli and found thirteen infected.[79]

During April 1901, the Board of Health sent medical practitioners a letter drawing their attention to the previously unrecognized phenomenon of "ambulatory plague." It appeared that this condition was frequently encountered among the Chinese, "who keep up much longer in severe illness than any other races here." A Chinese might fall dead in the street without evident cause, without obvious buboes — just as the rats were doing. "That such cases are true plague," the board reported, "is borne out by the recent investigations of the Board of Health, autopsies resulting in the finding of the plague bacillus and the characteristic pathological changes."[80] Laboratory investigation in some cases could now prove more sensitive than clinical observation and focus attention on hitherto unsuspected human elements. While the presence of buboes remained pathognomic, "the absence of buboes [did] not exclude plague."[81] Physicians were expected to watch out for meretriciously healthy Chinese and Filipinos and employ the bacteriology laboratory to reveal scarcely symptomatic carriers, who were "scattering and implanting the disease throughout the islands."[82] Where plague was involved, there would be no more amigos.

On March 21, 1902, Worcester heard that two patients at San Juan de Dios Hospital, both Filipino, were suffering from cholera—Strong had confirmed the diagnosis when he observed the comma bacillus in hanging drop slides in the laboratory. Within a day, another fourteen typical cases were identified, many of them dying soon after diagnosis. Official notification of the spread of the disease into Hong Kong had been received a few weeks before, so news of the outbreak in Manila was not altogether unexpected. In an attempt to block the entry of cholera into the archipelago, Dr. Victor G. Heiser, the chief quarantine officer, had prohibited the importation of green vegetables from southern China.[83] Whether unexpected or not, the new epidemic represented another serious challenge to the civil health administration. "Unfortunately," recalled Worcester, "there was no one connected with the medical service of the islands who had any practical experience in dealing with cholera, and we [would have] to get this as we went along."[84] In meeting this challenge, the public health administration was to assume a definite and durable form.

Cholera had visited the archipelago at regular intervals during the past hundred years. In response to the epidemic of 1882, the Spanish colonial authorities had stepped up the cleaning of streets, vacant lots, and public buildings and established four hospitals for the sick. Believing the disease to be miasmatic in origin, health officials lit fires with *tangal*, a type of mangrove bark, and tar at the foci of infection. Burial corps lurched through the mud of the streets, emerging out of the smoke with the bodies of the dead stacked on their carts. After a brief service, held outside the church gates, the corpses were covered with quicklime to counter noxious emanations and buried with haste. For personal prophylaxis, the mourners, priests, and those who labored to collect the bodies filled quills with camphor and placed them in their mouths. In the city and the provinces, the enveloping crisis mocked the government's plans for an orderly response. People fled in panic, hygienic

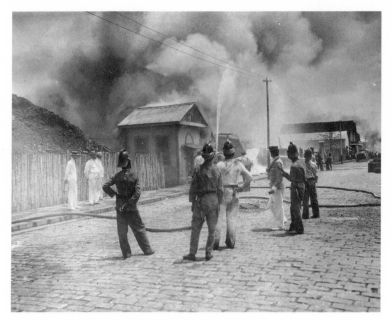

FIGURE 12. Burning the cholera-infected district of Farola (RG 350-P-E44.2, NARA).

precautions were abandoned, and few victims received medical attention. Eventually the epidemic had died down of its own accord.[85]

In contrast to the earlier Spanish response to cholera, American measures designed to suppress the disease in 1902 placed as much emphasis on controlling personal contact and social life as on a general cleanup and spiritual succor. With the development of bacteriology, health officials could trace the path of the cholera vibrio and use this intelligence to intervene in daily life and curtail its spread. Fears of diffuse emanations from the environment and the dead had lost much of their power. Instead, suspected cases and their contacts were isolated, removed from their homes, and placed in a temporary tent hospital on the grounds of San Lazaro Hospital, or else concentrated in the military "protection zone" at Santa Mesa Heights.[86] With quarantine strictly enforced around Manila, no one could trespass the city limits without written permission of the health authorities. Officers of the Board of Health went from house to house, day and night, rooting out cases, confiscating and destroying dubious foodstuffs. Nor were more general environmental measures neglected. Americans, too, lit fires, not mere bonfires to clear the miasmatic air but great consuming blazes that reduced to ashes the nipa palm houses at infected foci.[87] The "less dangerous" wooden houses of the more affluent

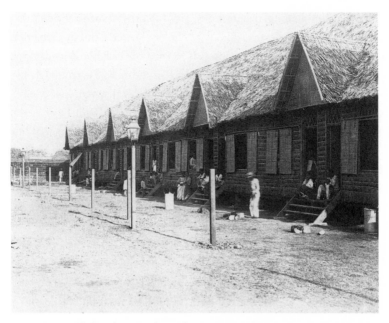

FIGURE 13. Cholera detention barracks, San Lazaro (RG 350-P-E42, NARA).

were simply whitewashed to disinfect them, and the inhabitants forcibly bathed in a bichloride solution. Patrols of sanitary inspectors and cavalry guarded the Marikina River, the main source of water for the city.[88]

But the comma bacillus continued to spread. From March 20 until the end of the month, 94 Filipinos, 6 Chinese, and 1 American were infected. By April, 15,275 cases of cholera had occurred within Manila, with 215 deaths, including 5 Americans.[89] Corporal Richard Johnson, with the 48th Volunteers, recalled that the cholera epidemic gave Americans "more scare than anything coming from the insurrectors, because with them we could defend ourselves with rifle and bullets, but cholera was an enemy whose presence we were unaware of until his fatal stroke."[90] More resources were committed to combat the disease. The Board of Health sought the advice of Munson, a military hygienist already famed for his "administrative and organizing ability, sound judgment, initiative, and forcefulness of an unusual order."[91] The Philippines division commander ordered 31 medical officers to report for duty with the civil health service. Some were detailed as sanitary inspectors or quarantine officers, others took charge of the cholera hospital and detention camps, and a few ventured out to the provinces to take control of the *pueblos* where the disease had broken out. Each sanitary inspector was supplied with a disinfecting spray pump, disinfectants, and "a corps of men versed in that special work."[92] Similarly, the staff at the cholera hospital and the detention camps would resort to internal antisepsis to treat the sick. Patients received enemata containing 1/1000 benzozone as well as the more conventional "hyperdermics of strychnia," hot water bottles, and general symptomatic remedies. Benzozone, an experimental drug discovered by Dr. Paul Freer at the Manila Bureau of Science, promised "excellent results in the treatment of this dreaded disease," but it was to prove distressing and useless.[93] Most cholera patients died, and their corpses were cremated, though some, as before, were covered in quicklime and buried in sealed casks.

Provincial centers invoked quarantine regulations in an effort to halt the spread of the disease, but postwar population movements and food shortages meant that protective barriers were constantly flouted. When cholera found its way to Biñan, the local authorities took to cleaning and disinfecting the victims' houses; they tried also to isolate all contacts for five days. But after a physician from the Board of Health came to set up a detention camp and a cholera hospital, the contacts "fled to all parts of the pueblo, and its barrios, taking the disease with them wherever they went."[94] To make matters worse, rumors about house burnings circulated. The public uproar caused the abandonment of plans for a detention camp. Surgeon George D. De Shon found "the sanitary work of combating this disease among an ignorant and superstitious people, impoverished by war, locusts and rinderpest, and embittered by conquest . . . an extremely difficult task."[95] In general, medical officers attempted, like Captain C. F. de Mey, "to rule with a rod of steel." While their power was never absolute, they expected to become "the commanding officer of a city when that city is threatened with or has an epidemic."[96]

Although cholera terrified the Americans stationed in the islands, it was principally a disease of the Filipino poor—and it was the poor, too, who endured the heaviest burden of American sanitary intervention. Fearing the destruction of property, the dissolution of bonds of family, and the infliction of painful and apparently pointless experimental treatments, many Filipinos tried to conceal suspected cases. Maus detected a feeling among the natives that "the disease was colic, probably resulting from the use of green rice, and that the Americans resorted to these extreme measures unnecessarily, and probably for purposes of revenge."[97] His wife complained that "one can scarcely realize what it meant to feed and water this horde of ignorant, panic-stricken people."[98] Luke Wright, the acting governor-general, reported that "ignorant natives resent our modern methods of dealing with cholera."[99]

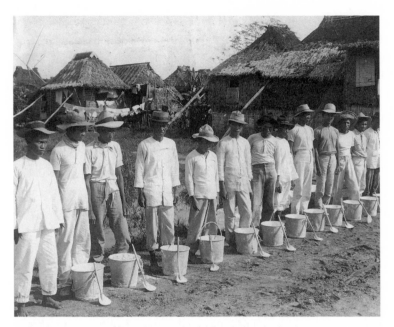

FIGURE 14. Line-pail brigade, Manila, during cholera epidemic
(RG 350-P-E44.21/2, NARA).

Rather than report a case, many Filipinos were prepared to take affected relatives or friends into the rice fields during the night, or occasionally they might dispose of the dead by throwing them into the Pasig River or burying them secretly. This resistance did have some effect. During May, Maus decided to abolish the detention camps and instead to isolate all contacts in their houses.[100]

The poor might resist "passively," but the Filipino elite, already accommodating themselves to the new regime, could voice their objections and make them heard. Evidently, the apparently arbitrary cruelty, accompanied as it was by restrictions on commerce, incensed Filipinos at all levels of society. Dr. T. H. Pardo de Tavera, one of two Filipinos on the Philippine Commission, wrote to Governor Taft, warning that "the people fear the Board of Health a great deal more than they fear the epidemic. The sanitary inspectors, white, brown, black, civil and military have committed and still commit all kinds of abuses." From the provinces he had heard complaints "against the barbarities committed by health agents." At Pasig, for example, the provincial treasurer "set fire to a house where a victim of the cholera had died and the flames extended to two neighboring houses," while the provincial inspector went about with "a gun on his shoulder in order to intimidate the people to make them obey sanitary laws."[101] Pardo de Tavera, as a physician, appreciated the need for such laws and supported their rigorous enforcement, but he could not condone the accompanying brutality and disruption. Like other Filipinos (and even Worcester), he had found Maus especially abrasive and severe; but Carter, following Munson's advice, would prove a little more conciliatory, at least toward local elites. It was later believed that Munson's style of dealing with "people of different races whose manners and customs are alien to ours" had enabled the Board of Health "to obtain active public support, instead of opposition, even for the extremely stringent measures which were necessary during the cholera campaign." This ability "to handle difficult situations without arousing opposition, and to secure not only acquiescence, but enthusiastic cooperation" would become an even more valuable quality, though still a rare one, in the health department after 1902.[102]

Americans frequently used their modern laboratory to confirm and further specify previously vague etiological suspicions. Regulations prohibiting the peddling of all drinks and cooked foods on the streets had come into force at the outset of the epidemic. Subsequently, Strong's laboratory examined many samples of food, along with some flies snared in infected dwellings. As expected, the microscope revealed cholera vibrios in much of the cooked rice that was left exposed and attached to some bluebottle flies. "These flies," observed Maus, "are commonly bred along the side of the esteros, which are emptying grounds for numberless private sewers and latrines. . . . Cases which have been observed along the banks of certain esteros may be accounted for by food infection from blue-bottle flies."[103] On the basis of this intelligence from the laboratory, the Board of Health inaugurated a campaign against insects and the unsanitary human practices, especially those involving defecation, that were allowing them to multiply and spread disease.

Within a year, the epidemic abated. After June 1902, the number of deaths in Manila from cholera steadily diminished; in January 1903, only 4 succumbed.[104] Before the disease finally was checked in Manila there were 5,581 cases and 4,386 deaths, while in the provinces more than 150,000 were infected and perhaps as many as 100,000 died.[105] Even in May 1902, Louis D. Baun, a teacher, wrote to his mother, "The cholera seems to be on the decrease, but the authorities look after every case closely. The Dr. said yesterday that the Spanish doctors claim it is not cholera at all; not enough people have died. They do not take into account all the means that the Americans have used to prevent its spread." He went on, "Another sanitary inspector just

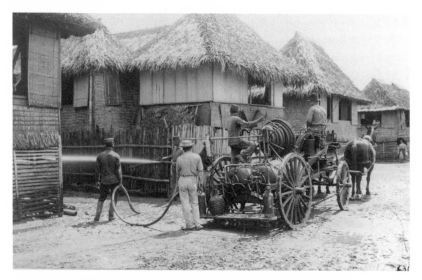

FIGURE 15. Fighting cholera with wholesale disinfection. Courtesy of the Rockefeller Archive Center.

showed up. . . . They certainly are doing enough inspecting."[106] As the morbidity and mortality from cholera fell during 1902, the quarantine around the city was lifted, and a number of sanitary inspectors left the health service. The Board of Health had by then developed a basic organization and mode of action — an administrative apparatus forged in the crucible of colonial warfare and melded with the new bacteriology — that would prove exceptionally durable.

"AN ENTIRE NATION HAD TO BE REHABILITATED"

"At the end of the Spanish-American War," Victor G. Heiser later noted, "the United States was confronted with large responsibilities in the field of tropical sanitation . . . an entire nation had to be rehabilitated."[107] It seemed obvious to Heiser, who was director of health in the Philippines from 1905 until 1915, that "as long as the Oriental was allowed to remain disease-ridden, he was a constant threat to the Occidental who clung to the idea that he could keep himself healthy in a small disease-ringed circle."[108] Thus he hoped to transform the Filipinos from "the weak and feeble race we have found them into the strong, healthy and enduring people they may yet become."[109] His method required the modification of personal habits of Filipinos — to render them more self-disciplined — as well as an old-fashioned attention to environmental nuisances. Heiser undertook the rigorous enforcement of vaccination, hygiene education, isolation of the diseased, quarantine, sewage disposal, improvement of housing, clothing, and nutrition, water and food examination. He introduced periodic health checkups and ensured the distribution of effective doses of quinine. By 1912, his Bureau of Health had a staff of three thousand, two hundred of whom were physicians. He had a small army of sanitary inspectors in the field preparing detailed reports on every town in the islands, daily during epidemics, weekly otherwise. In these circumstances Heiser boasted of his "almost military power" and pointed to his "sanitary squads."[110] "Necessarily," Heiser recalled, "we had to invade the rights of homes, commerce and parliaments."[111]

Heiser did not come from the military but from an institution in part modeled on it: the U.S. Public Health Service (PHS). An orphan who had lost his German-American parents in the Johnstown floods, Heiser put himself through Jefferson Medical College and then studied bacteriology and hygiene in order to pass the Marine Hospital Service (later PHS) examination. He soon made a name for himself devising a more efficient system for medical inspection of immigrants from southern Europe. An ascetic and authoritarian functionary, Heiser found the administrative goals and strategies of the PHS entirely congenial. He had entered a career corps with military ranks and uniforms and an emphasis on drill, hierarchy, and efficiency. Walter Wyman, the surgeon general of the PHS, had recently compiled a manual of procedure that reduced to writing every step in the handling of correspondence, accounts, appointments, and other administrative tasks.[112] Responsibilities and authorizations, whether for routine transactions or policy matters, had to be set down in detail, as they were in the military, and in the civil health service in the Philippines. Heiser was thus preadapted to the military model of the Philippine health service and would accept without hesitation the advice of more experienced medical officers like Munson, Maus, and Carter. For Heiser, the Philippines would prove "a huge laboratory in which my collaborators and I could work out an ideal program."[113]

The laboratory was emerging as an ideal discursive space, an exemplary colonial site—a symbol of control, purity, and precision that initially was far more significant than the routine practices of bacteriological investigation that went on within it. Colonial military tactics and protocols of population management remained fundamental in disciplining Filipinos, and the army camp still presented an appealing image, but the laboratory implied an even greater capacity for intervention and manipulation. For Heiser and his colleagues, their representation of the Philippines as tropical laboratory suggested an ability to vary scale from macro to micro: it meant they might treat its inhabitants as though they occupied the sterile, hygienic space of experimental practice. But the notion of the Philippines as a laboratory suggested a discursive possibility, not an accomplished technical transformation. Achievement of this ideal would still depend on their application of administrative techniques to manage colonial populations more than on expert knowledge of bacteriology and parasitology. Not that knowledge of microbiology was irrelevant to efforts to "wash up" the Orient. It would provide useful intelligence and determine the location and direction of public health maneuvers: microbiological reconnaissance identified the causes and carriers of disease, tested for compliance with the rules of personal and domestic hygiene, and registered populations. But laboratory science alone would not imply any one course of action. The Philippine health service remained, above all, an organization on the march: when cholera broke out, military administrative logic suggested it seek intelligence, send out sanitary squads, burn houses, and isolate troublemakers, in the same way the army had suppressed or diverted *insurrectos* in the archipelago.

Preventive measures also were markedly homologous. New doctrines of colonial warfare demanded intense surveillance and discipline of local populations: it was supposed that reform of the social and moral terrain, a policy of attraction and transformation, would pacify and subjugate the natives, turn supposed savages into docile, disciplined subjects. It was no longer enough to protect and bound, militarily and medically, a colonial garrison or enclave: the goal now was to occupy and organize a territory and a people, cultivating new forms of life, regenerating customs and habits within the new "protection zones." This did not mean coddling local populations, any more than military surgeons were coddling troops: the notion of attraction in colonial warfare did not connote enticement; rather, it implied an involuntary, magnetic force. "Health in the tropics," Heiser argued, "is largely a matter of observing simple hygienic rules rather than of climate."[114] Just as raw recruits to the army were trained and transformed into disciplined soldiers, so might the medical officer and sanitary inspector attempt to reeducate Filipinos, to make them proper, retentive colonial subjects. Through the discipline of hygiene, Filipinos might eventually become properly self-governing. Of course, there was little expectation that Filipinos really did possess the capacity for hygiene that even the most ignorant rural American troops could demonstrate; hence full hygienic citizenship would in practice be deferred, and colonial supervision and training continue indefinitely.

Colonial warfare was not the only influence on the emergence of American public health in the Philippines, but it was a powerful adjuvant, promoting the growth of features that might otherwise have turned vestigial. Since the 1870s, interest in social pathology had developed in North America and Europe at the expense of older concerns with geographical and climatic determinants of disease.[115] In the Philippines, the exigencies of colonial warfare would further focus attention on mobile human agency. Similarly, the optimistic interventionism of the military surgeon at the end of the nineteenth century should not be separated from the rise of Progressivism and social reform movements in the United States during this period.[116] But the medical officer's self-confidence and assertiveness would give specificity and added impetus to these more general, diffuse reformist trends. The increasingly widespread recourse to business models and programs for administrative efficiency also was mirrored in the transformation of military bureaucracy; but in the Philippines it was the military that became the sole direct means whereby these organizational changes generated a health service.[117] The idea of "the gospel of hygiene," the plan to evangelize a Catholic or heathen population, must have struck a chord with American colonial officials, most of whom were Protestant; but it was colonial warfare that made proselytization a military and medical necessity. Colonial warfare was, at least in part, a manifestation of broader social and political developments at the end of the nineteenth century, but it became the first major conduit channeling these general principles and practices into the Philippines health service.

There are perhaps many routes to modern tropical hygiene, each winding through a different colonial terrain. It is difficult, then, to generalize from the intimate symbiosis of public health and colonial warfare in the Philippines. Certainly the political, professional, and military situation in the Philippines was unusual. The United States was trying to set up its first colonial health service at the same time as it waged a war of progressive occupation; there were no enclavist medical traditions or existing colonial bureaucracies to overcome; and ambitious American imperialists regarded themselves as uniquely efficient, reformist, and scientific. It was not, as they frequently pointed out, the British Empire — it was especially not India. But American administrators worked hard to represent the Philippines as the model colonial health service. Worcester was delighted to observe "the impact of American methods on those previously in vogue in neighboring colonies. At first our efforts to make Asiatics clean up . . . were viewed with mild amusement, not unmixed with contempt; but the results we obtained soon aroused lively interest."[118] According to Heiser, it was "generally conceded that the medical literature produced in the Philippine Islands is more voluminous, and has a greater scientific value than that of all the other countries combined. These writings have also had an important role in molding opinion with regard to medical and sanitary matters of other portions of the Orient."[119] Thus Worcester and Heiser tried hard to make the colonial military diction of hygiene in the Philippines the lingua franca of modern tropical medicine.

Chapter Three

"ONLY MAN IS VILE"

When Andrew Balfour spoke to the London Society of Tropical Medicine and Hygiene in 1914, his subject was "Tropical Problems in the New World," and he had new information that would startle some of his audience and reassure others. Balfour announced that Captain Weston Chamberlain, M.D., of the Army Board for the Study of Tropical Diseases in the Philippines had recently reported on his investigations of the "physiological activity of Americans in these islands and the influence of tropical residence on the blood." It seemed probable that the tropical climate itself exercised no harmful influence on the white residents. "By far the larger part of the morbidity and mortality in the Philippines is due to nostalgia, isolation, tedium, venereal disease, alcoholic excess, and especially to infections with various parasites."[1] Chamberlain's laboratory studies thus challenged long-held medical theories of inevitable white degeneration in the torrid zone. During the military campaigns at the turn of the century and under the new civil regime, American physicians had carefully monitored their white patients for any signs of such deterioration. Public health officials and army surgeons sought to protect whites from insalubrious circumstances, regulating their clothing, diet, housing, and personal conduct. Now it seemed that such concern had been either redundant or remarkably effica-cious: whites were not — not yet, anyway — especially degenerate or unmanly in the Philippines. They either had been robust enough to prosper anywhere all along or were now insulated sufficiently well not to register the change in milieu.

In the new laboratories of the Bureau of Science in Manila, Chamberlain and his colleagues were translating colonial governance into the positive lan-guage of biomedical science, expressing their confidence in the racial resil-ience of white male colonialists, and their anxieties about the bodies and customs of ordinary Filipinos.[2] As they studied the blood and the physio-logical activity of white males in the tropics, scientists allayed older fears of physical (if not mental) deterioration in a foreign realm. Whiteness and man-liness seemed tougher, or at least more readily armored, than any of the army surgeons in the early days of the Philippines campaign had ever expected. At the same time, the modern laboratory was demonstrating repeatedly that alien blonds and brunets had more to fear from contact with a variety of native fauna — some evidently diseased and some meretriciously healthy — than from exposure to rays of the tropical sun. Scientists in Manila con-firmed and elaborated earlier concerns about the dangers of *insurrectos* and insects, giving further microbiological effect to their respective *bolos* (knives) and stings. Together, the Bureau of Science and the Army Board for the Study of Tropical Diseases produced a white male body that was more or less indif-ferent to tropical relocation and European and Malay racial bodies with ap-parently natural, though not necessarily fixed, differences in disease carriage and susceptibility. That is, science helped to reframe the boundaries of white-ness in the Philippines, neutralizing or overcoming environmental contain-ment and making racial contact ever more salient and medically significant.

It is important to give equal weight to these two trends in colonial bio-medical research: the exoneration of the tropical milieu and the racializing of pathogen distribution. Both emerged during the military period, the first a result of rising faith in the effectiveness of sanitary management of troops, the second a result of the strategic premises of guerilla warfare among settled populations. With pacification, both research programs were taken up and amplified in the biological laboratories of the civil Bureau of Science and the army board, the bureau mostly (though not exclusively) focusing on Filipino pathology and the board on white physiology. Colonial scientists like Cham-berlain sought to reconfigure environment and race in the tropics, helping to resolve old fears of racial displacement and to reinforce anxieties about racial contamination. When Balfour finished reporting to the Society of Tropical Medicine, Sir Ronald Ross, probably the most distinguished tropical scientist in the audience, rose to endorse Chamberlain's findings and to confirm that the white races, striving to conquer savages, need not fear foreign climates: the unsanitary ways of local inhabitants were far more menacing.[3] As Balfour observed, science might yet demonstrate the truth of the couplet "Where every prospect pleases / And only man is vile."[4]

THE WHITE MAN'S CLIMATIC BURDEN

During the American military campaign, fear of the deleterious effect of the climate on the white race was for a time expressed in an especially raw and accentuated manner. Such concern had earlier pervaded Spanish medical theory, and it lingered in the American colonial bureaucracy until well into the twentieth century. The Spanish colonial commitment to neo-Hippocratic doctrines, which assumed a dynamic interaction of human bodies and their environment, is not surprising. It was after all a commonplace of nineteenth-century European medical theory that a race's temperament and physiology were adapted to its place, and any dislodgement would imply hazard. This "ethnic moral topography," as David Livingstone describes it, accorded with popular beliefs about the need to stay in harmony with one's circumstances.[5] But the persistence into the twentieth century of this vision of races and proper places is perhaps more remarkable. Even as scientists were postulating theories of harder, more robust heredity and identifying microbiological rather than physical causes of disease, ideas of environmental fit and stress continued to appeal to the public and to many doctors. Thus the experience of discomfort and nostalgia in foreign lands for many years still popularly connoted pathological sequelae, whatever the staffs at the bureau and the board might say.

The Philippines had long ago established a reputation as an unsavory spot even for southern Europeans. In the middle of the nineteenth century, as the number of Spanish in the archipelago multiplied, some physicians speculated on the effect of the climate on Mediterranean physique and mentality. In 1857, Dr. Antonio Codorniu y Nieto, a sanitary officer with the military garrison in Manila, considered "the nature of the modification of the human body in the Islands" and especially the potential for "degeneration of the race."[6] He observed that "Europeans who arrive in the country as adolescents, full of virility, especially suffer the effects of acclimatization; new conditions modify their temperament in certain ways, generally in relation to the constitution, and influence their growth and development." For all Spanish sojourners, "acclimatization in the Philippines means alteration in the organism as it is tested in a trying, humid climate: the loss of digestive activity, diminution of respiration, impoverishment of metabolism, and in sum, a tiring of the blood that gives rise to nervousness, of the sort one sees in the local races." Codorniu was particularly worried about the insidious disease of nostalgia, "which consists of a state of moral suffering, of sadness and desperation, attacking most Europeans, but principally those engaged in a military career."[7] The precise outcome of tropical residence depended on the initial quality of the constitution and the part of the islands where one resided. Eventually, though, all aliens would degenerate unless revived in a cooler climate: "The European who decides to stay in this country for an indefinite period must do what is needed to refresh his blood, that is, he must move after six to eight years to a temperate country, staying there as long as necessary to restore his temperament; thus he will recover his dash and enough vitality to counteract another period of enervation in a hot and humid climate."[8]

When Fedor Jagor, a German ethnologist, traveled through the archipelago in the late 1850s he found the long-term Spanish residents "uneducated, improvident and extravagant." In the fertile, torrid zone—a "lotus-eating Utopia," according to the ethnologist—they had adopted the slack standards of the natives. The hospitality of nature had made them louche and dissolute. As the Spanish residents acclimatized to the Philippines, they were sinking into "a disordered and uncultivated state," gradually becoming indistinguishable from the natives. In Jagor's opinion, only the Spanish and Portuguese possessed the constitutional wherewithal to take root in tropical countries in this lamentable way; northern Europeans like him would sicken and die before they degenerated and so must limit themselves to brief visits.[9]

At the end of the century, just as they were about to be displaced from the islands, a few Spanish commentators would come to express greater confidence in their ability to withstand tropical circumstances. Dr. Victor Suarez Caopalleja, for example, still expected that dampness combined with high temperatures might produce "paludic" fevers and mental and physical fatigue in whites. He saw some of his compatriots become "pusillanimous," pessimistic, "pathologically selfish," and melancholy in the Philippines.[10] He could detect "modifications in the individual and in the race, characterized by indolence, submissiveness and laziness, which follow the febrile activity of the first few days, and a certain apathy especially for anything that does not lead to fortune." There were many cases of "facial pallor, sometimes earthy yellow skin tone; thinness, pronounced sunken eyes; loss of appetite; restless sleep; a general sense of fatigue that permeates all limbs." But Suarez now believed this doleful condition might be prevented or alleviated with proper attention to hygiene. "The fortified body subject to good methods of hygiene is a safe harbor undisturbed by common illness, and difficult even for epidemics to assault. Take care that the skin, which shields the organism," advised the doctor, "functions well—the result of plentiful water and a wise disposition."[11] Fortunately, the Philippines were not nearly as insalubrious as most other tropical countries and certainly not as uncomfortable for whites as West Africa was proving. For Suarez, writing in 1897, the biological prospects for Spaniards in the Philippines had never looked better.

On their arrival in the archipelago, American military and civil leaders reiterated older Spanish fears of degeneration in the tropical climate. The prospect seemed especially grim, as we have seen, for white soldiers, who labored hard in such hostile, foreign conditions. But even members of the executive government could feel imperiled. In 1902, Governor William H. Taft attested that "the tropical sun induces leisurely habits," and so was utterly antithetical to vigorous Anglo-Saxonism. It was "dangerous for Americans to expose themselves to the midday sun." For most of the day, the harsh tropical sun would "not permit the European or American to exercise under it with impunity. There is no doubt about that."[12] (Then again, Taft, a famously obese man, had never shown much inclination for exercise in his native Ohio either.) The governor was especially worried about the effect of the climate on white women and children: "The nervous strain upon adult females due to the high temperature . . . is great, and at the end of two years they ought to go and be refreshed in a cooler climate." He recommended too that white children head north to temperate lands after they reached the age of fourteen: otherwise they grew up "so rapidly that they become weedy in their make-up."[13] Evidently, Taft believed there was no hope of permanent white settlement in the tropics. Nature had decreed that white itinerants or sojourners, not settlers, would administer the American colonial state. In every picture of Philippine progress there would remain "a somber background of a baneful climate making it impossible for the American or the European to live in health and strength in the islands for any length of time."[14]

When Hubert Howe Bancroft surveyed "the new Pacific" in 1899, he observed that in the tropics "the heat is trying, being moist, and the air too often malarious." The historian of the American West concluded, "While for a time and with care the several races may live anywhere on the globe, unless it be at or near the poles, the white man cannot live and labor permanently in the tropics." Accordingly, "we may give ownership but not the occupation of the tropics to the white race."[15] Other commentators on the new empire echoed Bancroft's misgivings. Charles Morris, in his imperial handbook, announced that although no serious diseases were prevalent in the islands, "most of the deleterious effects upon whites are direct results of the tropical severity of the climate."[16] The Reverend William Elliot Griffis, an expert on Japan and the Far East, went further in climatic disparagement. "Many regions in the tropics," he warned, "are like a steam bath, and the heat and moisture together are oppressive beyond the power of the Anglo-Saxon to endure." Ever skeptical toward expansionism, Griffis thought it proved that "the tropics were never meant for the white man to live in or to greatly concern himself about."[17]

Some medical authorities initially endorsed Taft's pessimism. Sitting in a stuffy room of the Manila *audencia* in July 1899, the Philippine commissioners had questioned two visiting American medicos on the biologically correct form of American tropical imperialism. "We would like to know particularly," the commissioners asked Simon Flexner and Lewellys Barker, "what effect the climate and maladies would have on Americans coming here, whether they could endure the climate or not."[18] The pathologist and the physician, on leave from Johns Hopkins and still on their tropical tour, had bad news. "The climate," lamented Barker, "seems to affect Americans especially with regard to their assimilation. People who have lived here a long time grow gradually pale. . . . Women especially grow pale, and the European children have a tendency to anemia." White Americans might live in the tropics a few years, but they should never try to labor there: "I think a great many men would sicken, and if they tried it for two or three generations without replenishment from home, to use a slang expression, they would peter out." Barker had endured the climate for some months before giving his testimony and so could speak with conviction: "Someone had said that here the sun is always dangerous, and I am inclined to think so. I have felt it very much."[19]

For many Americans in the civil government, their experiences of discomfort and fatigue in the tropics still readily translated into portents of disease and degeneration. Typically, Herbert Ingram Priestley, a teacher in Nueva Caceres [Naga City], found he had "some little trouble getting acclimated."[20] Soon after arrival, he "went out a little too late and the heat was sickening. It makes one sick at his stomach," he wrote to his mother (November 10, 1901).

A year later he reported that "the doctor says the climate is wearing on me and I guess it is. I am down to 166 lbs and tho' I have a normal appetite and rest normally with a little aid from drugs, I have some very unpleasant half hours of profuse sweating, with nervous morbid apprehensions which are especially trying to a person of my sensitive temperament" (October 19, 1902). He felt that "the air seems to contain very little ozone, and the steady high amount of perspiration, with the never ending drag on one's vitality, seems to pre-dispose one to colds" (December 21, 1902). But he hung on until October 1904. A sense of discomfort and displacement also afflicted Emily Bronson Conger, an otherwise self-possessed nurse known appropriately as Señora Blanca. On first encountering the heat of the tropics "one gasps like a fish out of water and vows with laboring breath: 'I'll take the next steamer home, oh, home!'" The climate of the Philippines "seemed beyond physical en-durance . . . exhaustion without relief. The only time one could get a breath was about five o'clock in the morning; in the middle of the day the sun's rays are white-hot needles . . . and even if one carries an umbrella the heat pierces directly through." She felt the pores of her pale skin had been "weakened by excessive exudation," leaving her exposed to all the evils of the region.[21]

In 1905, Fred W. Atkinson, the superintendent of education, observed that long residence in the Philippines caused "loss of memory" and "loss of ability to spell." "Caucasians grow pessimistic and suspicious after a few years' stay; and those who do not stand the climate are apt to become hypersensitive and hypercritical." Dengue fever prevailed during the period of acclimation, and intestinal disorders were common thereafter. By eating good food, following regular habits, consuming no alcohol, and avoiding the midday sun, while at the same time limiting their mental and physical exertion, whites might live in the Philippines for a few years without too much suffering. But tropical condi-tions meant that "no extensive settlements of Americans in the archipelago are likely to be made for years to come, if ever; extensive colonization by us seems to be precluded."[22]

Major Charles E. Woodruff, M.D., confirmed the apprehensions of Atkin-son and other colonial bureaucrats. A disaffected and irritable medical officer, Woodruff dedicated himself to warning his more complacent fellows of the dangers of tropical light for blonds and brunets. He contended that exposure to the "actinic," or ultraviolet, rays of the tropical sun led to racial decay and degeneration. The actinic rays, he argued, produced "some kind of chemical breaking up which renders [the cell] paretic," leading at first to a misleading sense of "stimulation," but soon followed by a chronic "low vitality of tissues." Not surprisingly, then, the poorly pigmented "blonds suffer in the Philippines more than brunets, have higher grades of neurasthenia, break down in larger numbers proportionately, and in many ways prove their unfitness for the climate."[23] In an influential monograph, Woodruff explained that the white race should never live closer to the equator than fifty degrees: "Even in New Zealand and Australia the native white families are already dying out or kept alive by constant new importation from home."[24] Accordingly, the white man should not try to colonize the Philippines, for colonization was doomed to fail biologically. Instead, Woodruff advocated a "commensalism": a careful expansion into the tropics based on mutual aid.[25]

In 1913, soon after he arrived in the Philippines, Francis Burton Harrison, the new Democrat-appointed governor-general, received a letter from Woodruff warning him to stay out of the sunlight. "Mrs. Harrison and I," responded the governor-general, "are making it a point to keep indoors at least during the hours of noon and three o'clock, and to keep ourselves and our children out of the strong sunlight all the time that it is possible."[26] Mark Twain once had pilloried American efforts to shine the light of civilization on "the person sitting in darkness" — but now, ironically, it seemed it was the white imperialist who would be compelled to recline in the gloom.[27]

WHITE PHYSIOLOGY IN THE TROPICS

With longer tropical experience, some American medicos gained confidence in white robustness, or at least in the race's ability to insulate itself from insalubrious physical circumstances. Wallace de Witt, M.D., found the Philippines' climate "very enervating, lowering the natural resistive power against disease." But like an increasing number of his colleagues, the medical officer attributed most disease to failure to obey "a few simple sanitary laws" — especially those relating to contact with unhygienic Orientals — and generally exonerated climate as the prime culprit.[28] William S. Washburn, M.D., the chairman of the Philippine civil service board, believed that the archipelago was actually more "comfortable and hygienically favorable for the treatment of many diseases" than any other country at that latitude. In any case, he could cite a number of scientists who had argued that "the European may, under proper sanitary conditions, transplant himself anywhere."[29] Indeed, it now seemed that "evidence is accumulating that the rate of mortality among the white race now living in the tropics is less than that of the native population." In the past too much reliance was placed on military statistics. "Disease and death invariably accompany the invasion of an army into any country," he told the congress of the Philippine Islands Medical Association, "whether it be in the temperate or in the torrid zone." But as conditions stabilized and "hygienic living" became established, rates of white morbidity and mortality declined: "Regular habits, the leading of a temperate life, and the absence of indulgence in excesses, have much to do with one's health in any country."[30] In conclusion, Washburn quoted Major General Leonard Wood, M.D., the governor of Moro province and a former Rough Rider, who believed that "Americans can live and do good work where any other white race can. A moral life, with plenty of hard work, will be found to counteract in most cases the so-called de-moralizing effects of the Philippines climate."[31]

Laboratory scientists in the archipelago soon began to capitalize on the dispute between white racial possibilists and environmental pessimists. In 1905, Dr. John McDill, the president of the American-dominated Philippine Islands Medical Association, advocated further analysis of the "vast amount of clinical material under the control of the Bureau of Science" in order to determine if the tropical climate would undermine white physiology. For "if the United States is to continue its governmental relations indefinitely, the fact that Americans can lead healthful lives in the Philippines is important of itself."[32] Created in 1905 from a reorganization of the Bureau of Government Laboratories, the Manila Bureau of Science provided a haven for those medical officers who sought a career in research. From their headquarters in Manila, army and civilian scientists sought to reinscribe the archipelago, producing rigorous environmental descriptions, detailed ethnographies, laboratory reports, discussions of sanitary engineering and architecture, and extensive physiological investigations. Statistics and scientific rationality were supposed to supplant anecdote and mere experience. From 1906, the investigations of the second Army Board for the Study of Tropical Diseases supplemented the bureau's work. Until it was temporarily disbanded in 1914, the board would take advantage of "the vast field for original research which has been opened up for our medical officers by service in the tropics."[33] Its scientists undertook diagnostic work for the army, collected specimens for the Army Medical School, and conducted experiments on white soldiers and Filipino scouts, investigating unknown fevers, the microbial carriage of healthy men, and the acclimatization of blond and brunet recruits.

Scientific research in the Philippines contributed to at least a partial dissolution of the sense of tropical peril that had accumulated over the previous century. Some investigators at the Bureau of Science challenged directly the notion that the tropics represented a distinctive pathological site. They

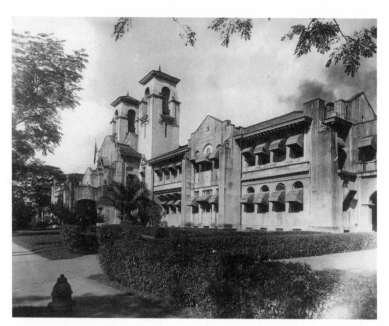

FIGURE 16. Bureau of Science, Manila (RG 350-P-E27-32, NARA).

decried Woodruff's theories of special actinic danger. Hans Aron argued that "the spectrum of the sun's rays does not extend much, if any, further into the ultraviolet in Manila than in Northern climates."[34] His colleague H. D. Gibbs concurred, having demonstrated that "when the normal intensities are compared, the light of the tropics is no different from any other region."[35] When Alfred O. Shaklee exposed his experimental monkeys to the sunlight of Manila he found they died from heatstroke after varying periods, depending more on the proximity of a fan than on any quality of the sun's rays. Evidently, exposure to direct sunlight caused such an increase in body temperature that the poor animals succumbed to hyperpyrexia, just as they would in temperate climates. In every case, Shaklee noted, those with darker pelts died more quickly than those with light fur, on account of their greater absorption of heat.[36] Therefore the "white organism" might not inherently be a transgressor against tropical nature.

Perhaps the most striking demonstration of the dangers of pigment envy was the remarkably influential test of colored underwear. In 1907, concerned about Woodruff's claims, Lieutenant Colonel W. T. Wood, the inspector general of the army in the Philippines, asked the army board to conduct a long-term study of orange-red clothing to see whether white Americans might artificially adapt themselves to tropical conditions.[37] The army had always been interested in sunstroke and fatigue on the parade ground, even in temperate regions, so the study of acclimatization in the tropics seemed an obvious outlet for its scientific energies. Over the following three years, James M. Phalen and his fellow investigators supplied five hundred soldiers with orange-red long underwear and compared their well-being in the course of a year with another group wearing conventional white undergarments. Each man had his own case record, detailing age, height, nativity, hair and eye color, complexion, and length of tropical service. The investigators regularly measured the research subjects' weight, pulse, and respiratory rate—while some recruits were followed more closely with blood pressure readings to determine the "effect of short exposures to the sun." Astoundingly, men attired in the orange-red lingerie, far from being protected, showed marked changes due to heat, such as loss of weight, and falls in hemoglobin and blood pressure, all worse than among achromatic controls. Moreover, most of the research subjects hated their colorful garb, finding it itchy and heavy, and tried to discard it altogether. Phalen concluded that colored underwear was more receptive to heat rays than white, since wearers had complained so bitterly of greater heat and perspiration. He expressed the opinion that ordinary khaki clothing provided enough protection from the sun's rays, without any of the evils of colored underwear.[38] In this case, to have color had actually been disabling in the tropics.

Until the board began taking the temperature of white men in the tropics, most authorities had believed that European metabolism increased near the equator. As early as 1839, John Davy published his observations of the mouth temperature of seven healthy young Englishmen on a voyage to Ceylon. He found that Europeans became hotter as they passed from a temperate zone into the tropics, and those long resident there generated abnormally high temperatures.[39] Thirty years later, Alexander Rattray confirmed the rise in metabolism, but he based this conclusion on recordings of the mouth temperature of only a few young men as they sailed from London to Bahia, Brazil.[40] Chamberlain, however, took three thousand mouth temperatures at quarterly intervals from six hundred healthy American soldiers in the Philippines and found no appreciable variation with season or complexion. The average temperature hardly differed from that of white men living in the United States. "The matter is of some importance," Chamberlain suggested, "in the selecting of recruits and civil service employees for tropical countries."[41]

The impact of white displacement to the tropics on blood pressure, or "tension," was more ambiguous. Evidently it was important that white men maintain their tension in a potentially depleting, relaxing tropical environment. As Phalen and H. J. Nichols surmised, "If loss of physical or mental tone is measurable in objective terms it has seemed to us that blood pressure readings should show it."[42] In 1910, W. E. Musgrave and A. G. Sison, from the Bureau of Science, examined 97 white Americans, 10 Sisters of Charity, and 40 Filipinos, all of them resident in Manila. The investigators concluded that a long stay in the tropics reduced blood pressure — Filipinos showed by far the lowest tension — perhaps as a result of decreased peripheral resistance.[43] But Chamberlain disputed these findings in the following year. He took the pressures of 992 American soldiers, making 5,368 observations, and he concluded that "the average blood pressure of 115 to 188 millimeters found in these large bodies of men differed little, if any, from the accepted standard among males of the same age in a temperate zone." The indefatigable researcher conceded that temporary variations might still occur, such as a rise on exertion or a fall due to flushing of the skin, similar to the effect of a hot bath in a temperate country. But these changes would prove evanescent and certainly not pathognomic of tropical life.[44]

Another commonplace of the old medicine of warm climates was that the "quality" of European blood deteriorated in moist heat. Europeans in equatorial outposts often appeared unnaturally pale and sallow, the likely victims of "tropical anemia." Most experts assumed that the "thinness and poorness" of the blood — an incontrovertible sign of racial degeneration — derived from climatic conditions alone.[45] But not until the early twentieth century was the microscope used to reveal the constituents of white blood in the tropics. After Chamberlain performed 1,718 red cell counts and 1,433 hemoglobin estimations from 702 American soldiers, he found that the figures "do not differ from the normal at present recognized for healthy young men in a temperate zone."[46] Most cases of anemia in the tropics were the result of malaria or hookworm, and with proper hygiene these parasites might be avoided.

Still, Chamberlain and Captain Edward Vedder did detect a few regional abnormalities in the blood of white soldiers and Filipinos. In each group, but especially among Filipinos, the total number of leukocytes, the white blood cells, was less than expected, while the number of eosinophils, yellow-staining blood cells, was higher than it should have been. Moreover, when the composition of the diminished white cells was analyzed, the investigators discovered that the "less-mature" polymorph fraction of the total count was greater than that found in healthy Europeans living in a temperate climate.[47] Cham-

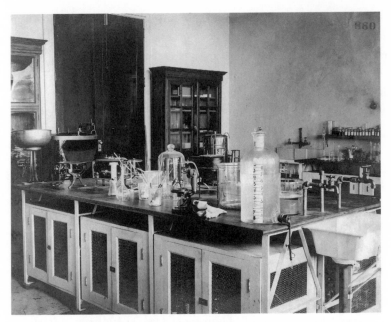

FIGURE 17. Biological laboratory, Bureau of Science (RG 350-P-E57-20, NARA).

berlain felt that this "disturbance of the normal proportions of different varieties of leukocytes is probably common to most primitive and semi-civilized
peoples in the tropics." He concluded, "We may therefore look upon Igorots
(and probably most Filipinos) as having a chronically increased percentage of
eosinophiles and small lymphocytes."[48] The coincidence of blood picture and
supposed racial morphology is marked: Filipinos showed an abundance of
yellow-staining cells and fewer white cells, which were in any case mostly
small or immature. But the scientists did not regard this pattern—unlike the
later discovery of the ABO blood groups—as a primary racial characteristic;
rather, they interpreted it as a feature secondary to disease carriage. Of
course, the behavioral propensity to acquire and spread disease organisms
might still have a biological substrate organized by race, but the emergence of
a similar pattern in whites suggested that blood picture was at best a very
unstable and indirect racial marker. Chamberlain and his colleagues chose to
regard this pattern not as evidence of degenerative change per se but as an
effort to cope with an increased load of specific pathogens. Thus similarities
in the blood pictures of Filipinos and whites resident in the topics merely
indicated that American standards of hygiene were becoming more lax or that
colonial emissaries were making too much contact with the locals—and not
that a process of irreversible climate-induced degeneration was under way.[49]

American scientists in the tropics were refiguring white males as resilient or well-armored bodies, surrounded by a relatively harmless, exploitable physical environment. The chief threat to their health appeared to come from contact with disease-dealing natives and insects — and, as army medical officers had shown, such proximity to potentially pathogenic local "fauna" might be limited or rendered innocuous through meticulous hygiene. This white corporeal self-assertion implied the production of an alienated, or denatured, type of body, one that was almost impervious to physical circumstance. The influence of climate on mentality, however, was not so readily dismissed: the specter of "tropical neurasthenia" would, as we shall see, continue to haunt even the most optimistic proclamations of a white conquest of the region and to menace the promoters of a global white civilization.[50] But the laboratory studies in Manila had at least discounted older anecdotal and crudely empirical accounts of inevitable European physical degeneration in the tropics.[51] In the tropical laboratory, the dirty, humid, complex environment, with its diverse animal and human populations, had been converted into controllable specimens and measurements, simplified and standardized, and then further consolidated as figures in the scientific paper. Bruno Latour, writing about Louis Pasteur, has observed that "in this series of displacements, no one can say where the laboratory is and where the society is."[52] But even as the laboratory suggested a variation in the scale of colonial society and environment, not everyone was convinced, or "enrolled" in the activity, and some hardly noticed what was happening. It was perhaps premature for Victor Heiser to claim in 1906 that already in the Philippines "the microscope supplanted the sword, the martial spirit gave place to the research habit."[53] The process of making the whole archipelago laboratory-like would continue for some time yet.

IMMUNITIES OF EMPIRE

In the early years of the twentieth century a new language of immunity largely substituted for increasingly discredited talk of the risks of acclimatization. Of course, older theories of racial acclimatization were, in a sense, already based on assumptions about natural immunity, or susceptibility, to place and climate. But *immunity* was a term rarely invoked in discussions of acclimatization. It was not until the development of germ theories in the late nineteenth century that the word *immunity* seemed to find the right culture medium and began to proliferate, giving rise to new variants such as *acquired immunity* and *sanitary immunity*. This *fin-de-siècle* mobilization of immunity did not, however, leave behind all racial traces: the supposition that racial difference would somehow shape disease occurrence and expression proved remarkably resilient. Whereas before native races had been deemed naturally fitted to their proper place and therefore normally in a state of health, now it seemed more likely that these races had acquired immunity — with some perhaps inherited — to the specific germs that happened to prevail there.

The novel idea that immunity might be acquired through exposure to a specific microorganism in infancy generally received a facile racial gloss.[54] Washburn discerned that "natives of the Philippines eat and drink with comparative impunity articles of food and water, the use of which by white men is disastrous."[55] Examples of such default from individual acquired immunities to broad racial typologies are legion. William B. Freer, a schoolteacher and occasional doctor to his charges, observed that smallpox "is never entirely absent from the Philippines, but so many generations of Filipinos have experienced it that it does not, as a rule, go badly with them. But woe to the American who contracts the disease. He invariably suffers severely, and the malady usually takes its most malignant form, that known as 'black smallpox.' Such cases are nearly always fatal."[56] Freer's brother, Dr. Paul C. Freer, the director of the Bureau of Science, explained the apparent immunity of Filipinos to local ailments as "a process of heredity [in which] the substances that confer certain types of immunity on individuals of a race have been produced by a course of development concomitant with the other manifestations of immunity."[57] Therefore, over many generations, the acquired immunities of the indigenous people to the diseases that surrounded them had in effect become natural, heritable, and racial.

The apparent racial homogeneity of lowland Filipinos aided early medical efforts to construct a simple dichotomy of white susceptibility and native immunity. The views of Colonel L. Mervin Maus on Philippine racial types were conventional in this regard. Apart from some highland, or isolated, "Negritoes" — the Igorots most famously — "the native Filipino belongs to the Malay race, or the Oceanic Mongols. . . . Ethnologically, the natives throughout the archipelago are identical."[58] Robert Bennett Bean, the professor of anatomy at the new Philippine Medical School, regarded Filipinos as a distinct type, though he quibbled about the presence of elementary "Iberian" and "Primitive" varieties. Unusually, Bean tried to differentiate disease proclivities within the race, observing that Iberian Filipinos, who demonstrated some Spanish ancestry, were "more susceptible to all diseases but especially to tuberculosis than the Primitive. This may be indicative that the European and Filipinos offspring of the Iberian type is less resistant to disease in the tropics than is the aboriginal type on its own soil and in its natural environment."[59] Bean expected that the Iberian element would therefore soon breed out and ultimately disappear. But to most scientists and physicians, the anatomist's distinctions shaded into pedantry: the polarities of white and colored framed their understanding of disease distribution.

Even as the absolute vulnerability of the white race to tropical disease — if no longer to climate — was repeatedly asserted, the absolute exemption of Filipinos from local ailments was soon questioned. With the consolidation of the U.S. hold on the archipelago and with burgeoning interest in developing Filipino labor, it was becoming clear that Filipinos in fact succumbed to tropical disease at least as frequently as white Americans, if for different reasons. Many medical officers had noticed Filipino frailty quite early. Nonetheless, a few commentators continued to dismiss concerns about native health. Ralph Buckland, for instance, asserted that "they are attacked by light illnesses of short duration, all of which worry the sufferers almost to distraction."[60] But Mary H. Fee noticed that her students were afflicted with "boils and impure blood and many skin diseases. Consumption [tuberculosis] is rife, and rheumatism attacks old and young alike."[61] Malaria was common, though often surprisingly mild, and when plague and cholera swept the islands, they scourged Filipinos more than Americans. The extent of Filipino illness and infirmity nevertheless came as a revelation to W. Cameron Forbes, the patrician governor-general. When Forbes visited the new medical school, Paul Freer showed him a "rather gruesome dissection" and then "pointed out that as a result of the first one hundred autopsies they could state positively that the physically diseased condition of the Filipino was such that he absolutely couldn't do the work that a well man could."[62] Forbes found this information on racial liability disconcerting.

Evidently Filipino racial immunity, whether innate or acquired was less absolute than many had first thought. William Freer gave a socioeconomic explanation for the peculiar Filipino susceptibility to local disease: with the decline in agriculture during the war, most people ate poorly, and "when attacked by disease they succumb quickly because, already weakened by hunger, their power of resistance is not sufficient to withstand the ravages of fever."[63] Such sensitivity to historical and contemporary misfortune is rare. Most others attributed this newly recognized liability to moral failings, which generally were framed as inherently racial, though perhaps not fixedly so. For if the locals were acquiring diseases that their race presumably had hitherto resisted, then they must surely have become very depraved indeed. After all,

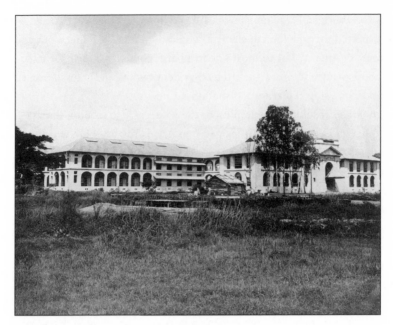

FIGURE 18. Philippine General Hospital (RG 350-P-E25.5, NARA).

Filipinos should have had a long process of exposure and adaptation on their side, unlike any whites that succumbed; Americans, in contrast, were more likely the innocent victims of immigration. To Señora Blanca and others, evidence of tropical disease among Filipinos implied that their naughty, child-like charges must have been wallowing in filth, enough to overcome their supposed racial immunity. "And I looked at them," she recalled, "saying to myself, as I so often did, 'You poor miserable creatures, utterly neglected, utterly ignorant and degraded'. . . . No wonder that the diseased, the de-formed, the blind, the one-toed, the twelve-toed, and monstrous parts and organs are the rule rather than the exception." The Ohio nurse wanted to "dip them into some cleansing caldron" but resisted the impulse, for "charity be-gins at home."[64] Others would more readily intervene, of course, though their methods were never quite so harsh.

Scientific evidence of Filipino disease carriage repeatedly reinforced fears of racial contact—a phobia that the guerilla war had already amplified, if not prompted. Laboratory intelligence was confirming again and again mili-tary suspicions that there were no amigos. Just as it became common knowl-edge that many Filipinos were manifestly unwell, scientists in the archipel-ago were also revealing more widespread and hitherto disguised carriage of microbial pathogens. Even healthy Filipinos might be spreading the local germs to which whites were especially vulnerable. The contraction of venereal disease from apparently healthy prostitutes provided an increasingly plausible model for the transmission of most tropical diseases. When Chamberlain reported on an outbreak of venereal disease among soldiers at Pangasinan in 1904, he observed that even prostitutes "listed as clean probably contained some gonococci, and that those who were marked as infected nonetheless were patronized by soldiers."[65] The germs or parasites for many other diseases might also be carried secretly. Malaria organisms could now be found "commonly" in the blood of "healthy" lowland Filipinos, especially children.[66] Chamberlain reported that 92.5 percent of Igorots showed enteric parasites in their stools, while 95.9 percent of Filipinos were infected, though usually asymptomatic.[67] P. E. Garrison claimed he had discovered "one of the most striking instances in the history of medicine of a population almost universally infested with animal parasites."[68] A local population, then, possessed at best only a limited clinical resistance to local disease — just enough to render a large number of them carriers, and a few of them victims, of surrounding microbial pathogens.

Major Charles Woodruff, as chief surgeon of the department of Luzon, in 1903 had issued a circular warning that perhaps one in five Filipino scouts carried the malaria parasite. Yet they "never had any symptoms of the disease whatever, the organisms apparently being harmless through racial immunity." Even though the Filipinos were unharmed, "they are a source of fatal infection to white men, who do not possess this racial immunity." "You are therefore to consider," Woodruff ordered, "all apparently healthy native soldiers as possible sources of fatal infection to whites." He went on to suggest that natives with malaria would not benefit from treatment with quinine, as the malaria germs in their blood lacked the vitality they acquired in nutritive white blood. Whites, however, always needed copious quinine.[69]

It was during this period that Patrick Manson, the founder of tropical medicine, changed his mind about liability to typhoid: in 1914 he decided that natives no longer seemed to enjoy absolute immunity, and the disease was "by no means uncommon among all classes."[70] In 1915, in his book *Infection and Immunity*, Victor C. Vaughan reported that evidence from the colonies suggested that "variations in susceptibility among the races is not so great as once believed": more thorough research had revealed that malaria was "highly prevalent" among Africans; and if there was any immunity to yellow fever, it was acquired by light exposure in early infancy.[71] By 1920

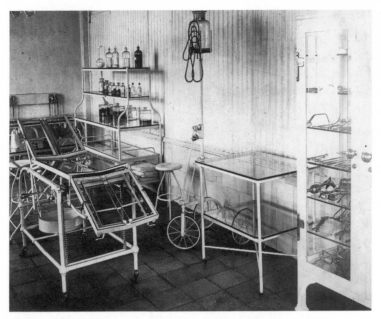

FIGURE 19. Operating room, Philippine General Hospital (RG 350-P-E28-6, NARA).

Aldo Castellani and Albert Chalmers had concluded that native races at best were "partially immune hosts [who] act as reservoirs or carriers," enabling "the parasite to complete its life-cycle without producing marked pathological changes in the host."[72] Racial immunity proved imperfect, thus fashioning native races as biological reservoirs to contain local disease organisms. Accordingly, we find emerging the figure of the meretriciously healthy carrier of disease — a condition of pathogenicity that in the tropics would always be associated with racial difference, however this was marked.

If previous subclinical exposure of individuals — or adaptation of the race's ancestors — had fashioned Filipinos as potential reservoirs of tropical pathogens, to white Americans it seemed that unhygienic racial custom and habit would ensure that this potential was realized. An appreciation of supposedly insidious cultural practices, especially those concerning defecation and eating, soon supplemented the emerging biological understanding of disease transmission and acquisition. Generally regarded as primitive and foolish, Filipino customs took on a more intimate and frightening significance. The race's patterns of behavior explained not only its unexpectedly vitiated immunity; they also suggested a source of danger for the utterly unprepared white immune system. Thus Filipino customs and habits would now prompt a sense of danger as much as thoughts of impurity. It appeared the natives were unable or unwilling to take necessary precautions against acquiring, transporting, and distributing the disease organisms most virulent to whites.

For James A. LeRoy, the Filipino's "shocking ignorance of sanitary principles as regards his house and community" was still chiefly a problem for the Filipino—it accounted for the evident impairment of the race's immunity to local pathogens. Although unhealthy habits might explain the deficit in Filipino labor power and attest to racial immaturity, they caused LeRoy no anxiety.[73] But other Americans felt more threatened by the proximity of diseased Filipino bodies and "disease-dealing" Filipino behavior. Edith Moses, the wife of the secretary for public instruction, found that rendering her house sanitary required "continuous oversight" of "twelve ignorant, superstitious Orientals"; when cholera struck in 1902, she "hosed off the 'China boys' and Filipinos with disinfectants" to prevent the spread of germs. "I made their eyes stick out with fright by describing a cholera germ. . . . They go about with their mouths shut tight, scarcely daring to open them lest a microbe pops into them."[74] Few accounts of domestic colonial life during this period fail to discuss the treacherous behavior and embodiment of servants.

The search for "healthy natives" as sources of disease—their microbiological interrogation—was intrinsic to the new tropical hygiene. If Filipinos once were thought to be completely immune to typhoid, now their race was prima facie evidence of germ carriage. When the disease appeared at Camp Eldridge between July and October 1909, the post surgeon attempted to determine the source of the infection. The first suspects were nearby natives, but the president of the local Board of Health, "an American resident of the town since 1902 and a physician," knew of no recent cases in Los Baños.[75] Attention then turned to the detection of "one or more typhoid bacillus excretors in the command"—but fecal specimens were negative. All the same, the post surgeon thought it wise to ensure that additional measures "were taken to prevent the contamination of food from excreta." Guards at the latrines checked that "all deposits are promptly covered with a liberal amount of dry earth and that each man washed his hands after defecation in a one percent solution of tricresol."[76] Dishes and food were screened from flies, drinking water was thoroughly boiled, the use of raw native vegetables was forbidden, and "two natives employed in the company as dishwashers were dismissed," although producing negative specimens.

In practice, the term *healthy native* referred to a deceptive appearance, not to any exemption from disease carriage. It usually implied a qualifier:

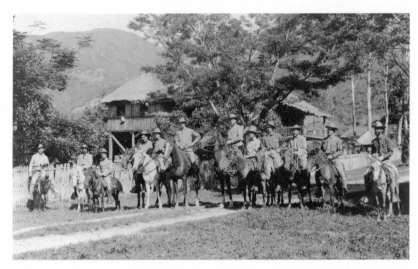

FIGURE 20. Dean C. Worcester with provincial governors and doctor "starting his trip through the wild man's country." Courtesy of the Rockefeller Archive Center.

apparently. When typhoid broke out at Ludlow Barracks, the post surgeon reported that "my first effort was to discover a possible carrier. The natives and kitchen force around Co. 'I' were tested for 'Widal' reaction and later the cooks of other companies were examined."[77] No asymptomatic carriers were detected. Yet the surgeon decided, regardless of any bacteriological result, to issue orders "forbidding natives, laundrymen, etc., to sleep under barracks. . . . Natives were prohibited from touching or eating from any dish used by soldiers."[78] Although it was later determined that the typhoid epidemic arose from drinking of contaminated water, and no native disease carriers had ever been identified, his report concluded, in part, that "natives are uncontrolled as to their personal hygiene and are undoubtedly a source of disease. Malaria, filarial diseases, cholera, dysentry [*sic*] and hookworm diseases as well as typhoid must be distributed by these natives who as laundrymen, kitchen and dining room servants, woodchoppers and private servants swarm around every barracks."[79]

Physicians did not hesitate to magnify the threatening microbial pathology that lurked within native bodies. Malaria, the most typical of tropical diseases, provides the best example. Wherever microscopy was undertaken, it revealed that many Filipinos harbored "so-called latent malaria."[80] Charles Craig, a member of the army board detailed to Fort William McKinley, sought out the cause of the high incidence of malaria among enlisted men at the post.

His suspicions led him first to examine blood specimens, taken "somewhat at random" from natives in a nearby town. These indicated that "the same general latent infection of Filipinos, both children and adults, which has been observed elsewhere in the Islands, exists in this community": 28 of 45 adult Filipinos and 87 of 180 children had latent infections.[81] Craig concluded, "In view of the well-known proclivity of the native soldiers for sleeping out of quarters and the convenient location of the native houses which shelter their wives and children, who take no precautions against mosquitoes, it is not surprising that latent malaria exists."[82] The results had confirmed the impression, now common, that "the greatest source of danger to the white man in a malarial locality lies in the native population, especially in the native children." Therefore, it would be "futile" to attempt to "rid any locality of malaria so long as the native element in the question is neglected."[83]

TOWARD A SANITARY IMMUNITY

What, then, was to be done? In theory, new research on the individual immune response to specific disease might be harnessed to confer on everyone an appropriate stock of antibodies and white cells. Paul Freer extolled experiments based on the idea that "a natural immunity may be increased or one which is scarcely existent may be rendered apparent and protective by the introduction of cells, or the products of these cells." In pursuit of this goal, the serum laboratories of the Bureau of Science produced an enormous variety of trial vaccines and sera — but their use remained limited.[84] Whether for technical, financial, or administrative reasons, colonial health authorities preferred to rely on sanitary engineering and stipulations of personal hygiene to control the transmission of pathogens. Automatic immunological protection might have made behavioral reform seem avoidable.[85] Until 1915, smallpox vaccination was the only large-scale program of biological protection in the archipelago.

In the early twentieth century, the enforcement of stipulations of personal and domestic hygiene was by far the major concern of the mature public health department. The basic assumption was that purer personal, domestic, and social life might confer on Filipinos a new sanitary immunity, augmenting the partial or inadequate physiological immunity that permitted disease carriage. Victor G. Heiser, for example, imagined himself "washing up the Orient" — and not just vaccinating it. Public health measures involving training, discipline, and surveillance focused increasingly on the regulation of personal conduct as a means to control the transmission of newly identified

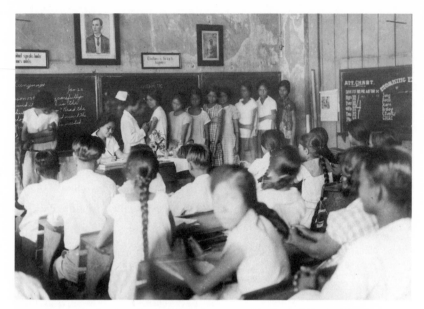

FIGURE 21. Vaccinating schoolchildren. Courtesy of the Rockefeller Archive Center.

microbial pathogens. But the peculiar and refractory social life of the Filipinos supposedly complicated the sanitary officer's task. Heiser lamented the profusion of their "incurable habits." He cited as obstacles the "unsuitable dietary of the people, their peculiar superstitions concerning the contraction of the disease, their almost unshakable fear of night air as a poisonous thing, a fear which has kept their houses tightly closed at night for generations past, their habit of chewing betel nut which has made the custom of expectorating in public . . . universal."[86] Without an acquired biological protection, "they will have to be first cured of their superstitions, which is as great a task as converting them to new religion; houses will have to be open at night, betel nut chewing gradually abolished, and then a gigantic anti-spitting crusade begun, and, last of all, comes the Herculean task of rousing them out of their inertia."[87] Health authorities reached out to those who had not yet contracted disease to emphasize "they live in constant danger of infection" and to point out that "the path of safety lies in the maintenance of good general health through the observance of simple rules of right living."[88] The prevention of infectious disease thus chiefly required the treatment of pathological social habits — not, primarily, vaccination or even the improvement of environmental, economic, or industrial conditions.

Colonial health officers in the Philippines were thus among the first advocates of what came to be known in the United States as the new public health. In 1902, on his return from Havana, Cuba, Charles V. Chapin, M.D., the influential superintendent of health in Providence, Rhode Island, deplored the fact that in the United States so "little stress was laid on *personal* uncleanliness" and too much still on "filth." Like many colonial medical officers, Chapin now believed that "personal cleanliness is the most important factor in the prevention of the infectious diseases."[89] A few years later, in the "Fetich of Disinfection," he pointed to the danger of the healthy carriers of disease, who ramified further the risk of contact between infected and uninfected. "It is our duty," he wrote, "to teach that hygienic salvation can only be attained through the good works of personal cleanliness."[90] Similarly, Charles-Edward Amory Winslow, another votary of the new public health, warned in 1914, "It is people, primarily, and not things, that we must guard against."[91] But this was old news in Manila. Gradually, in the continental United States too, the emphasis of local health work would shift from sanitation and environmental intervention toward a focus on the individual and the management of population. The discovery of "Typhoid Mary" in 1907 served to amplify concerns about the role of healthy carriers in the spread of disease.[92] But in the Philippines, the public health service had been almost from the beginning predicated on the identification and control of dangerous individuals and the regulation of social contact.

As president of the United States, W. H. Taft also tended to attribute the origin of reformist American sanitary science to the stimuli of the Spanish-American War and the need to pacify and purify the Philippines. Advances in the tropics "brought to the attention of the whole country the necessity for widespread reform in our provisions for the maintenance of health and the prevention of disease at home."[93] Having to deal with disease-carrying Filipinos, he told an international congress on hygiene in 1912, had made clear the need for "an additional branch of general education in the matter of the hygiene of the home and of the individual." Initially, the purpose was simply to make the region "habitable for white people." But now, colonial medical authorities were "engaged in the work of developing the tropical races into a strength of body and freedom from disease" — even though the Filipinos' "natural laziness and resentment at discipline make the enforcement most difficult."[94] Hygiene reform in the Philippines was nonetheless a model for what might yet be achieved in North America.

The new public health that emerged at the edge of empire was considerably more racialized in character and military in inspiration and style than the versions developing at a slower pace along the northeastern seaboard of the United States. The colonial Bureau of Health had absorbed the army medical department's commitment to drill, discipline, and bodily reform — and its disregard of the existing civic structures and sources of power. In the Philippines, the public health officer could generally work out an interventionist program with fewer constraints than in the major urban centers of the United States. Moreover, in the colony, the interventionist health officer would always be as sensitive as any southern U.S. physician to the boundaries of race — in this case, to the distinction of native and alien — as he campaigned against personal uncleanliness and sought to regulate social contact. Race was also a salient in the North American war against infectious disease, yet it seems rarely quite as pervasive and encompassing as in colonial skirmishes. In San Francisco, certainly, epidemics of smallpox and bubonic plague and fears of venereal disease and leprosy had since the late nineteenth century caused the public health department to focus on the dangers of Chinatown and later on the personal pathogenicity of Chinese bodies.[95] Some physicians, especially those in the South, worried too that African-Americans might be fearsome vectors of disease. In 1903, for example, William Lee Howard, a Baltimore physician, argued that "there is every prospect of checking and reducing these [infectious] diseases in the white race, if the race is socially — in every sense of the term — quarantined from the African."[96] Also, during the first decade of the twentieth century, U.S. immigration authorities became ever more likely to view the bodies of poor, non-Anglo immigrants as potentially diseased or as potential carriers of disease.[97] But in the Philippines, the race card had trumped all others — even class was secondary. In the United States, the patterns of disease carriage would often appear more complex, and still also more readily circumscribed by older methods of isolation and quarantine.

American medical efforts to inculcate civic virtue in Filipinos, to improve the race in order to limit disease transmission, should also be distinguished from the more conventional forms of colonial public health practiced in the region. The adjacent French empire in Indochina intermittently displayed an assimilationist sensibility, but education in hygiene did not really develop there until the 1920s, although the Saigon Board of Health, established only in 1907, did issue some health pamphlets before then. Despite the French republican substrate and some colonial "mimétisme," it seems that the "ré-éducation délicate" that Laurence Monnais-Rousselot describes exerted little influence on the local population until the 1930s.[98] Similarly, the British colonial medical authorities in Malaya and the Dutch in the East Indies demonstrated little commitment till the 1920s to health education and the modification of personal conduct. Although the Dutch had proclaimed an "ethical policy" for their vast territories at the beginning of the century, interest in "social evolution" and welfare remained scanty in the East Indies until after World War I.[99] Nearby Siam, later Thailand, was not formally colonized, but local officials observed British and American health policies closely and frequently sought advice from Malaya and the Philippines. Germ theories infiltrated Bangkok around 1901, yet for some decades they were adapted to an older tradition of environmental reasoning. No Thai texts on personal and domestic hygiene circulated before 1918, and attention to "population" and "national hygiene" languished through the 1920s.[100] Even Japanese "scientific colonialism" in Taiwan, north of the Philippines, avoided social engineering during this period, concentrating instead on the creation of "healthy zones" for vulnerable colonizers. From 1897, Gōtō Shinpei, a Japanese physician who had trained in bacteriology in Germany and come to admire Prussian state medicine, advised the colonial government on sanitation, but his "sanitary police" and surveillance system remained limited to the healthy zones. It proved hard to extend this infrastructure to rural areas until the 1930s.[101] British India, of course, was even more lamentably enclavist during this period: the leaders of the colonial medical service pressed for more efforts in health education and rural hygiene after World War I, but achieved little before the 1930s.[102]

In developing a distinctive new public health that would modify Filipino customs and habits, whether through education or regulation, the Bureau of Health was attempting to imbue a distrust of the body and its products, a dread of personal contact, and a respect for American sanitary authority. Health authorities targeted toilet practices, food handling, dietary customs, housing design; they rebuilt the markets, using more hygienic concrete, and suppressed the unsanitary fiestas; they assumed the power to examine Filipinos at random and to disinfect, fumigate, and medicate at will.[103] Strict enforcement of the rules of personal and domestic hygiene promised multiple benefits: local populations, less manifestly unwell, would work more efficiently and be less likely to carry disease organisms, and they would present fewer dangers to Europeans (whose own disease-carrying capacity generally was ignored). In this sense, tropical public health was principally a militarized form of industrial hygiene, first for the colonizer and then for the laboring colonized. And clearly the policy of education and supervision had other advantages. Its goal of nurturing self-control among Filipinos offered to

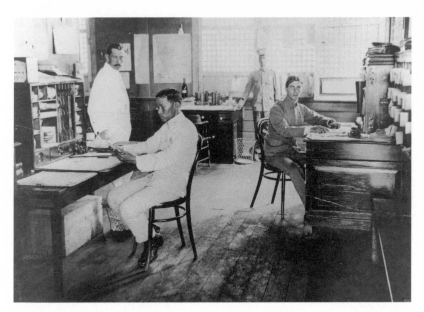

FIGURE 22. Interior of district health station. Courtesy of the Rockefeller Archive Center.

absolve the authorities from responsibility for both major environmental and social alteration, including the arranging of segregation — so promising the great financial savings never far from a colonial administrator's thoughts. Moreover, the reform of personal and domestic hygiene accorded in the most progressive style with the new science of disease causation, transmission, and acquisition.

Most Americans in the Philippines believed it would take many generations to replace traditional Filipino customs and habits — which seemed almost as characteristic of the race as any morphological feature — with the "spirit of *hygienic thoughtfulness*," as Dr. W. E. Musgrave called it.[104] It was hard enough to turn raw white recruits into disciplined soldiers — how much harder to make citizens out of supposed savages? The path of hygiene eventually led to civilization, but traffic along it would be slow. The good news was that Filipinos at least seemed to possess the biological potential to become civilized. When Maximilian Herzog, a pathologist at the Bureau of Science, weighed the brains of Filipinos who died in Bilibid prison, he found they were not much lighter than European brains. "As a race," he reminded the readers of the *American Anthropologist*, "they are of course less mature in mental, moral, and ethical development; they are more childlike, and their power of inhibition is not strongly developed." But his anatomical findings should encourage "those among Filipinos as well as among the American people who claim that the Filipinos as a people may be educated to the same degree of civilization as the Western nations."[105]

Observing the early failures to inculcate American excretory habits in Filipinos, Dr. Allan J. McLaughlin lamented, "It requires a long time completely to change the habits of a people and it will probably require another generation to complete the work."[106] When the "native custom" of eating with one's fingers was not easily suppressed, Heiser saw "years of discouraging struggle ahead of us before they can be broken of so fixed a habit, the menace of which as yet is entirely beyond their comprehension."[107] Dr. Thomas W. Jackson, having lived "surrounded by Filipino neighbors" in a provincial town, where it had been "impossible to avoid an intimate knowledge of their manner of life," endorsed the general pessimism. The first seven years of American control had seen only minimal improvement in the condition of the market, the disposal of garbage, and in "such personal habits as defecation, urination, expectoration, and eating with the fingers." Jackson concluded that the teachings of sanitary principles might be the "necessary and preliminary foundation" for disease prevention, but the introduction of such sanitary teachings "into the home by schoolchildren must be a slow and tedious process, unlikely to produce results within a generation."[108] Until then, close supervision and regulation would be warranted. In the opinion of an editor of the *Cablenews-American*, for the moment "only by force can the lower classes of natives" be made to abstain from food and drink "laden with germs." Despite noble educational efforts, "the densely ignorant adult native persists in compassing his own death" and the deaths of innocent Americans, although "with the coming generation this fatal ignorance will largely pass."[109]

IMMUNE CHILDREN OF THE TROPICS —
OR NATIVE DISEASE-DEALERS?

The change in the understanding of racial immunities and disease-dealing proclivities is perhaps most vividly illustrated in attitudes toward African-American soldiers in the tropics and Filipino scouts. In 1900, Nathaniel Southgate Shaler, a geographer and the dean of Harvard's Lawrence Scientific School, had proposed that the "troops which are required for Federal service in tropical lands might well be recruited from the Negroes"; with their families, these soldiers would soon become "permanently and contentedly established in Luzon and elsewhere in the colonies."[110] Shaler believed these "children of the tropics" would make excellent troops — "at least as infantrymen" — because the African-American constitution, unlike the white, was preadapted to the tropical climate.[111] In the Philippines, the distinguished geographer's advice was redundant. During the previous two years, the United States had already been using African-American and Filipino scouts to suppress resistance to its occupation of the archipelago. To Captain R. L. Bullard, one of the "white men of good standing" who commanded the 30th Alabama Volunteer Infantry (Negroes), it had long been plain that "Negro volunteers" were more immune to the regional ailments than white soldiers. Indeed, the disparities between colored and white were "so great that they almost require the naturalist and do require the military commander to treat the Negro as a different species."[112] And yet, even as black troops "could accomplish the most amazing amount of work" in such trying conditions, they unfortunately showed a natural tendency to "go in parties, they herd"; and "in the lonely duty of the sentinel this herding peculiarity becomes a positive fault."[113] Evidently, Negro troops, as children of the tropics, could never attain the civilized individuality of white citizen-soldiers. Filipino scouts proved more abundant and somewhat more independent, though similarly resistant to the tropical diseases and climate of their ancestral realm. Captain Charles D. Rhodes observed that local troops were "able to drink all kinds of water with impunity, and the common intestinal disorders are unknown"; they were susceptible perhaps only to "calentura or break-bone fever."[114] As the Filipino soldier "stands in the rice-fields, knee-deep in mud and water, during the working hours of day after day, one almost believes that years of exposure have made him amphibious. The factor of sickness among soldiers made of such material will not cause the surgeon much uneasiness."[115] And for a short time it did not.

Significantly, the enthusiasm of Shaler and others for "Negro colonization" of the Philippines proved evanescent. In the *Voice of the Negro*, T. Thomas Fortune had argued that black Americans could best hold up the flag in the new island possessions since, "all in all, the Afro-Americans in the Philippines stand the climate better and are on terms of better and more helpful understanding with the Filipinos than are white Americans."[116] But the belief that black Americans, like Filipinos, were naturally suited to the tropics and its disease environment soon became, for whites, more a cause of concern than an excuse for complacency. Increasingly, the old confidence in racial acclimatization, the notion of races and proper places, was giving way to fears that all allegedly tropical races lacked proper sanitary standards — they had not yet developed a "sanitary immunity." Doubts soon surfaced about the African-American soldier's "moral stamina" and a perceived tendency to "fraternize" with "native women."[117] Medical officers now pointed out that any natural affinity for Filipino customs and habits, combined with any residual inherited advantage in disease resistance, was likely to produce only more carriers of the diseases prevalent in the tropics. African-American troops within a few years had gone from being regarded as preadapted immune or acclimated children of the tropics to representing augmentations of the vast native reservoir of disease.

The enthusiasm of tropical physicians for hunting microbes, their preoccupation with tracing the distribution of the "exciting cause" of each disease, can obscure the persistence of hereditarian thought in medicine. But one finds, on closer inspection, that theories of racial predisposition and custom continued to suggest the contours for new disease maps, even if the lines so described by race have shifted. To be sure, immunity to local disease appeared more often to be acquired by exposure to specific germs during the individual's childhood; little was inherited solely through descent. And whatever immunity happened to be acquired was more likely to be partial than absolute. But the physiological adaptation of local inhabitants to surrounding disease seemed to have fashioned a natural reservoir for microbes, many of them entirely new to foreigners. The tendency of so-called primitives to acquire, to retain, and to spread portable pathogens—the racialization of pathogen distribution—appeared more important than ever before. Although cultural in character, this was regarded as a behavioral predisposition organized fundamentally by race. Thus it was the essentialized race culture—more than older notions of independent racial physiologies—that in the early twentieth century became the major salient in the war against disease-dealing native bodies.

Increasing confidence in science and hygiene was gradually helping to displace white somatic anxieties in the tropics. More and more it seemed that the alien race, following stipulations of hygiene—basically of the sort learned in the military—could survive near the equator without degenerating and perhaps without contracting, or at least without succumbing to, the local diseases. But this consoling routine was also part of a new political order, for medical optimism implied the need to intervene in the most intimate aspects of private life. If the great modern experiment in racial mobility was to succeed, Filipinos, even more than white Americans, would have to submit to reformation of personal conduct and social mores. In magnifying microbes as social actors, American physicians made Filipino bodies and Filipino behavior, both framed by adapted racial typologies, subject to ceaseless medical inspection, training, and discipline. Thus began the intimate workings of modern tropical hygiene.

Chapter Four

EXCREMENTAL COLONIALISM

Human wastes, the Bureau of Health warned Filipinos in 1912, "are more dangerous than arsenic or strychnine." Scientists had proven that "dysentery, typhoid fever, cholera, and kindred diseases are conveyed to a person, regardless of whether he be king or peasant, with minute organisms that, probably, have passed through the bowels of another person." Accordingly, all Filipinos should learn to treat their "evacuated intestinal contents as a poison," taking care to avoid contact with them or spreading them about.[1] Unlike Americans, Orientals seemed to lack control of their orifices. "The native and Chinese population," lamented Dr. Wallace de Witt, "tend markedly to decrease the general hygienic surroundings by reason of their unclean habits."[2] It was clear to Dr. Thomas R. Marshall, among others, that "the Filipino people, generally speaking, should be taught that . . . promiscuous defecation is dangerous and should be discontinued."[3] Ideally, Americans would train Filipinos to behave as meticulously and as retentively as any responsible white individual.

The importance of excrement in the modern medical calculus of risk is not surprising. Of all the manifold sources of germs — whether blood, urine, mucus, saliva, pus, water, air, or soil — feces appeared to public health officers the most abundant and most dangerous, just as to an earlier generation of physicians those places permeated by an odor of human waste had been the most feared.[4] Through much of the nineteenth century, medical officers demonstrated special sensitivity to excremental odors, and their twentieth-century successors, although discounting the morbidity of stenches in favor of the danger of germs, continued to identify human waste as a rich store of pathology. Only now, with the development of a bacteriological frame of mind, the dire consequences of feces would seem to derive more from direct physical contact than from any noxious emanation, that is, from any olfactory action at a distance. In the past, prevention of disease had mostly required avoidance of morbific sites or their cleansing and deodorization: the belated toilet training of adults had been rare and generally was regarded as unrewarding. Now, however, prevention usually would mean behavior change, improvement in personal cleanliness and the care of the body, as well as a shrinking from indiscriminate human contact. It meant reticence and containment, discretion and interment, more than simple deodorization and ventilation. But despite such permutations, the crucial link between excrement and danger proved remarkably resilient.[5]

When Charles V. Chapin urged health officers to trace infection not to things and places but to persons, he gave them special instructions to treat "all fecal matter as suspicious."[6] According to the new public health doctrine, feces provided a major conduit for germs from the manifestly unwell or healthy carriers to those previously uninfected. Chapin was demanding more attention to the personal element in disease transmission and greater efforts to reform the behavior of those who flouted the rules of hygiene. Of course, military hygienists had clearly anticipated both the civil health officer's interest in excrement as a vehicle for germs and his enthusiasm for behavior reform. The health officer in the Philippines did not need Chapin to tell him to treat fecal matter, especially that of other races, as suspicious; nor did he need instruction in the proper training of miscreants. The army surgeon's special preoccupation with the disposal of excrement and the need for discipline of new recruits presented a compelling model for colonial practice. Edward L. Munson had warned of "raw troops living like savages in their disregard of sanitary principles," spreading feces around the camp, but he expected that unremitting inspection and training would eventually reform them.[7] The same techniques might be applied to degraded Filipinos. Some of the more liberal and progressive colonial bureaucrats hoped that the race would respond to such surveillance and education, that it would eventually internalize the practice of personal hygiene and come to govern itself. Only it seemed the time frame for such response would have to be greatly extended.

In this chapter I want to consider the colonial health officer's obsession with ectopic excrement—with "matter out of place."[8] In the Philippines, American physicians used the body's orifices and its products to mark racial and social boundaries as well as to indicate how easy it would be to assail such enclosures. Waste practices became a potent means of organizing a heretofore diffusely threatening foreign population. That is, the colonial state came to be delineated on racialized bodies (Filipino or white) and behaviors (promiscuous or retentive); it was intimately reduced to orifices (open or closed) and dejecta (visible or invisible). In this new orificial order, American bodily control legitimated and symbolized social and political control, while the "promiscuous defecation" of Filipinos indicated their position on a lower bodily and civilizational stratum. As Americans issued formal directives and designed toilets, they imagined Filipinos inadvertently subverting their hygienic abstractions and defecating regardless. Such promiscuous defecation seemed potentially to mock and transgress colonial boundaries at the same time as it confirmed the necessity and value of such demarcations.[9] It was allowing germs to cross between the races in unsegregated Manila and thus to endanger lawful, innocent Americans. A sense of the porosity of the colonial membrane lent force to those health officers who sought to constrain the delinquent microbial traffic. Thus physicians extended their power to inspect and regulate the personal cleanliness and the social life of naturally erring Filipinos, whose toilet practices in particular seemed to require ceaseless supervision and discipline.

My argument is that through somatic control and moral training, the colonial state attempted to shape the bodies and conduct of Filipinos and Americans.[10] Racial type was manifested in bodily function and pathological potential, on which medicos put a gloss of civilizational status. If they wanted recognition from the public health department, Filipinos were expected to confess their uncleanliness, to voice their barbarity, and to make themselves available for hygienic salvation. Of course many either refused to do so or remained indifferent to medical opinion. Others, despite their misgivings, appeared to go along with the racialized performance of abjection.[11] After the confession of rottenness, Filipinos might eventually be raised and perhaps admitted to a sort of probationary sanitary citizenship.[12] Ideally, then, the colonizing process would resemble a civilizing process, a training of childlike Filipinos in the correct techniques of the body, rationalized as hygiene.[13]

White Americans, in contrast, would be obliged to perform a transcendence of their lower bodily stratum, to act as though they inhabited a more formal, expressive body. Their personal and domestic hygiene had to be immaculate. The labor of civilization called for constant self-discipline among American residents of the tropics: the rationale for territorial possession would thus be predicated on unsustainable self-possession.[14]

To attempt at this distance to determine the "true" pattern of Filipino and American excretory practices is unprofitable at best. Even if such a reckoning were possible, its results would contribute little to our understanding of the contemporary meaning of medical subject positioning in the Philippines. We may assume that Filipinos frequently transmitted pathogens — but so too did Americans; no doubt Filipinos, as much as Americans, constructed boundaries and transgressions with "matter out of place." But it is American assertion that suffuses the historical record. Here I would like to find out what was at stake politically in performing an American sublime and a Filipino abject. How was pathology embodied? How were excretory habits racialized? What did it mean to promote personal hygiene above environmental sanitation? And perhaps most important: in what productive forms might bodily control extend colonial modernity?

COLONIAL EMBODIMENT, FROM ABJECT TO SUBLIME

Sent to Surigao in 1902, Dr. Henry du Rest Phelan, a medical officer with the U.S. Army, found the town to be a "most charming and delightful spot" on a "picturesque" site. But its sanitary condition alarmed him. Filth abounded. The *tiendas*, or stores, were "all more or less filthy," the promenade in front of them "a lounging place for idlers of both sexes." The ground beneath the houses was covered with "filth of all kinds, human excrement included"; weeds had sprouted up in the streets; and garbage accumulated in vacant lots. That the islands had recently endured a brutal war and massive social disruption meant little to Phelan: the problem seemed one of innate Filipino fecklessness and lack of civilization. "They appear to me," he reported, "like so many children who need a strong hand to lead them in the path they are to follow." Filipinos were willfully polluting the soil, even around their own houses. Accordingly, Phelan, "necessarily somewhat autocratic," began his "crusade against filth." In a short time, "the roads were clean, the marshes drained, the houses purified, and the inhabitants impressed with the necessity of adopting new rules of hygiene." And when, despite this transition from squalor to cleanliness, the mortality rate climbed, Phelan wryly concluded that the transition itself "could have given the community a shock sufficient to cause such a thinning out of its ranks."[15]

Over the following decade, bacteriologists from the Bureau of Science and the Army Board for the Study of Tropical Diseases found widespread carriage of disease organisms among local inhabitants, even those who were apparently healthy. Filipino bodily wastes seemed typically to contain parasites and bacteria. In combating the cholera outbreak of 1915, Munson identified Filipino vibrio carriers as "not only the most numerous but the most insidious and dangerous sources of infection." His laboratory men had painstakingly collected and examined Filipino stools: the procedures for extracting these specimens gave even Munson pause: "The work meant invasion of the accepted rights of the home and of the individual on a scale perhaps unprecedented for any community. The collection of the fecal specimens necessarily might fairly be regarded as repulsive to modesty. Add to this the facts that the search was made among persons apparently healthy to themselves and others who could scarcely fall even within the class of suspects, and that those found positive were subjected to all the inconveniences of isolation, separation from family, loss of earning capacity, etc."[16] In 1909 alone, the hard-pressed staff of the Manila Bureau of Science had examined over 7,000 fecal specimens, almost all from Filipinos; and then in 1914, at the beginning of the cholera epidemic, they were overwhelmed by more than 126,000 jars of feces.[17]

Vulnerable foreigners would be wise, it was thought, to treat all Filipinos as potentially infected and dangerous and to limit contact with native bodies and their contents until the race was cleaned up. Yet avoidance of contact was not easy in the largely unsegregated colonial society; Filipino behavioral change, if possible, therefore seemed imperative.[18] When P. E. Garrison, for example, detected almost universal carriage of parasites among lowland Filipinos, he urged authorities to reform "the methods of the disposal of the excreta customary among the Filipino people."[19] Captain Benjamin J. Edger, M.D., recalling his sanitary experiences in the Philippines, observed, "Even in the houses of the wealthiest cities of Luzon, Lipa, Batangas Province, the lavatory and sink are in close proximity to the kitchen. Not until the American occupancy was the effort made to dispose of the excreta, even by the wealthiest classes."[20] An American physician declared that "the cleaning of the Augean stables was a slight undertaking in comparison with purifying the Philippines. . . . No imagination can make the Filipino customs with respect to [defecation] worse than actuality."[21] But reform there must be. In 1909, the model disease survey of the town of Taytay pointed to many

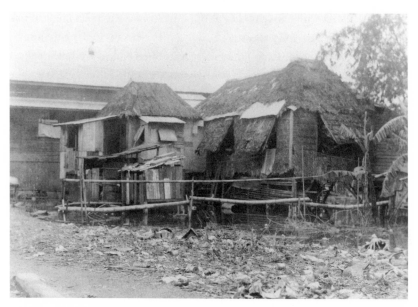

FIGURE 23. An unsanitary yard: "A home without a latrine causes the spread of many diseases." Courtesy of the Rockefeller Archive Center.

peccant waste disposal customs. Richard P. Strong and his colleagues reported that most residents in the mornings would empty, in any convenient place, vessels containing their excreta; or else they defecated in the bushes at the edge of town. Only a quarter of the dwellings had separate outhouses, and even these were generally holes in the floor, through which human waste dropped onto the ground, where the pigs scavenged it.[22] The investigators felt that modification of such customs and habits — a civilizing process — would take some time and effort, but still it must be attempted. Captain Edger claimed that "principally through American Army officers the Filipino race has been shown we are clean and mean to keep our surroundings clean." Although the struggle would be long and hard, he hoped, like Strong and others, that Filipinos might eventually follow the white American example. He reflected that "constant association and influence of Americans is bound to have its beneficial effects on the Filipino. He advanced from almost a savage state to the better advanced progressive Spanish methods by force. It is almost impossible to tell what he will do in coming years when given the advantage of free American ways and liberality."[23] American "liberality" would create the desire among Filipinos to imitate whites and seek self-government of their bodies and habits.

Since contact with native bodies or their excreta now implied medical risk for white Americans, servants warranted relentless scrutiny and regulation. At times, the "half-naked, dark-skinned creatures" employed by Edith Moses gave her the impression of being "trained baboons," especially a "monkey-like coolie" who polished the *narra* (hardwood) floors. On other occasions, however, her servants were simply "like children," fun loving and filthy. "In spite of all my lectures and my practice," she lamented, "our Chinese do not understand the first principles of sanitary cleanliness."[24] Nevertheless, Moses persisted in her efforts to teach her servants to avoid handling food, to set tables decorously, to dispose of their wastes fastidiously, and to wash their hands regularly. She house-trained them. Similarly, Emily Bronson Conger despaired that "it never occurs to [Filipinos] to wash their hands," and they never used soap or towels. "They rub their bodies sometimes with a stone," she noted. "It does not matter which way you turn you see hundreds of natives at their toilet. One does not mind them more than the caribou [*caribao*, buffaloes] in some muddy pond, and one is about as cleanly as the other."[25]

Conger claimed indifference to these infractions, but her peers did not: most were convinced that such uncivilized, indeed dangerous, behavior required reformation. Thus, in Lilian Hathaway Mearns's *Philippine Romance*, the heroine, Patricia, expresses the nobility of her character when she assures her suitor that "everyday I have made a visit to the barrio, and have preached soap and water without ceasing."[26] In the interests of hygiene and the American way of life Patricia was teaching supposedly barbarous Filipinos to contain their bodily wastes and not spread them around. Less noble, perhaps, were the methods of Mr. and Mrs. Campbell Dauncey. When they moved to Iloilo, Mrs. Dauncey was appalled to find that her new house was next to "a rabbit warren of low-class Filipinos, who keep all sorts of animals in the rooms, and throw all their refuse out into the narrow alley between this and the next house." She put out bowls of disinfectant to ward off her new neighbors, but to no avail. Far more effective was her husband's response to these "transgressions of the laws of cleanliness and decency." He followed the simple plan of "leaning out of the window when the people below do anything he does not like, and calling them '*Babuis*' [pigs], or '*sin verguenza*' [without shame] in a very loud voice, which they don't like at all."[27]

If the anus was a synecdoche for the medicalized Filipino body, the mouth just as surely symbolized American presence — in the case of the Daunceys, English presence.[28] In this sense, American physicians were doubly spokesmen for the body. Unlike Filipinos, they produced abstractions, by mouth and by hand, not waste — or, at least, not dangerous and visible waste. White Americans talk, write, report, police, supervise servants, hunt, fish, and fight: but after reading the medical documents produced in the Philippines in the first decade of the century, one suspects they rarely, if ever, went to the toilet. Whatever happened to *their* lower bodily functions? These retentive colonialists seem to imagine themselves to have achieved a sort of transcendence of the natural body. American bodies become abstracted from the filthy exuberance of the tropics, represented as truly civilized models for Filipinos.[29] But this American sublime demanded relentless self-discipline; and, in this sense, the disparagement and civilizing of Filipinos would also be a labor of American repression.[30]

THE LABORATORY AND THE MARKET

The medical laboratory in the tropics was as much sign as signifier of difference. In focusing on the laboratory as an idealized representational space, we are inclined to forget that this modern workplace had its own distinctively abstract spatial texture.[31] It was a delibidinized place of white coats, hand washing, strict hierarchy, correct training, isolation, inscription — in short, a place of somatic control and closure, organized around the avoidance of contamination. Just as the laboratory's spatial representations — its reports and scientific papers — reduced the tropics (the lower regional stratum) to a series of controllable, visualized specimens and abstracted intelligence, so the spatial practices producing these inscriptions depended on its workforce (mostly young, single males) transcending the lower bodily stratum, setting themselves apart from the filth outside. The laboratory thus became a distinctive and discriminating locus of colonial modernity.

As early as July 1901 the Philippine Commission had established a Bureau of Government Laboratories — the forerunner of the Bureau of Science — consisting, initially, of a biological and a chemical section.[32] The biological laboratory was expected to provide "adequate facilities for investigation into, and scientific report upon, the causes, pathology and methods of diagnosing and combating the diseases of man and of domesticated animals" as well as to perform any routine biological work required by other government departments.[33] The chemistry laboratory investigated food, drug, and plant composition and mineral resources. Paul C. Freer, the first director of the bureau, declared that the new Manila laboratories provided "a position for the higher type of educated American investigator, not only for the actual material results which he may obtain, but also for the benefit which will accrue by his very presence in the community."[34] Indeed, Freer never tired of extolling the value of scientific work in the Philippines. Nor did he hesitate to point out that "the work is of so difficult a nature, so important, and, if imperfect methods are used, so subject to error, that a poor equipment both in the literature of medical biology and in apparatus would be the precursor of failure." He thus presented his demands for "the highest type of trained investigators, a complete library, and exceptional facilities."[35] In 1904 he got his "properly equipped biological laboratory," with large rooms ("well lighted without direct sunlight") and a supply of microscopes, incubators, sterilizers, microtomes, glassware, stains, chemicals, and small animals. The new laboratory buildings, decorated externally in a modified Spanish style, occupied a fine site on the old Exposition Grounds near the heart of the city.

Laboratory design was predicated on a transcendence of the tropical environment. A modern power plant provided the rooms with vacuum, air pressure, and steam and supplied light to all the laboratory buildings. To ensure good ventilation and coolness in the two-story building, on each floor the rooms were grouped on either side of a large, main corridor ten feet wide and running the entire length of the building. When the hallway was open, Freer noticed that "a breeze is almost continually passing through it, generally supplying a suction as it passes the doors of the individual laboratories so that a constant circulation of air is produced."[36] The largest part of the building was the main laboratory structure, facing toward the south and divided into two symmetrical portions, one for the biological laboratory and the other for the chemical laboratory. In the rooms of the biological wing, a microscope table ran along the entire window front. So that "the strange breezes which prevail in this country" should not play havoc with materials on this worktable, the windows were placed well above the desks.[37] In the center of the room, two tables afforded ample space for the general work of the laboratory, particularly for heating, filtering, and distilling. Along another wall of each biological room was a chemical worktable furnished with gas, water, and vacuum. A hood occupied the opposite wall; its flue extended up into the attic and connected with the main exhaust tanks, producing a strong artificial draft. On the ground floor a special room was given over to the preparation of culture media: here steam was provided for sterilizers and the main autoclaves of the building. Each floor of the biological wing included a room for the refrigerating boxes and for the incubators, each heated by Bunsen burners. A separate house behind the biological wing held the cages of the experimental animals.

To assess accurately the tropical environment and to gauge the character of its inhabitants, the investigators, all correctly trained "higher types," needed to compare new specimens with standard reference material. The museum was therefore one of the more important sections of the laboratories. Typical examples of anatomical and histological pathology were carefully preserved, along with a collection of local parasites and insects.[38] But the scientific library was perhaps of even more use to investigators trying to formalize and abstract the apparent chaos of the tropics. The scope of the library meant that "no one need fear a lack of literature" in Manila.[39] This "central depository of scientific books for the entire Government" boasted an extensive holding of monographs and periodicals.[40] An assiduous researcher could find there all the major British, German, and French publications dealing with tropical science. But constant vigilance was required to protect this defining resource from tropical depredation. The environment it codified threatened constantly to consume it. "Books must be inspected daily," Freer lamented, "and wiped off very frequently during the rainy season, on account of the mold." Rapacious insects, particularly cockroaches, could destroy overnight the texts that stigmatized them. To protect the books, the covers were varnished, and the legs of the bookcases rested in cans of petroleum. Freer took comfort in the fact that white ants had never attacked the library, although they came very close.[41]

Colonial bureaucrats sometimes hopefully described the whole of the archipelago as a living laboratory; then again they might despair of ever achieving such control. "The Philippines may be considered today as a laboratory," declared James A. LeRoy in 1906, "where an experiment with important bearings of the 'race problem' is being conducted."[42] Decades later, Joseph R. Hayden, a vice governor of the islands, reflected that "one of the great achievements of the period [was] that within the Philippine government an essentially scientific attitude should have been substituted for the unscientific ways of Spanish days."[43] Americans hoped that with much time and effort the disorder and promiscuity of the islands might be subdued, so that colonial space might come to resemble the controlled conditions of the modern laboratory. Yet this expansionist trajectory, in which the laboratory is imagined simply as a territorializing technology, can disguise a more complicated scalar politics. At times, it was equally important to make a distinction between colony and laboratory, if only to emphasize the superior culture of American modernity and how much more progress Filipinos and their country had yet to make. The flexible scale of the colonial laboratory — its capacity to magnify and diminish its focus — allowed a play of differentiation and assimilation. At one moment the whole of the archipelago and its inhabitants seemed to constitute a living laboratory; at another, the place and its people were woefully unlike the conditions and the life forms characteristic of a modern laboratory. At one moment, no one knew where the laboratory was and where society was; at another it was all too clear.[44]

Indeed, outside the laboratory even higher types might still be contaminated and transformed. That most of the American laboratory workers, all college graduates, lived in small rooms and ate out at the local restaurants appalled Freer. After all, this risked exposing the Americans as slaves of intimate activities involving contamination and excretion. "In a country like this where hygienic surroundings are of the highest importance and where sickness causes such a large decrease in the normal efficiency of a working force, it is highly desirable that members of a staff should be able to find suitable and healthful accommodations upon their arrival."[45] Above all, it was imperative that young American scientists avoid the filth of Philippines' markets. Seen as a center of pollution and disorder, the market was evidently the antithesis of the laboratory. Regarded as a negation of American formality, the open market, like the grotesque Filipino body, appeared ever in need of scientific reformation.[46]

For many American colonialists, the Philippine marketplace conjured up fascinating images of chaos, sensuality, and danger, however bland the social life of these public spaces may in fact have been.[47] The marketplace, especially the large, overcrowded city market, Divisoria, was readily represented as a locus of promiscuous contact and contamination, a space quite unlike the ideal laboratory that was formally documenting its dangers. If Americans were scorned and ridiculed, surely they were most exposed — most open to such an inversion of colonial relations — in the marketplace. This necessarily perverted place was recognized as a place of risk, both symbolically and materially so. LeRoy found that "unless there be rigid and efficient supervision," the markets were "foci of infection." Whenever he wandered through these places, Nicholas Roosevelt assumed that "many varieties of intestinal germs and parasites may lurk in most foods." For Daniel R. Williams, the markets were simply "unwholesome and death-dealing plazas." "No one who has not traveled in the Orient can conceive of the noise and confusion," William Freer wrote of Manila's street life. "Words fail utterly to describe it."[48]

But how to render this teeming, promiscuous environment more laboratory-like? Just as the laboratory had constructed — or rather, informed and rationalized — the problem of contact, so it offered solutions. When Katherine Mayo visited the "Isles of Fear," as she called the Philippines, in the early 1920s she was pleased to note the strict control of potential "disease carriers" in hotels and restaurants: no servant could handle food "without a health certificate showing he was free from germs likely to convey disease."[49] Washing and disinfecting of hands were constantly emphasized. Governor James F. Smith was himself convinced that cholera attacked only those "people drinking from esteros, eating with fingers and refusing to recognize the importance of sanitary laws."[50] In order to protect consumers in the public sphere, new *sanitary* markets were constructed in Manila. The buildings, all of the supposedly hygienic reinforced concrete, were "supplied with ample water facilities, enabling them to be kept scrupulously clean."[51] Sanitary inspectors patrolled the aisles, checking regularly to ensure that the stallholders wore clean clothes, kept their hands spotless and their nails trimmed, and used only clean white wrapping paper.[52] To prevent shoppers from engaging in "the old custom of handling one piece of meat after another with the fingers," forks were provided. In case this was not enough, meat was placed in "substantial screen cages made of copper wire with sliding doors," in this way protecting it further, not only from "promiscuous handling but also from contamination by flies." Such modern markets, constructed throughout the archipelago, became "educational features . . . doing much to spread the doctrine of cleanliness throughout the Islands."[53]

Despite improvements to the water supply, sanitary inspectors still detected "bacilli of the colon type" in samples of drinking water dispensed in the *tiendas*. The director of health therefore stipulated that in order to be licensed each *tienda* must have a teakettle "for rendering water sterile." Instructions printed in Spanish, Tagalog, and Chinese required the kettle, filled from the city pipes, to "boil violently" for at least fifteen minutes before it was poured.[54] The Bureau of Health also recognized that the common drinking cup served to transmit several kinds of infectious diseases. In institutions and churches the necessity of the individual cup appeared urgent. A disposable cup was the only practical and progressive solution. The bureau suggested a method of making an individual drinking cup from a square sheet of tough paper. "Inmates of institutions soon learn to make their own cups," Dr. Victor G. Heiser reported, "and take great delight in the thought of protective cleanliness which is afforded by their use."[55]

When the author of *Interesting Manila* first visited the city in 1900 he observed that the *tienda*s were "so open to the street as to be practically in the

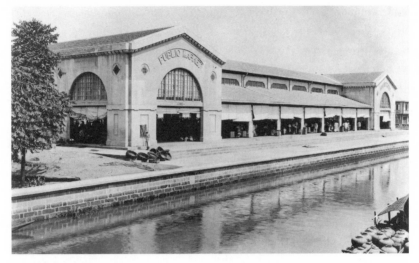

FIGURE 24. New type of concrete market. Courtesy of the Rockefeller Archive Center.

highway," and those of the Chinese were "always repulsive and dirty." But after ten years they were far cleaner, better enclosed — more safely "interesting." As for the markets, "before the days of American sanitation," he recalled, "the condition of these places was always indescribably bad, but modern regulations and efficient inspectors have changed all this to comparative cleanliness and good order."[56] Similarly, Frank G. Carpenter remembered that in 1900 the largest marketplace in Tondo "consisted of ten acres of rude sheds, roofed with straw matting or galvanized iron laid upon a framework of bamboo poles." But by 1920 it was a building of concrete and steel, hosed down every night.[57] It was nearly as clean and orderly as a laboratory.

THE TOILET IN THE TROPICS

To combat apparent racial obstacles to behavior change — to the civilizing process — health experts vigorously promoted educational and publicity projects in the second decade of the twentieth century. The Philippine health service began issuing a semiweekly bulletin, never more than a page in length, dealing with some topical public health question. This was published in all the daily papers in English, Spanish, and Tagalog and mailed to medical officers and other government officials throughout the islands. From 1915, women's clubs conducted pious discussions on maternal and infant welfare and issued their own bulletins. Sanitary commissions visited selected towns, surveying health conditions in the community; giving practical demonstrations of how to prepare balanced diets from the local food supply and instructing the local inhabitants in personal hygiene, home cleanliness, and the care of the sick. The health service also maintained permanent exhibits of model sanitary houses, sanitary methods of sewerage disposal, and sanitary and unsanitary *barrios*. Photographs, "moving pictures," parade floats, and (in 1921) a "health-mobile" that was sent out to fairs and fiestas illustrated modern methods of hygiene.[58] Cartoons in English and Tagalog also showed promise as effective means of persuading infantilized Filipinos to change their unhygienic habits. Warnings about the poisonous nature of fecal matter, the evils of handling food, the dangers of "the promiscuous spitting habit" abounded. No wonder, then, that when exercise was advised it was "for the purposes of enabling the body to eliminate its waste products and become clean."[59] The general message was that Filipino bodies were especially dirty and infected — had not the microscope shown it to be so? — and that personal contact and loose behavior would only distribute their filth.

The public schools became a major sanitary venue. Teachers compiled a "health index" for every child in their class. The Bureau of Education's idealized "healthy child" had a "well-formed body," "clean and shining hair," "a clear skin of good color," "ears free from discharge," "a voice of pleasing quality," "an amiable disposition," and so on.[60] A premium was thus placed on the Filipino child's formal, expressive qualities. Furthermore, every child was to be weighed once a month, and the height measured at least twice a year. If anything was amiss, the teacher reported it to the local health officer. But this was not enough. It was also the duty of a teacher to "instruct pupils to care for themselves and to put into practice both in the school and at home miscellaneous health principles."[61] The transcendence of the lower bodily stratum was also to animate everyday life. Through correct training, children would learn of the dangers of raw vegetables, impure water, poorly ventilated houses, a sedentary way of life, and deformed posture. Every child had to carry a clean handkerchief, drink at least a cup of milk each day, sleep from ten to twelve hours a night under a mosquito net, bathe daily, wear shoes, and wash his hands before eating — and never touch the food. So that the noncontaminating abstract space of the classroom should be faultlessly extended — to stabilize a new sense of embodiment and new habits — health experts urged that "the construction of a toilet, either in his own home or in that of a neighbor, be a project for each seventh-grade boy."[62]

Toilets soon were cropping up everywhere. The Bureau of Health from the beginning had urged all Filipinos to treat their "evacuated intestinal contents

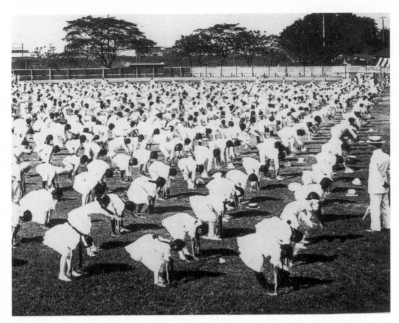

FIGURE 25. Calisthenic drill by three thousand children at the Manila Carnival, 1915 (RG 350-P-Cd-2-1, NARA).

as a poison," taking care to avoid contact with them. "Let those who are able to put in septic tanks and flush closets do so" — all others should install a pail closet, at a cost.[63] In the smaller communities in which cholera had prevailed in the early 1900s, sanitary officers had found the pail system to be effective, although it seemed initially that "the cost of maintenance and inspections as a regular measure is prohibitive and only warranted by emergency conditions."[64] In the poorer towns, which had no sewer or pail system, every householder had to "dig a simple pit closet and to cover each fecal deposit promptly with lime or fresh earth."[65] But public health officials hoped that widespread use of the pail could be made feasible and affordable elsewhere. Heiser suggested that a pail system might even be profitable in routine conditions if it was installed along "with an after-treatment of the night soil which would render it suitable for fertilizing mulberry trees, thus promoting the silk industry." He was, however, vehemently opposed to the plan "followed in many Oriental countries" of letting out private contracts for the collection of night soil from private residences, for it was "established custom" to use this untreated waste to fertilize vegetables — often with mixed cultures of amoebae, cholera bacilli, and other pathogens.[66] If the profit motive was insufficient, then taxation might make the pail system commonplace. Householders soon had to choose between paying quarterly charges of 7.50 pesos for individual pails kept on the premises or 1 peso to use the public pail system.

Much attention had been given to the design of a cheaper and more efficient "sanitary pail." The bureau recommended a raised frame of four posts set at a height that allowed an "ordinary five-gallon kerosene can" to be slipped under the bottom of the seat. By covering the hole with a self-closing, hinged seat, the designers had carefully ensured that no flies or other insects could gain access to the contents. But the "container for the can has the advantage of being entirely open, which fact secures good ventilation and leaves no opportunity for the collection and retention of disagreeable odors," an unfortunate consequence of the superceded boxlike designs.[67] The ordinary carabao cart could haul far more of the light cans than it could the old-fashioned wooden pails, so the costs of collection were also much reduced. With the savings, an attendant could be hired to supervise "a suitably located central pit" where the contents of the cans were dumped.[68]

Even after improvements in efficiency and reductions in cost, many years passed before the pail system was widely used. The poorer sections of Manila continued to depend on a few scattered public collections of "unsanitary closets" or none at all long after the more prosperous sections were sewered.[69] Until the 1920s, approved systems of waste disposal remained a rare sight in the provinces. When David Willets visited the Batanes Islands in 1913 he reported bluntly, "A suitable method for disposing of human excrement is lacking." Water closets were very rare, "and furthermore the people have not learned to use them."[70] But if the local inhabitants continued to disregard sanitary advice and regulation, sanitary officers could still, when emergencies arose, forcibly disinfect them and their surroundings. When Allan McLaughlin took charge of the sanitary response to the Manila cholera outbreak of 1908, he organized over six hundred men into disinfecting squads that went about spraying carbolic over dwellings and "liming all closets and places where fecal matter existed or was likely to be deposited." Each day in the "strong material districts," squads disinfected the closets, while "in the light material districts, the effort to disinfect the dejecta of the entire population necessitated the disinfection of entire districts. It was necessary to disinfect practically the whole ground area."[71] Anyone who tried to obstruct the disinfectors was arrested and fined. The amount of disinfectant dispersed was enormous: more than 150,000 pounds of lime and 700 gallons of carbolic acid were used. When the entire stock of disinfectant in the islands was gone, supplies had to be ordered from Hong Kong. When they ran out

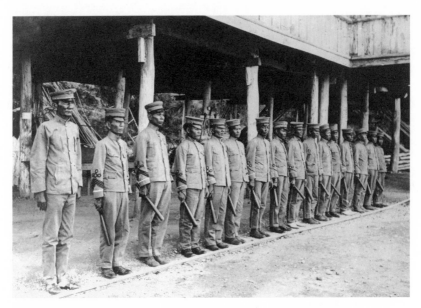

FIGURE 26.   Filipino sanitary inspectors (RG 350-BS-1-4-175 [BS 9834], NARA).

of lime, squads took to digging ditches and cleaning up the yards until new stocks came in.

By 1920 forcible disinfection was no longer a major part of the sanitary response to enteric diseases. Filipinos were generally obeying the provisions of sanitary code that required "any building of whatever character" to include "adequate privies or toilet accommodations, constructed according to plans approved by the director of health." A sanitary inspector could now demand to see, at the very least, "a pit not less than one and a half meters in depth, securely covered by a slab of stone or concrete . . . a seat, provided with a cover, so devised to close automatically when not in use; a vertical conducting pipe . . . leading from the seat to within the pit; and a vent pipe not less than ten centimeters in diameter leading from the pit to one meter above the eaves of the building." The capacity of the pit was set liberally at one cubic meter for each resident. Though "adequate facilities for ventilation" were crucial, this "Antipolo toilet" was not permitted to "communicate" with any other room and had to have "a tight-fitting door."[72]

FROM FIESTA TO CLEAN-UP WEEK

José Rizal has provided us with an almost rhapsodic account of a Filipino fiesta in the 1890s. To the community, on the eve of the fiesta, it seems "the air is laden and saturated with gladness." And on the day, while "everything is confusion, noise, uproar," it is an amiable confusion, not at all contaminating or threatening. Banners float and wave in the streets as processions pass by; the community gathers to watch, join in the parades, sing, dance, and attend the cockfights and the games of chance. People saunter about at will. In the plaza, on a bamboo stage, the comedy from Tondo begins its songs, dance, and mimicry. Members of the audience are dressed in their best clothes, and, according to Rizal, a scent "of powder, of flowers, of incense, of perfume" permeates the town. If, in the pushing and the crush of the crowd, one caught a whiff of "human animal," this contact with one's fellows was more to be cherished than feared. And so the romance of the fiesta continues, until at the end of the day "the lights and variegated colors distracted the eyes, melodies and explosions, the ears."[73]

But Mrs. Dauncey had quite another impression of the fiesta of 1904 that commemorated the death of Rizal. The crowds "swarmed out" into the town of Iloilo in the evening. "They hang out flags and lanterns," she reported, "and every Filipino knocks off what little work he ever does, and crawls about on the streets and spits . . . while the women slouch along in gangs with myriads of children."[74] To her eyes it was a time of promiscuous, animalistic contact. In June 1900, Edith Moses, newly settled in Manila, had heard of the dangers of such gatherings. "Many officers seem to think that the fiesta is a mask for an uprising on a large scale," she wrote, "and all American women and children have been warned not to go into the streets." Clearly the fiesta represented a challenge to the American control of colonial public space, if not to the actual institutions of government. And though skeptical of the "dangerous fiesta," Mrs. Moses later imagined "insurrectos whispering under my bed and coming up the ladder," invading even her domestic refuge, her personal enclosure.[75] Thus the communal fiesta appeared an earthy, open site for the subversion of American colonial modernity.

To the materialists in the Bureau of Health the uncontrolled fiesta meant principally a concentration of "an extraordinary amount of foodstuffs, most of which are improperly prepared and handled, and exposed to contamination."[76] It sometimes involved the congregation of sick, often infected, people at some religious shrine. The "lack of sanitary preparation to accommodate the crowds" thus dispersed diseases across the archipelago. In order "to meet this menace," the Bureau of Health demanded that local authorities provide "clean, disinfected, and otherwise supervised" convenience stations where people concentrated, a clean water supply, and food prepared and served "in

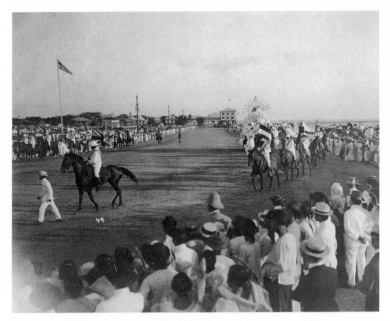

FIGURE 27. Parade, Manila Carnival, 1908 (RG 350-P-Ua-14, NARA).

a cleanly manner."[77] To ensure this occurred at Antipolo during the pilgrimage to the shrine of "Nuestra Señora de la Paz y Buen Viaje" in 1915, the Bureau of Health had dispatched an auxiliary corps of sanitary inspectors. As a result, "instead of proving a menace to the people of the town," the event became "a means for educating and improving them."[78] But the bureau did not have the resources to supervise all the local fiestas.

In 1907, inspired by the success that year of Major General Leonard Wood's Wild West performance in the capital's streets, the colonial government decided to establish an "institutional Carnival" in Manila as an alternative to insidious, uncontrolled fiestas. The first such "Oriental adaptation of the far-famed customs of the south of France, of Italy, Spain and Latin America" occurred in February 1908. Conceived as an allegorical event, the theme of the pageants, displays, sports, and revelry was the visit of the Monarch of the West to the Monarch of the East. The latter, played by young Manuel Gomez, "with his gorgeously attired court and retainers, embarked in gaily bedecked and richly ornamented barges and water craft of all description" to welcome the Occidental potentate, Captain George T. Langhorne, who stormed into Manila Harbor accompanied by the American fleet.[79] Over the following days, revelers participated in parades along with the monarchs and the non-

Christian tribes, attended sideshows and circuses, danced at balls, and engaged in sporting contests. According to G. A. O'Reilly, the director of the carnival, it was evident that "the Oriental . . . does not, as the Occidental, merely PLAY a carnival part, but actually LIVES it."[80] Harry Debnam recalled that on the arrival of the Monarch of the West "the spirit of carnival seemed to take hold and intoxicate with its queer and enticing flavor of mirth and good-fellowship. No one was offensive; no one too boisterous." The festivities culminated in the crowning of the king and queen of the carnival on the last night. Few would have been surprised to find that no persons were better fitted to take up these duties than the Monarch of the West and his captivating consort, Miss Marjorie Colton. The dancing continued till dawn. "Never before in the history of the islands," gushed Debnam, "had anything been so magnificent, so thoroughly cosmopolitan, and so successful."[81] Smith, the retiring governor general, also felt the carnival was a "magnificent success," with 128,000 paid admissions: he was especially impressed that "perfect order prevailed."[82]

In the following years, however, the carnival became ever more commercial, educational, and martial; industrial displays, military parades, and athletic contests came to dominate proceedings. Thus the prospectus for the carnival of 1909 states, "It has definitely been decided by the Carnival Association that, while the Carnival features proper shall be brought out in their most attractive form, the great effort of the Carnival . . . will be along industrial lines." It was above all an opportunity to illustrate how "there has been planted in Manila a government machine in which the most modern ideas have been incorporated."[83] The incoming governor general, W. Cameron Forbes, thought that Filipinos still enjoyed themselves and behaved "in a most orderly and decorous manner, in spite of the fact that fancy masks, disguise, and the throwing about of confetti permitted a license in conduct in which one might have expected a letting down of the barriers of convention to a degree which might have proved disagreeable." All the same, he went on, "next year it is proposed to limit the masking, confetti, jollification and entertainment features of the Carnival to the last three or four days and to devote the first four or five days to an industrial, agricultural and commercial exhibit."[84] In fact, the most significant aspect of the carnival of 1910 was the presence of soldiers. Forbes believed the review of eight thousand troops at the conclusion of festivities "ought to be quite impressive and not to any harm, as it is advisable to let the natives know that the troops are here."[85] Indeed, the military procession turned out, he wrote to the secretary of war, to be "a beautiful affair, beautifully carried out, and I think most opportune."[86]

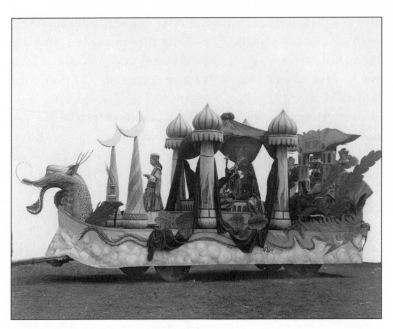

FIGURE 28. King of the Orient, Manila Carnival, 1908 (RG 350-P-Ua-6, NARA).

Despite the wishful thinking of its promoters, initially it proved difficult to interest Filipinos in the annual carnival. In 1908, only the American press gave the event much coverage. The Spanish and Tagalog newspapers took a few years to recognize its news value. At first, the carnival publicist was unsure whether this inattention derived from "lack of appreciation of the importance of the carnival to Manila, or . . . lack of sympathy or hostility to the carnival project."[87] In later years, hostility was clearly evident. In 1911, for example, an editorial in *La Vanguardia* condemned the imminent carnival, which, "rather than the celebration of the memory of the pompous festivals of paganism adopted frantically by all people, appears to be and is an outpouring of positivism and speculation" dominated by a search for profit. "It is truly marvelous simplicity to see in the carnival of the Americans one atom of [Filipino] energy and activity." The radical paper urged its readers instead "to hold a great purely Filipino carnival festival."[88] A few days later, however, the more moderate *La Democracia* argued that an alternative carnival was far too provocative and would fail without majority support.[89] The Municipal Board refused to let any alternative carnival take place in 1911. In the following year, hostility focused instead on the repeated exhibition of "savage tribes" at the carnival, a reminder of Dean C. Worcester's shaming display of Igorots at the St. Louis Exposition of 1904.[90] *El Ideal* complained that "the public will be obliged this year like previous years to witness the not very edifying spectacle of a legion of savage men, torn from their forests and haunts to be the object of derision and ridicule of 'civilized people.'" The pavilion of the Mountain Province would again become "The Temple of Nakedness."[91] The editor of *La Vanguardia* was even more incensed:

> Without them [the mountain people], the wise ones and the pontiffs of coloni-
> zation do not feel themselves satisfied with their profound anthropological
> investigation. Without them, in brief, the general level of our life would be
> uniform, monotonous, and entirely equal to the lives of cultured people, and
> this is not good, nor does it serve the theory of the ineptitude of the [lowland
> Filipino] people, nor does it consecrate the principle of the superiority of races,
> nor can it in any manner excite the curiosity and fondness for novelties of the
> tourists.[92]

Forbes soon relented and insisted on clothing the visiting Igorots, but the newspapers continued to express their disgust with the efforts of the administration to lump Christian Filipinos with mountain heathens.[93] In later years, hostility to this Wild East show became more muted, though there remained many Filipinos who found it demeaning or just plain boring.

By February 1918, the reformed "big fiesta" was a lavish occasion, a Red Cross Carnival resembling a small city. Designed to "combine pleasure with the noble spirit of business and democratic understanding between all who live and trade in the Orient," the carnival now consisted of a patriotically decorated piazza, commercial establishments, including a few "curious Chinese concessions," a motor industry display housed in "buildings constructed in Roman style," a merry-go-round, some instructive government exhibitions, and an auditorium "where the Queen of the Great Festival is crowned."[94] The "atmosphere of patriotic solemnity" was supposed to "convince people that the Red Cross Carnival was not merely an occasion for mirth and frivolity." One imagines that after watching the parade of Red Cross women who reflected on their faces "the beautiful rays of Christian charity and unbounded patriotism," the "martial columns" of school cadets, and "the allegorical floats of the different establishments, institutions of learning and bureaus of Insular Government" the attentive crowd found its sense of frivolity was indeed suitably muted. But just in case, the eager revelers had been told to wait until the end, "when they could throw confetti right and left without offense or undue familiarity and when they could feel to have come in tacit under-

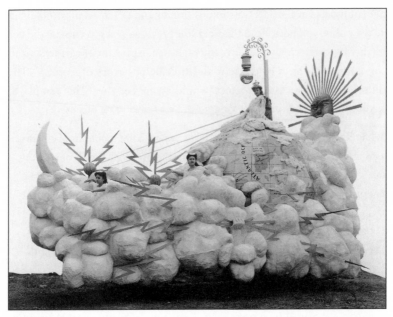

FIGURE 29.   Queen of Electricity, Manila Carnival, 1908 (RG 350-P-ua-2, NARA).

standing to enjoy themselves without encroaching the unwritten code of good manners." Not, one suspects, a carnival Rizal would have appreciated. Indeed, one irreverent reporter observed that the conspicuous presence of recruiting stations "gave the general atmosphere of merriment an aspect of the grim reality of life in army camps."[95]

Of all the exhibitions, perhaps the most elaborate and the most telling was the Philippine Health Service's display of a Sanitary Model House, complete "to the minutest detail" with an exemplary water closet: "Beautifully surrounded by a flower and vegetable garden, [the model] made a lasting impression on thousands of home lovers."[96] Perhaps more reliable is the description of the carnival as "one big gambol" — even if such unadulterated pleasure was illicit — followed by a dutiful admonition to "those of us who have spent the last eight evenings dancing, throwing confetti and visiting side-shows" to take a little time to view the government exhibitions. These were as "instructive" as ever, the breezy report noted, which "leaves very little to be said."[97] More prudish commentators lamented the behavior of dedicated revelers. While many of the subversives who took part in "the hubbub, the jollities, the fooleries, and the emptying-purses" were students, it seems they had little time for the edifying structures of the Red Cross Carnival. Rather, students went straight for the "hurly-burly dancing, pitching handfuls of confetti at some giggling lasses" or they strolled "around the city of mirth throwing a few centavos here and there . . . to the fake freaks of nature exhibited in the side-shows." Evidently this institutional carnival could in reality scarcely contain the carnivalesque, let alone reform it. As a result of such "unbridled plea-sure," the students awoke the next morning "haggard-looking," with "a dull head, unable to concentrate their minds on their lessons."[98] If only—one hears the reproach—they had lingered longer at the Sanitary Model House.

While the Manila carnival occurred in February each year, Clean-Up Week, the other alternative to the traditional fiesta, usually took place the week before Christmas. Promising "the sanitation and the beautification of the Philippine towns," it was chiefly a time for "the cleaning of private and public premises, the gathering and burning of rubbish . . . the construction of drains, the repair of fences, the trimming of hedges, the construction of toilets."[99] In the past, it had been "the custom to have a municipal clean-up before town fiestas"; but what used to be merely preparation for a festival had become the raison d'être of community activity.[100] In this sense, it was promoted as a "nation-wide" revival of a "good custom of our grandfathers, only to be done in a more systematic way."[101] The first such celebration of Hygeia took place in 1914—to a "distinct lack of cooperation and interest on the part of every-body."[102] But eagerness picked up after 1920, when the government began offering one hundred pesos to any "charitable or social institution in a town in each province, which will make the best effort to have the greatest number of houses and lots cleaned and improved."[103] By 1922, Clean-Up Week was well observed. It had been divided into special days, including weed-rubbish day, draining day, privy day, repairing day, scrubbing day, and house furnishings day. On privy day, of course, all were expected to build or repair their toilets. The week opened with decorous parades and band music and closed with speeches and prizes. A policeman, often assisted by a teacher or councilor, went about with standardized forms scoring all dwellings and shops in the district. "Line up, folks," the Filipino townspeople were exhorted. "Roll up your sleeves. Get ready for the great national event."[104]

By the 1930s, the institutional carnival and Clean-Up Week, along with the laboratory, the concrete market, and the flush toilet, had come to repre-sent sites of civilized public and private life in the Philippines, special places of nation building.[105] As Nick Joaquin put it, "How could a silly old fiesta or a superstitious procession be culture at all? In the 1930s culture was the 'streamlined,' the 'up-to-date,' jitterbugs and jive, Mickey Rooney slang,

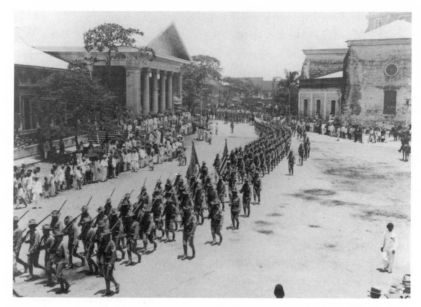

FIGURE 30. Parade of American troops in Manila. Courtesy of the Rockefeller Archive Center.

Flatfoot Floogie with the Floy-Floy, swing music and the rhumba, and every-thing ge-noo-wine made in America."[106] Nevertheless, many Filipinos, like Joaquin, continued to find a useable past in the bowels of Manila's Intra-muros, in the older local and Spanish traditions, while addressing Americans in the special civic terms they understood and rewarded.

THE COLONIAL LABORATORY AS RITUAL FRAME

American physicians in the early twentieth century sought to ensure that the colonial Philippines was inhabited with propriety. The new tropical hygiene, informing an expanded apparatus of surveillance and regulation in the archi-pelago, worked to reproduce in parallel the formalized body and the abstract space of colonial modernity. The enforcement of this imperforate orificial order would lead, ideally, to a seamless reformation of supposedly grotesque, open Filipino bodies and to a reterritorialization of the marketplace and the old fiesta, both of which had figured in the American imaginary as places of promiscuous, threatening contact. As Americans attempted to erase or ab-stract their corporeality, Filipinos had become the chief and most generous sources of contaminating matter. Represented as uncivilized, even bestial, Filipinos often were seen as "promiscuous defecators," transgressing colonial safe havens, imperiling the innocent Americans who were trying valiantly to transcend their lower bodily stratum.

How convincing was this assumption of transcendence? Americans clearly were still fascinated by defilement and the boundaries, both social and spatial, it marked in a manner so excitingly assailable. Much as they denied it, Americans were themselves victims of the abject, for even as Filipinos were isolated and disinfected, the rejected Other could never be radically excluded from the colonialists' own embodiment. This secret rottenness remained a "non-assimilable alien," an abiding structure within even the most apparently abstracted of bodies, always there to disturb and unnerve as much as to constitute American identity. And so it was that the effort to suppress this abject Other, this alter ego, required relentless self-control and sublimated productivity — the development and further expansion, that is, of a conflicted colonial modernity.

American scientists, as we have seen, collected obsessively any specimens of Filipino feces they could lay their gloved hands on. Indeed, for scientists in the Philippines native excrement was as practically creative as it was potentially destructive. If Filipinos could not spread their feces on their fields, and ordinary Americans could not touch the stuff, the "ritual frame" of the laboratory permitted accredited scientists to smear the pulverized, reduced material on their microscope slides and agar plates with abandon. Thus when E. L. Walker and Andrew W. Sellards conducted their investigations into the etiology of dysentery, they did not hesitate to feed their Filipino "clinical material" with organisms cultured from the stools of acute cases and carriers of the disease and to analyze their subjects' feces for the answer to the problem.[107] The decent, delibidinized, closed space of the modern laboratory had conferred on shit the "epistemological clarity" of just one more specimen among many. On the resulting abstractions and inscriptions depended the colonial scientists' reputation and career prospects. "Within the ritual frame," Mary Douglas reminds us, "the abomination is . . . handled as a source of great power."[108] Not surprisingly, it would propel Richard P. Strong from Manila, where he had helped sort out the cause of dysentery, to the first chair of tropical medicine at Harvard.

Chapter Five

THE WHITE MAN'S PSYCHIC BURDEN

For all their polo playing, sweaty tennis matches, consumption of red meat, and celebrated dedication to the strenuous life, senior American colonial administrators in the Philippines could still discern in themselves great vulnerability and tenderness. While it now seemed that with proper hygiene their bodies might resist physical decay and degeneration in tropical climes, their mental apparatus continued to appear distinctly fragile. Preoccupied with fighting germs and disciplining Filipino cleanliness — with disseminating civilization and republican virtue — most Americans nonetheless remained convinced that tropical displacement might destabilize their minds and morale. Few of the outwardly hardened white bureaucrats did not at some point break down or become "unnerved" and thus "unmanned." Nearing the end of his term, Governor-General W. Cameron Forbes, a former Harvard football hero and a commanding number 2 on the polo team, had to retire to his sickbed "worn out." "I had worked my head until I had what they call brain-fag," he scrawled in his journal. His physician, Richard P. Strong, known as "medico stocky" and a dashing number 1 at polo, thought Forbes's condition serious.[1] But Strong had been suffering too. "Dr. Strong ought to have quite a rest from his arduous service of nearly 14 years in the tropics,"

Forbes wrote. "He broke down under the strain last year."[2] Also in 1912, Dr. Percy Ashburn of the Army Board for the Study of Tropical Diseases noted that "it is a matter of common belief that men, as well as women, do 'go to pieces,' and become neurasthenic in the Philippine Islands."[3] Even those tropical physicians who had come to scoff at the notion of a physiological degeneration of the white race still conceded, reluctantly, that some mental and moral deterioration might occur. Their white patients never doubted it. The Americans' overpowering sense of mental stress in alien and disagreeable surroundings was not easily dispelled. As late as 1926, Nicholas Roosevelt warned his readers that "there are certain psychopathic and neurasthenic effects of living in the tropics," the results of "nerves frazzled from heavy, hot moisture." "In Manila," he wrote, "there is a disease called 'philippinitis' or forgetfulness which makes many persons unable to recall common occurrences within a few hours."[4]

As a novel and at first distinctively white American disease syndrome characterized by a depletion of "nerve force," neurasthenia had gained in popularity since the late 1860s.[5] In 1867, George M. Beard, a New York neurologist, offered a plausible materialist explanation for the plethora of vague symptoms, from fatigue to dyspepsia, that afflicted Americans in their efforts to cope with modern civilization (epitomized for him by steam power, the telegraph, the periodical press, the sciences, and the mental activity of women). The mechanistic metaphors initially invoked to explain the condition suggested that the human organism produced only a limited amount of nervous force: if the capacity was low or the demands excessive nervous function could become overloaded, and the system would then break down. The precise quantum of nerve force an individual possessed was a function of a hereditary endowment organized by race and gender. The disease seemed to attack the most refined and productive members of society, the caretakers of civilization: Beard thought Anglo-Saxons and non-Catholics in the prime of life were particularly susceptible. In general, men became neurasthenic from overwork, competition, and economic acquisitiveness; and women succumbed through dissipating their more limited neural vitality in study or excessive socializing.

The nervousness of American men in the tropics (whether "tropical neurasthenia" or "philippinitis" or "brain-fag") was formally recognized soon after 1898; during the next decade it became commonplace among senior colonial officials; and then in the 1920s it mostly burned out.[6] Its history parallels the establishment of the civil government in the Philippines, reaching epidemic proportions when the expatriate colonial bureaucracy was most extensive and declining with the eventual Filipinization of the service. Thus the framing of tropical neurasthenia in the Philippines affords us an especially revealing view onto the contours of American colonial culture.

This chapter builds, in the first part, on the history of nineteenth-century colonial psychiatry, and, in the second part, on the history of colonial psychoanalysis. Tracing the self-reflections of Lieutenant Colonel Fielding H. Garrison, M.D., I draw together these separate histories, as he did, and suggest more broadly how these disciplines may have shaped perceptions of colonial placement. Most accounts of early colonial psychiatry have focused on medical constructions of native insanity or on Europeans interned in colonial asylums, but tropical neurasthenia has not fitted easily with either of these historical interests.[7] Neurasthenia was deemed, at first, a normal consequence of white displacement; and it rarely required admission to an asylum, although repatriation might be recommended. In effect, it potentially rendered all colonialists outpatients, not inmates. But the ambulatory character of this psychopathology, its distance from outright lunacy, later made it the ideal subject for psychoanalysis, which was spreading through the tropics during the 1920s. A reformulated neurasthenia thus figures in historical accounts of colonial psychoanalysis, although even in this literature the primary focus has more often been the psychoanalysis of native elites and cultures.[8]

The medical shaping of nervousness, initially mechanistic in character, later psychodynamic, contributed to the cultivation of whiteness and masculinity in American colonial culture. The new American colonies in the tropics, as we have seen, presented both a special resource for white male self-fashioning and its testing ground.[9] In this novel setting, the convergence of ideas of bourgeois masculinity with ideas of whiteness and civilization becomes startlingly obvious, even as the nervy instability of the combination is revealed with equal clarity. American males, drawn often from the expanding university system (especially from Michigan, California, and Johns Hopkins), argued that they were fit to govern Filipinos because they were racially superior and more manly and, it followed, more civilized than their charges.[10] This is hardly surprising: such connections between masculinity and empire have become a postcolonial commonplace. Ashis Nandy has linked the British obligation to fashion a more rigid masculinity with colonial domination in South Asia; for Ronald Hyam, the British Empire demonstrated a "culture of the emphatically physical"; and Mrinalini Sinha has described "the imperial constitution of colonial masculinity."[11] In a series of essays on the "cultivation of whiteness" in the Dutch East Indies, Ann L. Stoler studied the colonial production of bourgeois civility through discourses of race and gender. She emphasizes the diversity within the category of the colonizer and the attendant "problematic political semantics of 'whiteness' " in colonial society. While not explicitly addressing the framing of colonial masculinities, Stoler observes that "degeneracy characterized those who were seen to veer off bourgeois course in their choice of language, domestic arrangement, and cultural affiliation." Poor whites were the failures of empire.[12] In this chapter, though, I argue that the term *degenerate*, usually indicating a discomposing of white masculinity, attached not just to subordinate and marginal colonialists: even the more civilized and apparently masterful of white men might break down and lose their nerve.

Colonial insecurities cannot be isolated from the uncertainties of those white bourgeois males who remained in the United States during this period. Historians of the Progressive Era have attributed American obsessions with manhood, the frontier, the strenuous life, and the great outdoors to a "masculinity crisis" that developed at the end of the nineteenth century. In the face of increasing dependence on bureaucracies, more opportunities for leisure, working-class competition, and the rise of an assertive women's movement, many middle-class men found it hard to affirm the manly ideals of self-mastery and restraint.[13] Yet it could also be said that manhood was not so much under threat during this period as being remade. Gail Bederman, for instance, suggests that the moral dimension of manhood became muted as anxieties about fin-de-siècle social change amplified a fascination with male aggression, muscularity, athletics, and virility.[14] Although it is tempting to follow Bederman and infer a tension between the ideals of manly self-restraint and masculine virility and to recognize a trend from one to the other, in a sense these tropes of masculinity were fashioned as a physiological amalgam. According to conventional wisdom, a strenuous life built up the nerve force necessary for the maintenance and advancement of civilization. A failure to develop physical force thus led inevitably to neurasthenia, the result not of civilization, but *overcivilization*, the exclusive focus on brain-work at the expense of body-work. Elemental simplicity — "intrepidity, contempt of softness, surrender of private interest, obedience to command," as William James put it — might correct the vices of overrefinement and overcivilization.[15] Not surprisingly, the rising concern with the dangers of overcivilization presented special difficulties in the new U.S. colonies, where white males regarded themselves as emissaries of civilization in an environment inimical to both mental

and physical exertion. Thus colonial breakdown, labeled tropical neurasthenia, came to represent the true, protracted weight of the white man's
burden.[16]

It is tempting, then, to find in the notion of tropical neurasthenia, with its
unsettling of ideals of masculinity and whiteness, the beginnings of an auto-
critique of colonialism. The recognition of white male nervousness in the
tropics would seem to suggest an ambivalence toward colonial expansion and
the civilizing process, a discomfort or anxiety that must be somehow as-
suaged. But the political and social meaning of this colonial ambivalence is
not self-evidently subversive. Mechanistic and, later, psychodynamic explanatory frameworks recognized the contradictions of colonial displacement,
gave them a voice, and in expressing these conflicts often managed also to
contain or deflect them. Psychology (in this period, anyhow) was more a
salvage operation than critique. A diagnosis of tropical neurasthenia began
the process of reconditioning failed colonial identity, not subverting it. Vicente Rafael has described a masterful "white gaze" in the Philippines: "spa-
tially it is a gaze that surveys and catalogs other races while remaining un-
marked and unseen itself; temporally, it is that which sees the receding past of
non-white others from the perspective of its own irresistible future."[17] Although I would argue that this white masculine gaze was often more a nervous glance than a commanding stare, it would be all too easy to overstate the
political significance of this white American admission of fragility and ambivalence.[18] My main concern here is not the distilling of any subversive potential
from colonial breakdown; rather, it is to see how the medical framing of
colonial nerves allows us to sample "empire as a way of life" — with all its
normal heterogeneity and instability built in.[19]

"IT IS NO LIGHT BURDEN FOR THE WHITE MAN"

Even at the Army Medical Library in Washington, D.C., Lieutenant Colonel
Garrison sometimes felt worn out and nervous. From the beginning of the
century, he had spent long hours compiling the *Index Medicus* and in the
evenings wrote historical articles — his *Introduction to the History of Medicine* was for many decades the most authoritative survey available in English.[20] Garrison regarded his correspondence with his friend H. L. Mencken
as a respite from all this wearying bibliographic drudgery. Through classical
allusion, disquisition on music, and reverence for German culture, he tried
to demonstrate in these strangely ornate and coquettish letters that he was
not just another physician with an "unfurnished mind" (July 4, 1925). An

unlikely Bohemian, Garrison shared Mencken's admiration for the German composers and a worship of Friedrich Nietzsche and even at one point dared to recommend Sigmund Freud to his skeptical correspondent (August 21, 1921). His ambitions always thwarted at the library, Garrison came to feel he needed a change of scene. When ordered to the Philippines in 1922, he assured Mencken it would be "a nice vacation after 31 years of official drudgery, and a good chance to see the East and come back via Europe." As he was attached "as literary scribe to the Board to Investigate Tropical Diseases," he expected, through his clerical duties, to learn something about tropical medicine too. Garrison was fifty-one years old. "I think the change will give a sort of goat-gland stimulation to the poor worn-out bean or cerebrum," he wrote just before departing (April 13, 1922).[21]

He was sadly mistaken. "I am stacking up fairly well," he noted in his first letter from Fort Santiago, "but perspiring as I do, the Klima is a sort of Shylock that exacts a pound of flesh a day, while the humidity and monotony are so depressing that I am 1/16 what I used to be mentally. I do all the military work satisfactorily — anyone could — but have to take calomel weekly, as being of the perilous disposition described by fortune-tellers: 'no sense of humor, homicidal tendencies and an overly conscientious disposition.' I feel quite homicidal most of the time, but Bilibid prison is a dreary sort of place so I will postpone action until I get back to the States" (May 3, 1922). Although the facetious tone soon vanished, he remained "utterly worn out and neurasthenic" for the rest of his stay in the Philippines. "When I struck this place," he recalled, "I was totally unacclimated to that old bromide, the humidity, and the tedious period of getting the body temperature adjusted to the beastly outside atmosphere, or rather lack of it, [so] my reaction was one prolonged, unintermittent growl at being badly stung" (December 11, 1922). He found it "impossible to do anything worthwhile in this strange devitalizing climate. It inhibits thinking of an orderly kind, and, worse still, it superinduces a lethargic forgetfulness" (March 24, 1924).

But the climate was not the only provocation. Filipinos got on his nerves, and Americans were not much better. "The average American hombre," he declared, "is either a lean reflective pig or an unreasoning fanatic" who "wouldn't know Schiller from a wombat" (April 28, 1924). The climate and the banal social life together seemed to "corrode" his nervous system. "Were it not for the liquid refreshment available hereabouts, which, as in the case of Themistocles, 'makes us forget,' life would be diabolically unendurable" (December 11, 1922).[22] Toward the end of his stay in the Philippines, Garrison

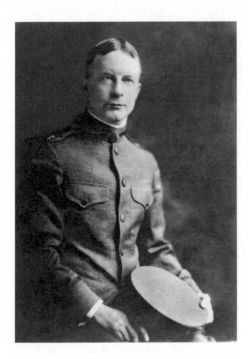

FIGURE 31. Fielding H. Garrison, 1917. Courtesy of the National Library of Medicine.

mused yet again on his "sufferings" in the tropics: "I have lived from day to day in this environment in a state of lowered vitality, like the man in Edgar Poe's poem who felt his life ebbing and oozing away as he poured out sand on the seashore, but even so, that is due to my age and metabolism, and when the foaming beakers of spiritus cerevisae are brought up in the siesta hour, I can say, with my old Bremen acquaintance, 'Ich habe gutes Bier zu trinken.' Better come over and try it" (May 12, 1924). Mencken wisely declined the offer.

Garrison was one of the last American males to admit to neurasthenia in the tropics: though the formulation of his symptoms is conventional, his clinical course was not. Usually it had taken a few years to become neurasthenic. David P. Barrows, the superintendent of education in the Philippines and a keen anthropometrist, remained vigorous from 1903 until 1906. Then, aged thirty-three, he found he was more irritable, with poor concentration: "if a good vacation in a cool climate restores my endurance," he noted in his journal, "I shall be content." But the next year was no better. "In my office work my dictating is now halting, confused and badly put together—a great change from say 1903–4–5," he wrote. "This is in part due to the nervousness which assails me at my work and sometimes makes clear thinking and expression almost impossible for me." Despite hiking, riding, and reading Rudyard

Kipling, the future president of the University of California was "consistently not in very good health" throughout 1908 and so returned to Berkeley the following year.[23] Nerves in the tropics could mean anything from Barrows's lack of concentration to Herbert I. Priestley's disabling morbid apprehensions. As a teacher in Nueva Caceres [Naga City], Priestley began having "morbid spells" in October 1902, but he quieted down with bicycle riding and bromides. "The doctor says the climate is quite wearing on me, and I guess it is," he noted. "I am worn thin, and my nerves are a little out of gear from the climate but I believe that if I hadn't been so foolish as to wear nainsook and cotton I wouldn't have felt my nerves so much." And soon after the new year, he observed that "of course I am nervous and upset tonight, and my notion is pessimistic, but I don't recover from my nervousness as fast as I should like." Priestley, who thought his "sensitive temperament" set him apart from many of the "hard, sporty" Manila types, left the next year.[24]

Colonel Valery Havard, M.D., in reviewing the effects of the Philippine climate on Americans soon after their occupation of the archipelago, had been especially concerned that the atmospheric humidity prevented free evaporation of perspiration, forcing the white organism to reduce its production of heat in order to maintain a physiological equilibrium. The result of "this necessary tropical regime" was a loss not only of heat, but of nervous energy too. "The loss of energy," he observed, "is chiefly felt by the mental faculties: there is a diminution of capacity for intellectual labor, an inability to do work requiring continued concentration." Although the northerner might carefully avoid the recently identified tropical pathogens, he must "resign himself to the loss of more or less of his bodily and mental activity."[25] Thus for an older generation of physicians, who still assumed some responsibility to observe and aid the body's regulation of intake and excretion, the inability to dissipate heat from the closed bodily economy implied a compensatory scaling down of energy production.

Younger medical colleagues, trained in a more reductionist method, had a more tenuous attachment to the notion that disease might derive from such mechanistic mismatches of racial constitution and alien environment. Their ontological orientation drove them to seek out a particulate cause for every disorder.[26] Major Charles E. Woodruff, M.D., as we have seen, warned "blond races" of the specific dangers of concentrated light. The complex and fragile mental apparatus of blonds and brunets seemed especially susceptible to the noxious actinic rays that pervaded the tropics.[27] In its later, more sophisticated form, Woodruff's argument would echo the militant degenerationism of

Bénédict Augustin Morel and Cesare Lombroso.[28] "The instrument for extinction of men in unnatural climates," he declared in 1909, "is degeneration in its modern sense, and it is brought about in the tropics by nervous exhaustion." The white man might now be able to avoid tropical infection, but he would always be prone to nerve weakness, flippantly called philippinitis. The causes of this debility were "overwork, vicious conduct, and the thousands of things which lower vitality." As a result, "low tropical savages are the fittest for their environment, and the strenuous white man is the unfit."[29]

When Woodruff sought to explain with reductionist solar and racial theories the epidemic of neurasthenia he witnessed among white males in the Philippines, he was also trying to fashion a coherent, appealing hypothesis for his (and many others') experiences of despair, illness, and incompetence in the tropics. Woodruff, who, as noted, was an irascible man frequently admonished by his superior officers, had himself been repatriated from the Philippines in 1904 suffering from chronic amebic dysentery and neurasthenia. Ordered back to the Philippines in 1909, he again developed there a "mucus colitis" and neurasthenia ("cerebrospinal type"), and consequently he demanded a posting to a more temperate climate. But in 1910 Percy Ashburn examined him back in San Francisco and found him in good physical condition. The medical board commented, rather snidely, that "in view of Lt.-Col. Woodruff's well known opinions as to the injurious effects of tropical climates upon white men and his marked disinclination to expose himself to such influences, it is appreciated that a return to Manila might result in a considerable degree of mental perturbation and distress." They sent him back anyhow, for a "trial," and he was repatriated again in 1912 and retired for disability in 1913. He died two years later, in his fifties, no doubt convinced that in doing so he was proving his hypothesis.[30] Although his theories and his experience had been unusually extreme, Woodruff's forebodings would continue to haunt even the most confident of tropical hygienists. Ashburn himself eventually conceded the dangers of tropical neurasthenia, though he thought it always preventable.

Like many others, Dr. Louis Fales found Woodruff's theory of actinic agency "perhaps a little indefinite" and was not ready to discard entirely Havard's physiological explanation, but he too had no doubt that, whatever the cause, after a few years' residence in the tropics "the white people become a race of neurasthenics." Fales had observed for himself how Americans in the Philippines soon fell into "a state of semi-invalidism." Brain-work in these circumstances seemed an especially effective means of further depleting the tropical resident's climatically diminished reserves of nerve force. American males in the Philippines "cannot easily concentrate their minds on their work," he declared; "they become easily fatigued, and they cannot do the efficient work they were formerly capable of doing." The syndrome was recited as a litany: irritability and peevishness; troubled sleep, bad headaches, and poor appetite; a lack of concentration; an inability to plan for the future; molehills became mountains; urgent matters were deferred indefinitely; and morbid introspection eventually prevailed. The symptoms resembled those of neurasthenia in the United States, except that vasomotor signs, such as "angioneurotic edema," were more common in the tropics, and neurasthenics from the Philippines recovered as soon as they moved to a temperate climate.[31] The future looked especially grim for white children, who were recklessly endangered by long residence in the torrid zone: "Born of neurasthenic parents, they will inherit an organism lacking in nerve force; being forced to live in an enervating climate, their small reserve will be still further drawn upon, and in a generation or two there will result a race with little resemblance to the mother stock, small, puny, weak-minded, in fact a degenerate race which would soon cease to exist if new stock did not continually come from the home land."[32] Thus in Fales's opinion, degeneration challenged any fond hopes for permanent white American control of the tropics.

When Ellsworth Huntington at Yale proposed his "climatic hypothesis of civilization" as the core of the "new science of geography," he drew in part upon the research of Woodruff and Fales. They had used medical science to show that the environment could influence the global distribution of "human energy." In particular, Huntington identified the deterioration of character they had described — "weakness of will" — as a crucial problem for the white man in the tropics. This fecklessness led frequently to a "tropical inertia," typically manifested as "lack of industry, an irascible temper, drunkenness, and sexual indulgence." If any should try to work too hard, they became "nervous and enfeebled."[33] Thus male nervousness in the tropics came to be represented (and, to an extent, exonerated) as an unfortunate but understandable failure of character — letting down the side of manly civilization, but perhaps the side was physiologically a forlorn hope in such a climate. In the early twentieth century this failure meant, in effect, the lack of exercise of the will over habit, a temporary slippage of racial and manly duty.[34] Formerly disciplined, strenuous Anglo-Saxon males routinely became enervated, louche, and irresolute in the tropics. And yet reproach was always mixed with sympathy as the process was represented as basically a natural one, though on occasion complicated by personal recklessness.

Both Fales and Woodruff had also speculated on the delicate constitutions of white women, which evidently rendered them especially vulnerable to the alien tropical environment. Most American women in the Philippines, according to Fales, "become nervous, irritable, anemic, lose weight, suffer with neuralgia, spells of faintness, sleep poorly, and almost invariably are troubled with menorrhagia and dysmenorrhea."[35] After a year in the archipelago, Francis B. Harrison, the new governor-general, reported, "My wife has stood the climate as well as any American woman can, but that is not saying much; I consider this climate an unqualified detriment to American women and I believe that a year is about all that any of them should stay here without taking a more or less long vacation leave."[36] As men succumbed to the climate and the onerous demands of administrative duties, women like Mrs. Harrison were victims of the climate and their excessive sociability and depletive reproductive tract. In theory, then, degenerating women should have abounded throughout the American tropics. Dr. W. W. King in Puerto Rico thought, for example, the tropical humidity inevitably caused a special "atony" of white female bodies. It was because American women in the tropics "menstruate more abundantly" than in the United States; they felt the lack of "accustomed society, pleasures and diversions" more keenly than the men; and "housekeeping where customs and language are strange and where servants are inefficient and uncleanly has its thousand and one little difficulties and worries that need to be seen to be appreciated."[37]

Yet accounts of tropical neurasthenia among women are surprisingly rare. Described in medical texts — and sometimes by their husbands — as pallid, weak, and nervy, without exception they appear in their own personal recollections as robust and competent.[38] Perhaps white women were reluctant to admit to a nervousness that was formulated (for them) so explicitly as an index of biological and intellectual inferiority. White American men in the tropics evidently could attest to the mental strain formalized in their diagnosis of male neurasthenia and so ratify an etiology that suggested their superior status. American women were understandably less ready to assent to a condition that marked principally a disorder not of an overtaxed mental apparatus but of a leaky reproductive tract. Female neurasthenia in the tropics signified a basic biological maladaptation that could not possibly be circumvented. A white man could rest from brain-work or mitigate it through exercise, but a white woman could not avoid her uterus. In medical treatises on neurasthenia, she thus became a physiological pariah in the tropics: biologically, this region was no place for a white woman or for the style of domesticity that her presence signified.[39]

A neurasthenic disposition was less commonly attributed to the military in the islands, perhaps because regular exercise and other virile activities compensated for what little brain-work they had to do.[40] Only a few officers, the self-consciously intellectual ones, were prepared to assert their nervousness. Lieutenant Colonel Eli Huggins, a convinced anti-imperialist and a poet, was appointed military governor of Ilocos Sur in 1901 after a distinguished Indian-fighting career (during which he had compelled the surrender of Rain-in-the-Face). "I am not in harmony with my environment over here," he lamented. "In fact there is a horrible jangling discord." Fortunately, the translator of Théophile Gautier and Alfred de Musset was sent home within the year.[41] More commonly, young (and less civilized) soldiers developed mild psychoses, nostalgia, or *delerium tremens*. Thus a private in the 19th infantry was repatriated in 1901 with "paranoia," believing his officers had been persecuting him. He was excitable, with "an abnormal development of Ego" and a "fixed delusion of his own ability," telling everyone about his ideas for a machine of perpetual motion and an "absurd" plan for "rifles which should fire some chemical preparation the gases from which would overpower the enemy."[42] A private in the 5th infantry was "excellent" until he went to the Philippines, where he "indulged excessively in alcoholics" and began to "labor under delusions of persecution" and develop an "acute melancholia."[43] It seems that when an enlisted man was exposed to the tropical sun he was more likely to show melancholia or paranoia than neurasthenia — a flattened affect or a psychosis, but not an overcivilized nervousness.

Filipinos, typically, went mad or ran amok. Conventionally, the "Malay race" was prone to disorders of emotional repression followed by excess and abandon, in contrast to the elite white colonialist's exhaustion of emotional expression and lack of "nerve vigor." In 1901, John D. Gimlette described the male native's tendency to succumb to homicidal mania after a period of depression and brooding. This disorder was triggered by a realization that his life had been beset by misfortune and insult. It culminated in the hypersensitive sufferer running amok, killing anyone he met, until he was slain.[44] Most commentators on amok regarded the condition as revealing a combination of infantile misjudgment, deficient self-control, and primitive reflex. It demonstrated the Filipino's vanity and immaturity, his racial jealousy and pathological sense of honor. Waves of passion eroded the rudiments of rationality, leading to an impulsive, random killing spree. Some Muslims in the southern Philippines, called *juramentados*, seemed especially susceptible to losing their wits and running amok.[45] This tendency to go on a rampage suggested to many white observers that most Filipinos, especially Moros, lacked the sustained self-control and capacity for reason necessary to become fully civilized.

Speaking in 1909 on "the nation and the tropics," William Osler impressed upon his audience that "it is no light burden for the white man to administer this vast trust." Despite the great advances in tropical sanitation and the consequent reduction in transmission of the region's disease organisms, Osler, that model physician, doubted that the higher-order transplanted Anglo-Saxon, laboring to impose order on the "blossom-fed Lotophagi," could maintain his characteristic "hardy vigor."[46] The white man might live among the banana palms — he might trade and, for a time, even fight boldly — but it was likely that the manly character of the white race would degenerate, and civilization would not thrive in the tropics.

HIJINKS AT BAGUIO

Foreigners in India, in Java, in Ceylon during the nineteenth century had felt their strength and their sense of physiological balance restored in settlements where the "conditions approximate in atmosphere and climate those of the temperate zone." Americans in the Philippines therefore counted themselves fortunate in gaining access to Baguio, a town at an elevation of approximately five thousand feet in the mountains of Luzon, "a rolling country filled with groves of pine trees and grass, in which the temperature rarely goes below 40 degrees and never goes above 80 degrees in the shade."[47] Finding the prospect enticing, the government in the early years of the twentieth century had extended the railway north of Dagupan and from the end of the line constructed a road to Bagiuo, at a cost of over two million dollars. To take advantage of the "health-giving influence of the climate," it established a sanitarium, a number of hospitals, and Camp John Hay, a brigade post "for the recuperation of our soldiers." Americans in the islands found these institutions furnished "for a very moderate cost a healthful regimen and diet."[48] Cameron Forbes regarded Baguio as "a place to which people exhausted or debilitated by their sojourn in the heat below may come and renew their strength and vigor and increase the number of their red corpuscles."[49] He helped set up a country club, which boasted a golf course and a polo field. Fred Atkinson, the secretary of public instruction, praised this "summer resort for the recuperation of those government officials who from the effects of the climate become run down." He had noticed that the "cooler, cloudier atmosphere makes outdoor life and exercise possible and furnishes just that stimulating force which is never found in the capital."[50] John F. Minier, a

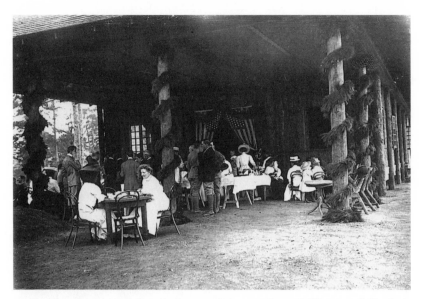

FIGURE 32. Dining at the Baguio Country Club, 1908 (Dean C. Worcester Collection). Courtesy of the University of Michigan Museum of Anthropology.

supervisor of schools, found that "the cool climate caused me to gain several pounds which I lost as soon as coming back to the lowlands."[51] Some were more eloquent. According to Frank G. Carpenter, in the mountains "every breath is filled with champagne, and so invigorating that new blood seems to flow through my veins."[52] On arriving in Baguio, Dean Worcester, the secretary of the interior, observed that "this climate always does wonders for me when I have been or am ill, and I do not see why it should not keep me well if I could have more of it."[53] So sure was he that the "delightful coolness and bracing air afford heavenly relief to jangling nerves and exhausted bodies, worn out by overwork and by a too prolonged sojourn in tropical lowlands" that he later retired permanently to the hills. "No development which has occurred in the Philippines during the past thirty years," he concluded, "rests upon a sounder foundation than Baguio."[54]

The indications for treating sick white Americans in the hills, initially so broad, soon became more limited. Not all cases benefited from elevation. Between October 1905 and January 1908, seventy cases of refractory dysentery came to Camp John Hay.[55] Forty-four of these returned "apparently cured"—with those whose disease had progressed least responding more promptly to "the stimulus of the climate." "On the other hand," H. R. Hoff reported, "in cases of long standing where often pathologic changes have

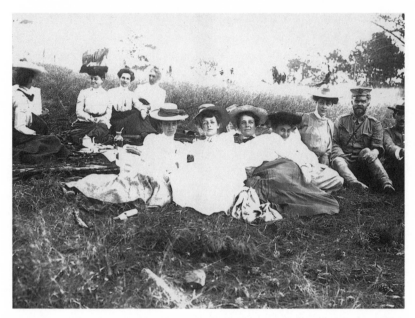

FIGURE 33. Baguio picnic party, 1904 (Dean C. Worcester Collection). Courtesy of the University of Michigan Museum of Anthropology.

occurred in the intestines improvement has been slow, as indeed would be the case in any climate."[56] A visit to Baguio seemed rather more permanently favorable for malarial cases: of thirty-seven cases treated, thirty-six returned to duty with no relapses. Anemia secondary to other diseases also appeared to benefit from treatment in the equable environment of Camp John Hay. But the most dramatic improvement often took place in cases of neurasthenia, with twelve out of seventeen patients returning to duty during this period, even though most of these later suffered a relapse. Hoff concluded that "neurasthenia developed under climatic conditions incident to the Philippine Islands is very apt to recur when the person affected returns to the place in which the disease first originated."[57] Most of these patients would recover completely only when permanently repatriated.

While a sense of the deleterious effects of a tropical climate was never entirely erased, over the next decade or so other factors such as the irritation of colonial social life would come to appear as more important contributors to bad nerves. Not surprisingly, public health officials increasingly emphasized those aspects of the problem that were most preventable or treatable. It would, of course, be infinitely more easy to reform negligent conduct or to circumvent the multiple vexations arising from racial proximities than to alter the climate. When Victor G. Heiser broke down in 1908 after suppressing a cholera epidemic in the islands, he identified the immediate cause of his illness as "the continuous efforts over the past five years of overcoming the passive resistance of the Oriental to health measures." The mental effort of dealing with the natives, he complained, had left him "mentally fagged out and physically weak."[58] Heiser later concluded (without recalling his own susceptibility) that philippinitis — the "mental and physical torpor, forgetfulness, irritability, lack of ambition, aversion to any form of exercise" of which so many of his compatriots complained and which they blamed on climate — was in fact the result of the "direct violation of hygienic laws, especially those governing the production and dissipation of body heat."[59] The answer to his own nervousness had been a better diet, more tennis, and opposition to the irritating Filipinization of the health service: he did not choose to leave the tropics for another seven years.

By the 1920s, the years of Garrison's neurasthenia, medical officers in the tropics had become convinced that relentless supervision and regulation of personal and domestic hygiene, with emphasis on manly restraint and strenuous exertion, promised to prevent or limit any local pathology, mental or physical. Colonialists thus tried, more optimistically than ever before, to build up hermetic microenvironments, enclosures that allowed free play for the masculine virtues. It seemed likely that such an iatrocratic colonialism might circumvent tropical neurasthenia, making it little more than an object lesson, a token of pessimism. In effect, the diagnosis had become a means of containing or disciplining breakdown, a means of recovering a faltering civilized identity in the tropics. By attending to the rules of personal, domestic, and public hygiene and carefully regulating social life, complete acclimatization of the American male was possible; and if acclimatization was possible, so too was a manly white civilization.

It is therefore hardly surprising that within a few decades few extolled the *curative* properties of Baguio's climate, even for nervous conditions. Many did, however, continue to believe that manly activities in the bracing air were effective *prophylaxis* against tropical neurasthenia — but it was the activity and not the air that seemed to do the trick.[60] While patients with chronic dysentery, malaria, and anemia still filled the wards of Camp John Hay, their conditions seemed to respond better to specific therapeutics than to any meteorological adjustments to constitutional tone. Baguio had become principally a place where senior colonial administrators might renew their strength and vigor through a combination of rest and exercise and so harmonize their

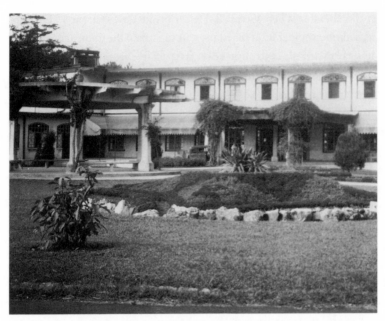

FIGURE 34. Officers' Club, Camp John Hay, Baguio (RG 350-P-Qa-1-5, NARA).

jangling nerves. Much as it may have provided some relief from a disagreeable climate, Baguio came to represent above all a deliverance from colonial responsibility. The perceived advantages of Baguio derived as much from its distance from the bureaucratic routines of Filipinized Manila as from any avoidance of humidity or actinic rays. When managerial force began to fail, the discipline of strenuous activity in the open air seemed to offer hope of recuperation. Playing polo and tennis, hunting and fishing still gave many Americans a visceral sense of their regenerating an overstrained, depleted nervous economy. The annual regimen of diet, rest, exercise, and cleanliness, often supplemented by nerve tonics such as strychnine and bromides, seemed immensely restorative and toughening. Forbes, Atkinson, Worcester, and others all felt themselves becoming more decisive and resolute after a month of the moderately strenuous life in the hills. Charles Burke Elliot noticed an improvement in his mood a few days after reaching Baguio: "As my head ceases to ache my ambition returns and I am already planning many things which are to be done on my return."[61]

How then to justify the expense of a hill station after the *tropical* in tropical neurasthenia has largely become vestigial? As climate gradually loses medical significance, even for nervousness, so too does the rationale for manly society in the hills become susceptible to challenge and ridicule. In 1911, the editor of *El Ideal* decried the excesses of "Baguio the sublime." "Baguio is sublime because of its geographical isolation," he wrote, "it is sublime because in it dwell the intangible ones, because the plebeians do not get there, because the voice of the people which is raised to those heights is lost in space." It was not therapeutic; it was not even toughening: "The high dignitaries of [the] regime" found there "a wide field for spiritual meditations and the full satisfaction of their bodies. Power is fond of softness."[62] Recourse to Baguio had become a sign of individual weakness, and although represented by Americans as a recuperative site and disciplinary locus, the hill station came instead to resemble a haven of dissolution. The strenuous life had turned into white mischief. The governor-general and other members of his Buccaneers Club engaged happily in song, fancy dress, and gay repartee. While Americans "brag of Puritanism," their actions belied any ideals of character and manliness. When Forbes held a party for some British visitors "it took the form of an *impromptu* carnival, circus and sports in the field, and people prominent in Baguio society entered for all the events on the program. Clowns were provided in the persons of Richard P. Strong, Captain Mitchell, and Messrs P. G. McDonnell, Edward Bowditch and Conrad Hathaway, and a clown polo match was played. . . . Major General J. Franklin Bell joined the governor general and many society people in a race in which eight men sat astride a large pole, to the huge satisfaction of the large crowd."[63] Activities at Baguio had become a caricature of manliness; and if they were therapeutic at all, then it was the sort of remedy that better disclosed weakness than repaired it.

FROM DEPLETING MILIEU TO ROTTEN CORE

Fielding Garrison's breakdown had always suggested more to him than the temporary overstrain, in a depleting climate, of a refined mental apparatus. Its meaning was not fully contained in the notion that one was manfully, if with faltering steps, trying to carry the burden of civilization. Not simply a potentially avoidable physiological failing of the white race in an alien land, neurasthenia became for him a sign of willful individual disaffection with modern life, evidence of deep-seated mental conflict, of the family drama. Secretly, he came to suspect that his nervousness indicated not an overpermeable outer membrane, but a rotten core—his own internal tropics. And yet, Garrison's Freudian revisions of the meaning of his tropical nervousness illustrate further the complexity and redundancy of any mental derangement. No one frame, mechanistic or psychodynamic, would fit permanently his disorder.

To the skeptical Mencken, Garrison had rendered his nervousness in terms consistent with earlier environmental etiologies of tropical breakdown, even though he, being better informed than most of his military colleagues, must have known how dated such materialist assumptions had become. Humidity and social frustration clearly retained some conventional and phenomenological appeal as causes of devitalization, and perhaps he thought Mencken would appreciate their literary resonance. But Garrison himself was too sophisticated to believe the theories he proffered; or, at least, too taken with a new psychological formalism to regard physiological disturbance as sufficient explanation for fragmentation of identity. In an extraordinary memorandum book he wrote while in the Philippines, he interrogated his own internal psychological processes, his "unconscious." But he kept this self-analysis to himself. Scrawled across the lines in pencil, the memoranda are a potent, disturbed, and disturbing pastiche of quotation, précis, statistics, confession, and philosophical speculation. Each note merges with the next: "thyroid in myxoedema" runs into Mendelism, into "causes of low blood pressure," into Ezra Pound on democracy, into the *Golden Bough*, Baudelaire, "Masochismus in Am. male," somatotypes, syphilis in the Middle Ages, "schizoid types," "schizothymia," homosexuality, Jews as "hereditary profiteers," frigidity in albino women, impotence, marriage, "Wundt and Freud on tabu," Manila, racial types, infantile sexuality, the Oedipus complex, penis size, ideas as "sublimated sex instinct," D. H. Lawrence, Sherwood Anderson, Frank Harris, and Gertrude Stein—an intertextual series delivered in precisely that order. There are few discernable boundaries: quotations end as vehicles for self-revelation without any indication of the point at which Garrison's thoughts began to wander; Latin, Greek, French, German, Spanish, and English often cluster on one page; the line breaks are erratic; banal self-assertion is mixed with complex and innovative historical analysis, all within the space of a few pages. Through this stream of consciousness, Garrison was seeking a new formulary for his disorder.[64]

The first memoranda are mostly medical and literary. And then, after fifteen pages or so: "I wish to be protected from my enemies but from myself, my vices and passions, *no!*" There follow a few more pages of clinical notes, and then:

Look out for the stenographers the
cuties sit in your lap and invite you by their
willing manner to take them out to dinner
& first thing you know along comes a shyster

lawyer with a breach of promise blackmail
prospectus
didnt fall for a skirt but for a mesh-bag
[x] being raped
Villa Palagonin
Chinese musical records
— "the undiscovered secret of perpetual
motion might after all be lust."

This merges into a summary of an article on "Heredity of homosexuals," signaling the beginning of Garrison's sexual reflections, which soon come to dominate the text. Often he will begin with a quotation or a synopsis, but after a few lines "one" will be crossed out and replaced with "I":

offshoot of an outworn and inbred
stock, the son of a mother who was
physically gummy and mentally
asthmatic — aunts ~~one~~ I damned
puffballs, rickety

This is followed by "a clever practical race the Jews," and a little later, "I fear my mother — makes me feel inferior in intelligence — a shriveled old woman nearly mad with an image of human futility." And then:

Callow idealist — American
whipping post of sadistic Puritanism
she cat —

At the end of a summary of E. M. Forster's *A Passage to India*, Garrison writes, "Letter: Dear Dr. Aziz: I wish you had come into the cave. I am an awful old hag and it's my last chance."

In fracturing Garrison's racial, sexual, and professional identity, the memoranda seem at first to frustrate any effort at coherent reconstruction. Where has the manly white physician gone? Who is it that scribbles, "Creative minds opposed to the Army regimen the creative ones go morbid. Scares you when you stop long enough to think. The answer is: don't stop long enough to think; just whistle in the dark . . . The skin of which you think so highly is no good. It smells disagreeably to my nose. I knew in the dark that your skin was white. caliente cubierto nagging woman." And who, then, launches into an account of a prostitute with a fur coat who resembles "a rabbit who has had an extensive career"?

I've needed my body so little in my career.

Where does she act?

In an old-fashioned piece of furniture with 4 posts.

I ate so much rabbit I hopped just like a kangaroo.

I said kanga

I mean roo

This leads inexorably to a discussion of Hippocrates on humors and, later, to a recounting of a biological classification of races, followed by Isadora Duncan and Freud again on "pansexualism." For Garrison,

sex knowledge is the key to the world

Erotic periods are also the most inhibited (erotically)

Inhibited periods are the most erotic

why because there is ambivalence

shameful and erotic feeling in us.

Bibliographic drudgery — brain-work — did not mean an excessive drain on a limited supply of nervous force: Garrison was trying to get it to mean a destabilizing and unsustainable repression of the sex instinct, but experience and fantasy repeatedly exceeded his explanatory capacity. If Garrison could recognize himself at all, it was as one of civilization's discontents, not as a dutiful representative of the white race vulnerable to nervous depletion in a steamy, sunny environment.[65]

THE WHITE MAN'S DIRTY SECRET

Garrison may not have understood himself, or entirely recomposed himself, but at least he thought he knew there was "no individuality as a unity but complex," and repression was never complete. He could privately invoke the new psychoanalytic theories to explain, or work through, his sense of mental fragmentation. The psychodynamic formula he turned to offered a more complex structuring of identity than the conventional diagnostic complex of tropical neurasthenia, yet both descriptions presupposed a mental apparatus of superior refinement, and both offered hope of its eventual reconditioning through individualizing therapeutic interventions. Although altered in form, from materialist to psychodynamic, the recourse to psychological explanation continued to erase the colonial specificity of his disclosures and thus displace the social and political setting of the breakdown. In Garrison's letters to Mencken, a frustrating military relocation had merely exposed an over-civilized white male's physiological settings to a devitalizing climate; in his memoranda, he revealed a complex internal psychopathology, probably dating from infancy, that again attested to his cosmopolitan overcivilized condition. The former was probably more respectable; the latter was increasingly legitimate for an intellectual and thus not particularly reassuring to most colonial officials.

Garrison's tentative Freudian speculations prefigured a more general psychodynamic understanding of tropical nervous breakdown. Before leaving for Manila, his bibliographic duties and literary ambitions had exposed him to Freud's work on the neuroses, at a time when few colonial medical officers would have understood the first principles of psychoanalysis. Some elite practitioners in the United States had become interested in Freud's ideas after his visit to Clark University in 1909.[66] But it was not until World War I that psychodynamic explanations—usually emphasizing notions of the unconscious, repression, and mental conflict—began to supplant the older mechanistic theories of constitutional degeneration. The scale of the problem of "shellshock" had been crucial in unsettling physicalist etiologies and substituting for them a relatively autonomous complex of psychological causation.[67] By the middle of the 1920s, a number of younger colonial psychologists were prepared to draw an analogy, perhaps one of dubious legitimacy, between shellshock and tropical breakdown.

Increasingly, it seemed that most examples of tropical neurasthenia were to be counted among the psychoneuroses, with their underlying causes located in internal mental conflict. In 1924, Commander Joseph C. Thompson, recently stationed at Guam, declared that so-called tropical neurasthenia was "the result of a conflict in the patient's mind. This conflict is regularly between the desires created by the repressed libido and the demands of the cultural environment of the individual."[68] When a person encountered the demands of social life, he could react in two very different ways. The "reality method" was to "attack the problem at hand, bring to bear upon it all the conscious efforts of training and education," and so dispose of it with "virility, efficiency and happiness." The other type of behavior was a "flight from reality," leading to "the entire gamut of human frailty and neurotic symptoms" (322). These unvirile symptoms were "compensations on the part of the organism for a repressed wish," a longing which relates "invariably and inexorably to unsated desires and mismanagement of the procreation instinct of the individual, in that no neurosis ever takes place in a person whose sexual life is normal" (323). To control these boiling internal pressures, Americans in their own land had become dependent on such diversions as "five-o'clock teas, large moving picture productions amid certain chair comforts and organ or orchestral accompaniments, theater going, terminating in cabaret climaxes, and ball-room dancing" (323–24). But in some parts of the tropics they were deprived of these distractions and so "there comes to the surface a curious set of what Adler terms ready-at-hand neurotic symptoms" (324). The "picturesque" terms previously attached to this "deprivation neurosis" should now be abandoned. To attribute "philippinitis" or "guamitis" to "physical material situations . . . would in itself be a flight into phantasy of so extravagant a nature that no medical officer in the Navy could be counted upon to concur in the concept" (322). Instead, patients should now have their internal psychological disorder explained to them, for a "psychoneurosis only thrives in a mind that is ignorant of the underlying unconscious motive for the ailment" (327).

Thompson urged his fellow tropical physicians to avoid the old diagnosis of neurasthenia, as Freud had decided to reserve this term for actual neuroses in which somatic pathogenic agents act at the same time the symptoms are manifested. Neurasthenia, warned Thompson, was now frequently attributed to "overindulgence in the sexual act, and a medical officer should be very careful in appending this diagnosis to a health record, especially in the case of bachelors."[69] But this caution was not always heeded. Thus in response to Major Hugh W. Acton's spirited, if conservative, defense of the humidity hypothesis in 1927, Major V. B. Green-Armytage daringly asserted that there were in fact three main causes of tropical neurasthenia in the British Empire: masturbation, *coitus interruptus*, and sexual starvation. The notion that it was due to "not wearing a solar topee" was "drivel." He was sure that over 70 percent of white males in the colonial service were masturbating regularly; and it was "extremely common in females in hot weather." *Coitus interruptus* was also lamentably widespread. Sexual starvation developed when happily married men were separated from their wives. "Under such conditions," Green-Armytage wrote, "when a married man tried to lead a 'straight life,' he became the subject of an inferiority complex, which resulted in psychic trauma."[70] Lieutenant Colonel Owen Berkeley Hill, one of the founders of the Indian Psychoanalytic Society, later commended Green-Armytage for his appreciation, unsophisticated though it may have been, of the "sexual factor" in the etiology of neurasthenia. "From my own experience, as well as from much study of neurological literature" he wrote, "I have reached an almost unshakeable belief in the correctness of the Freudian theory that real neurasthenia arises solely through a conjunction of an excess of efferent stimulation."

But he wanted to distinguish the new "real neurasthenia" from "all those subjective feelings of physical ill-being" — from the more prevalent psychoneuroses — which "arise secondarily from a repercussion of thwarted *libido* upon secondary erogenetic zones."[71] Thus tropical neurasthenia was a psychoneurosis, not a real neurasthenia, and it had little to do with the tropics per se.

These images of the variously sexualized and repressed white male, while not calculated to reassure worn-out colonial administrators or to impress local nationalists, still worked to erase, or at least to exonerate, the colonial setting of a breakdown. There is nothing distinctively colonial about these individualized psychopathologies: they are everywhere abstracted from social and historical determinations. And even though psychodynamic theories could be taken to indicate a less homogeneous identity, to locate, in effect, the destabilizing tropics within European mentality, it was evident that white male subjectivity, if sadly conflicted, was still of the greatest complexity. White males at least possessed something — civilization — that repressed their primitive sex instincts: that is, unlike most natives (as yet) they had a superego. The medical challenge was not how to remove the supposed repression, but how to manage this internal binary opposition, just as previously the goal had been to cope with the external depletive climate. If some white males proved maladapted to their higher tasks, then they must be retrained.

As nervousness increasingly was associated with sex, a diagnosis of tropical neurasthenia, whatever the theoretical associations with the burdens of civilization, became for its sufferers less a mark of mental distinction than a badge of personal shame. The white man's dirty secret was replacing the white man's burden. *Tropical neurasthenia* was acquiring a rather smutty ring, and no amount of clinical detachment could cleanse it. It is therefore not surprising that many attending physicians and their patients (especially more prudish and prudent Britons) continued to affirm the older, more comforting physical explanations. When the bishop of Singapore wrote to the *British Medical Journal* in 1926 wanting to know the cause of the "upset of mental balance" so common in the tropics, fourteen medical men offered answers, all different and none with a Freudian taint. The physicians cited humidity, strong sunlight, eye defects, worry, hyperemia of the brain, north wind, barometric pressure, electrical content of the atmosphere, food, alcohol, constipation, native servants, and smoking. Moderate exercise remained the best prophylaxis.[72] But Berkeley Hill and other modernist psychiatrists derided such old-fashioned, materialist explanations. Berkeley Hill thought this sophistry indicated just "how almost hopelessly ignorant we are about a state of affairs which no one can deny is of some considerable importance." He personally was convinced that Europeans in the tropics were prone to "a neurotic syndrome, the central symptom of which is a state of hyperexcitation manifested in a general irritability or a condition of morbid anxiety." The prime etiological factor in this anxiety-neurosis was a voluntary abstinence from sexual intercourse. If this could not be remedied (through concubinage, for example), then psychoanalytic treatment was indicated. Freud was right, and persisting with physicalist euphemism did no more than assuage mentally unbalanced patients with unscientific and misleading consolation.[73]

Psychodynamic theories did not produce anything like the earlier, pre-Freudian collective repertoire of assumption about the mind and the body. Indeed, the new psychological speculation rivaled microbiology in its alienating lack of self-evidence. The causes of mental disease had become as arcane and insensible and internal as the minute organisms that were supposed to be causing physical ailments. At the same time, theories of unconscious mental conflict did provide a body of specialized knowledge around which a psychiatric profession could organize itself. As this specialty became increasingly autonomous during the 1920s and 1930s, its reference group was more likely to include international colleagues than colonial officials. Articles on mental disorders in the tropics began to appear in general psychiatry journals, not in colonial medical publications. Experts on nervous diseases in the colonies had realized that their postcolonial future depended more on professional legitimacy than on local administrative service. If they must choose between offending colonial bureaucrats and appearing old-fashioned and ignorant, then they would jettison their soothing function in the interests of intellectual respectability. Since most psychiatrists had no intention of hanging around colonial outposts, during their brief tropical sojourns they did not see any need to show special respect to the modesty of their fellows. Increasing independence had allowed them to locate sexual ambiguity and otherness deep within the personalities of colonial administrators, even as they promised through psychotherapy to discipline the conflict they had discerned between civilization and the savage within.

THE TRUE TERRAIN OF CIVILIZATION

Breaking down in the tropics had once indicated an ephemeral failure of the will: a depletion in the racial allotment of nerve force that was not altogether discreditable in such trying circumstances. If the climate's burden on race and gender proved unendurable, those who succumbed could console themselves with the knowledge that they were, for a short time, the innocent victims of an inexorable biological process. Try as they might to avoid it, decay would still lurk in the humidity and actinic rays of the tropics. Unless they had flagrantly disregarded hygienic stipulations, the temporary victims of tropical neurasthenia could be absolved of blame — if anything, they had fulfilled their civilizing duties too meticulously. But in the 1920s tropical neurasthenia came to signify a pathology of the will itself, an actual deformity of personality: the destabilizing tropics had, in a sense, become internalized everywhere in the minds of white men. No longer was the main problem a physical mismatch between the white male's refined mental apparatus and an alien, depleting climate; the predicament was by then represented as a personal maladaption to civilized social life. Once a discomforting, though temporary, mark of distinction and self-sacrifice for tropical white men, a diagnosis of nervous debility now more likely signified an individual's internal psychological ambivalence and conflict.

Although considerably different in form and consequence, both mechanistic and psychodynamic theories shared during this period an assumption that the true terrain of civilization was the mind of the bourgeois white male. The threat to civilization might come from outside (the tropical climate) or from inside (the unconscious), but the locus of its target did not change. The medical problem was how best to educate or to discipline this civilized mind, how to harden it against internal and external enemies. The widely dispersed followers of Beard and Freud aimed to maintain or to recover, in significantly divergent ways, an exemplary colonial identity at once manly, white, and civilized. But in admitting a sensitivity or fragility of the generic white man (if chiefly to mark his superiority and retrieve it), psychological theories might now seem to prefigure a critique of colonial modernity. Like all family romances, however, such a genealogy should be received with skepticism. If there is a critique of colonialism within colonial psychology in this period it is a muted one, with the specificity of colonial history and politics conveniently erased. The stimulus to breakdown is repeatedly displaced onto the environment or internalized; its signs and symptoms are structured as manifestations of a personal crisis, not as evidence of political or social disorder. White men might become destabilized, but their problems were not allowed, in any serious way, to subvert the civilizing process, even in its colonial setting.

All the same, these medical efforts to codify and contain disturbed identity did still permit some play in many Americans' understanding of their colonial placement. For example, one might conclude with Woodruff that tropical neurasthenia allowed only a political commensalism and doomed to failure any direct colonial presence; or one might argue, like Heiser, that unrelenting self-discipline would circumvent the condition and so permit high-quality American brain-work in the tropics. It was a question of *how* white males, resident or distanced, might civilize the tropics and of whether that region deserved their best efforts — they remained the best possible agents of civilization. When Colonel Joseph R. Darnell saw James Fugate, the governor of Jolo, in 1926, he observed a "thin nervous man of middle age" who "seemed to dissipate energy in a nervous haste to accomplish things, as though fearing that the passage of time would find him less capable of carrying on." Colonial optimism always won out over colonial pessimism during this period, but it was nevertheless an endlessly prevaricating sort of optimism. "There was something pathetic about the thin, wistful white man," Darnell recalled, "almost alone in a brown man's country, standing on the dock and waving us goodbye."[74]

A diagnosis of colonial nervousness was never likely to generate coherent resistance or subversion. Far from providing an independent oppositional discourse, tropical neurasthenia did more to recuperate than to decompose colonial authority. And yet, it must be assumed that the practice of breakdown often exceeded the framing capacity of theory. The full meaning of colonial nervousness might sometimes be deferred by eloquent materialist analogy or psychodynamic speculation, but never indefinitely. Such formulas, whether conventional or novel, provided Garrison with only transient satisfaction: his memoranda are abundant, irreconcilable supplements to his tightly drawn theories of mental derangement. When an American man in the colonial Philippines broke down, he experienced himself as multiply fragmented, gone "to pieces," his carefully nurtured identity as a manly white colonial emissary fractured. What, then, was happening in his moments of fragmentation, before the re-collection of himself as a recovering neurasthenic or neurotic? The answer, if there is one, is probably inimical to history, for any narrative of breakdown will seek to find coherence where there may be none.[75] We lack evidence of embodied memories of colonial culture and cannot now observe directly the signs of the body, although we still might read Garrison's memoranda, in their deranged social and political specificity, their disjunctures and excesses, as constantly exceeding the reach of his recovery.[76] Of course, even this bizarre testimony, given all its disturbance, has emerged already heavily medicalized. But when Garrison notes that the white skin which he and many of his colleagues paraded was no good — "it smells disagreeably to my nose" — neither the mechanistic nor the psychodynamic theories he favored could fully account for such an incident of putrescence.

After the 1920s, reports of tropical neurasthenia among Americans in the Philippines are rare, mostly because few white males remained in the archipelago, but perhaps also because those who stayed on were reluctant to translate their experiences of disorder and nervousness into Freudian terms. If breakdown had to be articulated it was generally managed through casual recursion to the mismatch between mental apparatus and climate.[77] At the same time, an epidemic of neurasthenia was now recognized among another group in the colonial Philippines, one hitherto racially exempt from any diseases of civilization. The diagnosis was made available as an object lesson to "educated natives." When W. E. Musgrave, the director of the Philippine General Hospital, discussed his "clinical notes" on tropical neurasthenia, he emphasized for the first time the special susceptibility of elite Filipinos. "Few natives," he had determined, "are mentally constituted to withstand the normal stress of Western civilization which so many of them adopt." This was strikingly illustrated in the Philippines, where twenty years of inculcating "Occidental methods" of hygiene and conduct had led to widespread neurasthenia among the "younger generation of more progressive Filipinos." The imitation of "Western methods of energy, application and efficiency" came at great cost. The local race had been happier in a state of nature. For the native, Musgrave concluded, prevention of nervous debility "consists in holding his ambitions and energies within his natural bounds and resting before the breaking point is reached."[78] While adapted to manual labor in the topics, Filipinos evidently did not yet exhibit the mental discipline or self-mastery required to manage civilization in such a climate. According to doctors like Musgrave, civilization in the tropics would, for some time yet, remain the white man's special burden.[79]

Chapter Six

DISEASE AND CITIZENSHIP

In May 1906 the Coast Guard cutter *Polilio* passed the massive limestone cliffs of Coron and negotiated a channel through the Calamianes Islands to the new leper colony at Culion, an isolated outpost in the far west of the Philippines archipelago. Almost 400 leper pioneers disembarked there; mostly they were young adults, some were adolescent. By the end of 1910, a further 5,000 had followed the same route, though more than 3,000 died soon after arrival, and another 114 somehow escaped their doleful exile.[1] Inevitably, some leper women gave birth in the colony — sometimes the father was unknown, but more commonly after 1910 the coupling was sanctioned by marriage at the old Culion church. American colonial officials had structured the leper colony as a laboratory of therapeutics and citizenship, a place where needy patients were resocialized, where they performed somatic recovery alongside domestic hygiene and civic pride. Thus Filipino leper families lived in small houses in the new "sanitary barrio," washing and scrubbing, tending their gardens, voting in local elections, making cheap goods for export, participating in baseball games, receiving regular injections of chaulmoogra oil for their disease, and having nonleprous children.

For a while the medical authorities kept these exemplary families intact.

But evidently fears of contamination had not completely evaporated in the tropical theater of hygiene, and from 1915 nonleprous children lived apart from their families at the Balala nursery. After 1927, efforts intensified to remove children at a younger age, though separation at birth remained rare. Every Sunday, leprous parents could view their separated offspring through a glass barrier, until at the age of two the infants were either adopted or sent to the Welfareville Institution in Manila. Estela A., for example, was born in 1925, the daughter of two inmates, and in 1927 a middle-class Filipino family in Manila adopted her. A few months later her adoptive father wrote to the Protestant minister at Culion to reassure him that Estela was healthy and happy and that they were bathing her twice daily.[2] In the interests of medical and civic reformation the state had taken lepers from their families and loved ones, subjecting them to a combined regimen of treatment and educational uplift; now it removed their nonleprous children and sought to give them ready-made hygienic identities in Manila.

The Culion leper colony demonstrated a distinct political rationality: it was predicated on a form of biological and civic transformism in which the contaminated became hygienic, and "savages" might become social citizens. In the ritual frame of the colonial, or protonational, institution, liberal medicos amalgamated corporeal deficiency with perceived cultural failings, in particular a lack of civilization. They then sought to treat these fused conditions, to set their charges on a single trajectory from illness to health and from primitive to civilized.[3] That is, the identity of inmates, or patients, was assigned to one pole of a dichotomy or, more ambiguously, to the ground between, and these figures were expected dutifully to traverse toward the further pole. In a sense, American officials were staging a binary opposition between themselves and the "typical leper" and then asking the leper to resolve this typological difference through a personal conversion, so demonstrating that the affliction, the failing, was not absolutely irredeemable. Of course, the end point of this imagined trajectory was in practice unreachable: the leper was only ever in remission. Despite its professed goals, the colonial reformatory thus produced — not eliminated — the in-between. It excelled in fashioning estranged, marginal men and women, in making contaminated bodies and second-class citizens. It was, in this sense, the place for an asymptotic projection of cure and citizenship. Only bourgeois white males were qualified truly to reach the end point of civilization, and even they, as we have seen, might occupy it nervously in the tropics.

Identified as lepers, banished from their communities, the colonists of

Culion became the improbable subjects of intensive medical reformation and retraining in civic responsibility. Individuated through treatment protocols, lepers were expected to work diligently, tend their gardens, perform in brass bands, play baseball games, vote responsibly, and police themselves. Long-standing intimate relations were to be abandoned and reforged as abstract attachments to categories of progress, modernity, and nation. This was what the emancipation of lepers at Culion really meant. Medical officers urged their inmates or patients to forget traditional affective ties to family and community; they warned against nostalgia and praised those who looked forward to the hygienic future, to incorporation into a whitelike, though allegedly generic, citizenry.[4] Leprosy itself thus was translated into a language of modernity, of civic consciousness, of public interest — a vocabulary that both imperial officials and many Filipino nationalists could share.[5] In the late colonial reformatory, civic performance became more important than blood ties, hygiene more significant than kinship, or so at least the liberal medical vanguard in charge of these institutions would claim. In fact, neither the medical officers nor their charges could ever jettison completely their older — in a sense nonmodern or at least *völkisch* — attachments to community and race.

The new affective ties to state abstractions, or to the agents of the state, were rarely as intense as the progressive colonial intelligentsia had hoped. When Dr. Victor G. Heiser began his leper-collecting trips in the Philippines he claimed there was little resistance to the removal of the afflicted, in part, he thought, because of the successful inculcation of fear of the "loathsome" disease. "When it is remembered," Heiser wrote, that removal "often involved the lifelong separation of wife from husband, sister from brother, child from parents, and friend from friend, it will be appreciated that forbearance was necessary under such circumstances."[6] After having abducted them, Heiser regularly sought out the company of those lepers he meant to reform. On the day he left the archipelago, he confided to his diary his feelings for those he had so assiduously classified and displaced: "There is much sadness," he wrote, "that as yet I do not live in the hearts of the people . . . I wonder if I will ever be understood and if the lepers will sometime look upon me as their friend."[7] His regret is a vivid expression of the pathos of the progressive colonial bureaucrat.

Ann L. Stoler has recommended that we examine the ways in which "intimate matters, and narratives about them, figured in defining the racial coordinates and social discriminations of empire."[8] In this chapter I consider the

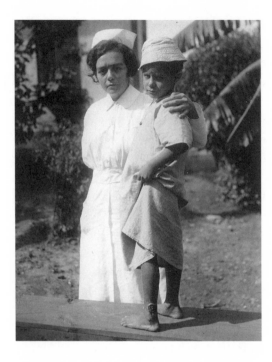

FIGURE 35.
Leper child and nurse at
Culion (RG 350-P-J6.1, NARA).

institutional management of probationary national subjects as an example of
"the distribution of appropriate affect."[9] This requires an expansion of the
historical understanding of the making of intimacy to encompass the expert
and habituated benevolence of the state. It is often forgotten that in the
name of public health the state is licensed to palpate, handle, bruise, test,
and mobilize individuals, especially those deemed dangerous or marginal or
needy. Moreover, in the twentieth century, an emphasis on personal and domestic hygiene allowed an exceptionally intense surveillance and disciplining
of subject populations, and this in turn involved a refashioning of interactions
and intimacies within these populations. Much of the prevailing attention to
the quantity and quality of population—of which eugenics was just a small
part—can thus be viewed as an effort to reshape identities and relationships,
to reforge affective ties. Accordingly, I want to consider leper treatment in
terms of the making of intimacy *with* the colonial state and the making of
intimacy *for* the colonial state.

THE LEPER COLLECTION

Michel Foucault has described how, gradually, "an administrative and political space was articulated upon a therapeutic space; it tended to individualize

bodies, diseases, symptoms, lives and deaths; it constituted a real table of juxtaposed and carefully distinct singularities."[10] He was referring to the development of the modern clinic; lepers remained for him representatives of the unproductively confined: "While leprosy calls for distance, the plague implies an always finer approximation of power to individuals, an ever more constant and insistent observation."[11] Foucault wondered what would happen, though, if one were ever to "treat 'lepers' as 'plague victims,' project the subtle segmentations of discipline onto the confined space of internment, combine it with the methods of analytical distribution proper to power, individualize the excluded, but use procedures of individualization to mark exclusion."[12] At Culion, for the first time, lepers did become subjects of such intensive surveillance and discipline. In the past, lepers might be segregated and excluded from civil society — the colony at Molokai, Hawaii, established in 1866, represented the best contemporary model of unproductive isolation. Once isolated, lepers at colonial institutions of this sort generally were neglected, except by missionaries who quickly discerned they might be especially susceptible to the gospel. According to Megan Vaughan, leprosy in Africa had "offered to missionaries the possibility of engineering new African communities" for the performance of collective, tribal identities.[13] Such collectivization would seem to present an impasse to the engineering of individualized leper-citizens. The progressive medical officers who established the Culion colony tried instead to deregionalize and abstract Filipino lepers as separate national subjects. They fought against any grouping of lepers into Visayans, Tagalogs, Moros, and so on, preferring to figure their patients as individualized, if standardized, cases of leprosy. Rita Smith Kipp has remarked that during this period "new therapeutic approaches to leprosy lessened the evangelical uses" among the Karo people of Sumatra.[14] But in the Philippines, the production of the individual civic subject — surely a form of evangelism — was predicated on such medicalization, on the spread of the "gospel of hygiene" and modern chemotherapeutics.

For most of the Spanish colonial period in the Philippines, medical authorities had assumed that leprosy was hereditary. Accordingly, the rare instances of isolation of sufferers occurred more often for aesthetic and social reasons than for medical purposes. The disease was identified in the archipelago in the early seventeenth century, and since then it had spread rapidly. The Franciscans took charge of charity work among lepers, building several asylums and hospitals for the severely afflicted. Institutions such as the San Lazaro Hospital, north of the old walled city of Manila, and the Cebú Leprosarium offered a refuge for those who sought it, along with palliative care in the last stages of their illness. In some of the larger towns groups of lepers often lived together in separate bamboo and nipa shacks. But the Spanish colonial regime did not try to isolate lepers from their communities in order to prevent the spread of the disease or to eliminate it.[15]

Toward the end of the nineteenth century, as we have seen, most medical scientists and clinicians came to favor social explanations of disease transmission, though hereditarian assumptions were never entirely abandoned. Sickness might now appear to spread from person to person, but the hereditary proclivities of certain groups still seemed to make them more likely to participate in this process. Thus germs to which one group of people appeared especially susceptible might lodge covertly in the meretriciously healthy bodies of another group or race. One race might demonstrate some immunity, relative or absolute, to a disease; another would seem utterly vulnerable to the same microbe.

G. A. Hansen's announcement of the discovery of the bacillus of leprosy, *Mycobacterium leprae*, in 1873 signaled the entry of leprosy into the emerging etiological mainstream. Its presence in the nasal scrapings of suspects — regardless of clinical signs — came to suggest, to the more scientifically inclined of medical and civic authorities at least, the need to isolate the victim, or carrier, and to engage in relentless efforts to remove the contaminating germ from the population. When Dr. N. C. MacNamara described leprosy in the early 1890s he emphasized that the old assumption of the ailment's simple hereditary nature had been discredited over the past few decades. "Pathology," he declared, "has at last led us to recognize the fact that leprosy is the effect of a micro-organism." Most physicians now believed that the disfiguring and disabling granulomatous disease was communicable, though not readily so. Therefore, MacNamara concluded, "strict isolation of lepers must be the proper and only way of stamping it out." Yet his experiences in India had suggested that "the religious feeling, customs and habits of the natives, as well as the number of lepers . . . all prevent the government from attempting to introduce a system of compulsory segregation in that country."[16] When Dr. James D. Gatewood reported to the surgeon general of the U.S. Navy in 1897 on the latest international conference on leprosy, he assured his superior that no one doubted any longer the disease's cause or its contagiousness. All therapeutic experiments so far had failed; the general opinion was that "in isolation is found the only safeguard" against what he called "the hideous sister of syphilis and tuberculosis." Only the English resisted isolation, regarding it as impractical in their colonies.[17] In 1898, Sir Patrick Manson agreed that leprosy was basically a "germ disease," although he suspected that "bad food and bad hygienic circumstances" were predisposing influences. Transmission of the mycobacterium probably required prolonged and "intimate personal contact." In the first edition of his classic text, Manson paraphrased MacNamara's apparently quixotic call for rigorous segregation of sufferers.[18] And in the 1914 edition not much had changed, except that Manson began to cite medical authorities who had "very sagaciously and truly remark[ed] that leprosy is more especially a disease of semi-civilization"; that is, "when the savage begins to wear clothes and live in houses he becomes subject to the disease." Thus the best way to control the condition was either to complete the civilizing process or never to begin it. If the goal was acceleration of the evolutionary trajectory from tribal to peasant to proletarian, then ideally this should be attempted in an isolated colony.[19]

As commissioner of public health in 1902, L. Mervin Maus had led the campaign to find a distant island on which to establish a leper colony. A committee of inquiry, including Dean C. Worcester, studied a number of locations and concluded that Culion "afforded an ideal site for the proposed colony, and furnished abundant and suitable lands for agriculture and stock raising." Water was available, and the harbor was extensive and safe. The population of three hundred or so nonleprous "poor day laborers" could be moved to an adjacent island. The committee believed that "nowhere else in the archipelago can there be found an island so healthful, extensive and fertile, which has so small a population." It urged the government to preserve the island for lepers, with land "to be set apart for every leper willing and able to cultivate the soil" and houses to be built for the accommodation of male and female lepers in "two widely separated areas."[20] At this stage, Worcester insisted that the "leprous women will be kept by themselves and an effort made to keep the men from getting at them."[21] The work of constructing an entire new town suitable for two or three thousand lepers took time. The dormitories, the hospital, the school, the theater, the dining halls, and kitchens were not ready until 1906.

Heiser, on assuming control of public health in the Philippines in 1905, urged all medical officers to take a census of lepers in their region and report their findings to him. He estimated there were more than six thousand lepers distributed over the archipelago, and each year some twelve hundred more contracted the disease. A review of the recent medical literature convinced him that only isolation and experimental treatment could accomplish the

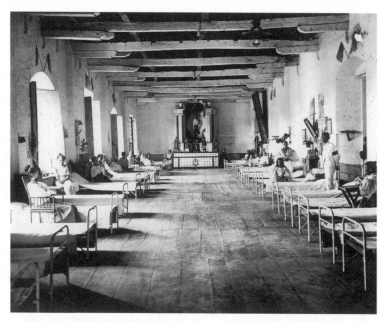

FIGURE 36. Leper ward, San Lazaro (RG 350-P-E38.2, NARA).

eradication of leprosy in the islands. "This policy," he observed, "at first sight seems to impose many hardships upon the lepers themselves and their imme-diate relatives and friends, but it is believed to be fully justified not only by the fact that hundreds may be annually saved from contracting leprosy, but also that the victims may be given as pleasant a life as possible."[22]

The lepers at the San Lazaro Hospital in Manila and at the Cebú Lepro-sarium awaited the completion of Culion with trepidation. In 1903, Dr. H. B. Wilkinson at San Lazaro reported that his patients "rarely or never get well, but are usually fairly content and happy, especially since the rumor of their transfer to Culion has faded away."[23] Over two hundred lepers occupied an ample, clean building — they saw no reason to move to some isolated island. But their departure had merely been delayed a few more years. Among the earliest of the inmates consigned to Culion was a "Spanish-mestizo" boy, Eliodore G., who had entered San Lazaro in 1901, at the age of seven. Two of his brothers and two sisters had died of leprosy. Eliodore had noticed a red spot of his left hip, and later other spots appeared on his cheeks and ears. The lab-oratory determined that he was "positive microscopically" for leprosy. Like many others in San Lazaro he had no one willing to care for him in his *barrio*. Treated experimentally with radiation and medications, the reluctant colonist remained positive microscopically after his transfer to Culion and died there within ten years — as one of Heiser's "prisoners of hope."[24] The formulation of the boy's record is conventional: Eliodore G. has been abstracted from his surroundings as a leper, and his life is further translated into a medical vocabulary. He has been silenced in the medical narrative, his existence reduced to a diagnosis. And yet, the same case record has made him visible; it has mobilized him as an individual in need of bodily and social reform.

Once all institutionalized lepers such as Eliodore G. were transferred to Culion, Heiser began to collect those still living in their local communities. A year or so before the visit of the "leper ship," the government began an education campaign in each region to inform lowland Filipinos of the "manner in which leprosy spreads and the improved conditions under which lepers themselves would live at Culion." Doctors from the Bureau of Health gave lectures on leprosy and showed photographs and films of the colony. Teachers discussed the government's leprosy work with their students and encouraged them to identify hidden cases.[25] Heiser was convinced Filipinos must be taught that "the leper who concealed his disease was a constant and deadly menace to the community in which he lived."[26] In his journal, he noted that "the keynote to success [is] to educate the masses to a fear of the disease."[27] It is hard to know whether he succeeded. When Charles Everett MacDonald, an unusually curious medical officer, asked people on Samar how leprosy was acquired, they attributed it to dependence on a diet of fish. No one believed it was infectious. The inhabitants also observed that it made the afflicted immune to cholera, tuberculosis, and some "strange fevers." The lepers MacDonald encountered there, though "much deformed," seemed "happy and content."[28] On the other hand, Corporal Richard Johnson of the 48th Volunteers reported that Culion was "a dismal word to the people of the Philippines," and lepers dreaded their exile "more than they dreaded the disease itself." "Sometimes the unfortunates were hunted down like criminals," Johnson wrote, "and it was a sad experience to relatives and friends to see them taken away to a living death among unsympathetic strangers." An easygoing "drifter," Johnson had docked with supplies at the colony on Christmas Eve, 1907. That year he would spend a "gloomy Christmas day at Culion."[29]

Beginning with the outlying islands, Heiser and his colleagues proceeded to examine and classify suspect lepers. At an arranged date, the provincial governors and municipal presidents would gather all known lepers to meet the ship at the harbor. The district health officer usually had made a preliminary diagnosis. The leper boat always brought at least three physicians, one of

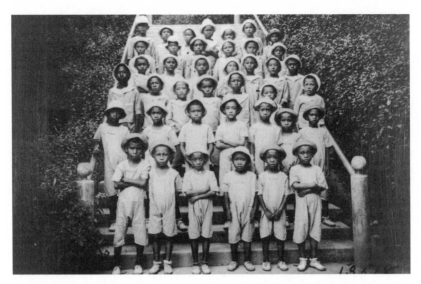

FIGURE 37. Leper boys at Culion, 1920s. Courtesy of the Rockefeller Archive Center.

whom was especially qualified in the diagnosis of leprosy, and all of them had to be satisfied that the label was correct before a leper was taken to Culion. In addition, a microscopist from the Bureau of Science examined the nasal scrapings of each leper, seeking to identify *Mycobacterium leprae*. After these precautions had been taken against error, the boat loaded the confirmed cases and sailed toward Culion.[30] By 1913 Heiser could claim that every recognizable leper in the archipelago was confined; over eight thousand had been sent to Culion, and thirty-five hundred were still alive. As the incubation period for the disease might last as long as twenty years, new cases would continue to develop. Nonetheless, the Philippines "enjoy[ed] the distinction of being the only oriental country where complete segregation is being attempted."[31]

"They say of Doctor Heiser," Eleanor Franklin Egan wrote in the *Saturday Evening Post* in 1918, "that he has handled with bare hands from two to three thousand lepers in all the horrible stages of that most horrible of all diseases; and I myself have seen him pick up a helpless leper in his arms and carry him aboard the leper ship to be taken to Culion with as little apparent concern for his own safety as he would display under the most ordinary circumstances."[32] Fashioning himself as a secular and uninfected Damien, Heiser regarded the scientific treatment of leprosy at Culion as his major legacy to the islands. "As long as [the leper colony] remained in his care," wrote a fawning Katherine Mayo, "it challenged the world's admiration."[33] Heiser spent a large part of each year between 1905 and 1914 sailing from port to port, collecting leper suspects, examining them, and exiling the confirmed cases at Culion. As he put it, "Some people collect postage stamps or cloisonne. I started collecting lepers."[34]

THE PERSONAL HYGIENE OF THE MICROCOLONY

In the Culion "museum" today one finds thousands of case histories, now dusty and insect ridden, piled on benches and on the floors. Each is prefaced with a photograph, followed by an account of the initial presentation, the family and social history, and progress, which was correlated with treatment, usually with chaulmoogra oil, and laboratory findings. The case record of José E. tells us he was admitted to Culion in 1913, at the age of twenty-three, having suffered from leprosy for eight years in Ilocos Sur. His signs were the white patches on his back and arms, thickening and contractures of the fingers, and an ulcer on his left foot. After receiving chaulmoogra oil for a decade he became "bacteriologically negative" and was paroled two years later. Or take the case of Marcelo A., who in 1909, at the age of fifteen, was taken from Batangas. He had nodules on his back, shallow scars on his legs, a fallen nasal bridge, and no eyebrows. For awhile he was bacteriologically negative but in his early twenties showed more "activity." After treatment with chaulmoogra oil and two years of negative findings he was paroled in 1926 — but he had nowhere to go and was soon readmitted. Then there is the case of Alfredo F., who was born at Culion after his parents were sent there and soon acquired the disease, developing reddish patches on his cheeks and lower abdomen. In 1926, after years of chaulmoogra oil injections, Alfredo, now an adolescent, was ready for discharge — but he too had nowhere to go. Each person has become a distinct case; each has acquired a standardized individuality in the medical record. And in each of these cases, the future has been structured as a prognosis. The Culion leper colony had thus become a total institution.[35]

In the hermetic world of Culion, in that infinitely detailed colonial miniature, lepers would repeatedly reaffirm their diagnosis and demonstrate their rectitude, in the hope of gaining the recognition that might confer both further medical relief and further moral elevation. Culion combined features of an army camp with aspects of an American small town. The government built a town hall, a store, a general kitchen, a jail, a school, and the Leper Club, which contained "a piano, a pool table, and many newspapers, some recent, and miscellaneous discarded 'charity' magazines and books unintelligible

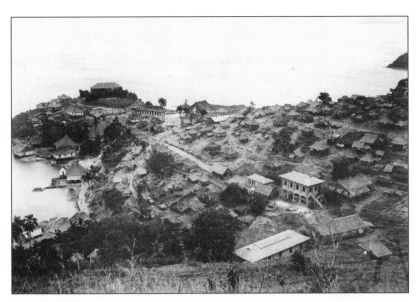

FIGURE 38. Culion Leper Colony (RG 350-BS-1-4-169 [BS 12675], NARA).

except for the pictures."[36] Visitors approaching the town by water received "a most unfavorable first impression of a dreary, parched, poverty-stricken settlement on stony, unproductive hillsides." But the physicians who worked at Culion, while conceding some "distinctly unfavorable features," felt that the "simple, orderly, not uncheerful lives of the inmates" greatly modified the visitors' initial misgivings.[37] Moreover, Culion soon became, according to Heiser's successor, J. D. Long, "the most sanitary town in the Philippines."[38] Life in the island reformatory — whether in the male and female dormitories or the "sanitary barrio" — was organized around the routinized, yet individuated treatment of leprosy. Every week the inmates went dutifully to the clinic, where they received an injection of chaulmoogra oil.

Culion became famous as a laboratory for the chemotherapy of leprosy. In the 1890s, MacNamara had achieved only poor results treating the disease in India: he had tried moving lepers to a "healthy and bracing district," improving their sanitary condition, and even rubbing chaulmoogra oil into the skin two or three times a day — to no avail. Nerve stretching and tubercle excision provided local amelioration at best. "Efforts must be directed," MacNamara concluded, "to discovering some chemical substance which will kill the leprosy bacillus."[39] A few years later, Manson enjoined "scrupulous attention to personal and domestic hygiene," frequent bathing, and "the free use of soap."[40] Although many of his colleagues had favored doses of chaulmoogra oil, and others had recommended ichthyol, hypodermics of perchloride of mercury, and thyroiden, Manson could not help wondering if the success they claimed for these remedies had derived instead from a remission in the disease's naturally fluctuating course. In his opinion, there was nothing yet specific for leprosy "in the sense that mercury and iodide of potassium are specific in syphilis."[41]

After 1910, Heiser and his colleagues in the Philippines were trumpeting the effectiveness of a new preparation of chaulmoogra oil that could be given by hypodermic injection. Although it would take "many years and exhaustive experimentation" to establish the fact definitely, it appeared this gift of "Western science" had relieved at least a few dozen lepers in the islands. Uncertain still if this was the true specific for leprosy, Heiser nevertheless believed it promised "more consistently favorable results than any other that has come to our attention."[42] Dr. John Snodgrass, the colony's resident physician, could cite the case of a twenty-seven-year-old Filipino admitted to Culion in May 1909.[43] Smears made from lesions on the nose and ears showed leprosy bacilli. Beginning in August 1909, he received "vaccine therapy" for one year but showed no signs of improvement. Between September and November 1910, he took crude chaulmoogra oil by mouth until he could no longer tolerate it, after which he was tried on the new injectable form. His condition improved dramatically, all the lesions disappearing by May 1911. For the next year "he remained negative microscopically."[44]

By 1914, even Manson was extolling the benefits of chaulmoogra oil when given hypodermically, as in the Philippines. He had seen the marked clinical improvement — but other laboratory studies had tempered his confidence in the drug's true specificity. Reports indicated that bacilli were "just as abundant in the nodules during and after as before treatment."[45] A new drug, nastin in benzoyl chloride, had promised more etiological specificity in laboratory investigations, but so far the clinical effect was "dangerous to life," a problem that unfortunately "imposed limitations upon the general use of the remedy."[46] Indeed, limitations were so severe that its use was restricted to a few painful clinical trials. Thus in 1918 Heiser could claim, with a degree of self-satisfaction, that "chaulmoogra oil alone has stood the test of time."[47] Having unrivaled clinical experience of the drug, he was convinced that its hypodermic administration, though it might occasionally cause "fever and cardiac distress," offered lepers their best hope of continued remission. All the same, he insisted that his patients take 2 percent hot bicarbonate baths every other day.[48] If lepers still could conventionally be classed as unclean and dangerous, then medical treatment might eventually remove their taint and purify their bodies.

Rituals of modern citizenship, closely bonded to therapeutic protocols, pervaded the leper colony. "The lepers," Heiser observed, "are given all possible liberty, and are, to a large extent, controlled by regulations which they themselves make."[49] Medical facts and social potential were amalgamated: as part of the treatment, the diseased were supposed to govern themselves. Heiser regarded the leper colony as "a microcosm, but on a very small scale indeed."[50] The community elected its own mayor and council; from 1908, women voted, the earliest female suffrage in Southeast Asia. Leper police saw that the town was "kept in good sanitary condition" and made "arrests of offenders against their own ordinances."[51] Leper sanitary inspectors, under the command of a nonleprous chief, also helped to maintain sanitary order in the colony. A leper brass band greeted new arrivals and gave occasional concerts—Heiser once joked that they were so enthusiastic they "literally played their fingers off."[52] Several times a year, the lepers put on a play; indeed, they "took eagerly to dramatics," recalled the director of health.[53] And twice a month in the large concrete theater, patients would dress up to watch "very cheap films."[54] "The disease does not deprive its victims of their desire to look well and to please," observed Dr. Alan J. McLaughlin. "Lepers love neckties and handkerchiefs, and things that are pretty and attractive."[55] Athletic gatherings, though held rarely, elicited considerable enthusiasm for baseball. "That they possess the true American baseball spirit," wrote Snodgrass, "was demonstrated at one of the games when both teams attacked the umpire with ball bats."[56]

The tiresome emphasis on performance animated social life and medical protocols throughout the colony: lepers at Culion were regularly on stage in therapeutic and civic dramas. The diseased body was repeatedly exposed to public view, as if to justify the disciplinary apparatus of the colony. Testing and treatment (especially injections) were generally performed on these bodies as a display of sovereignty for an audience of other lepers. And if medicine had to be seen to be done, so too did citizenship: treatments of the body and of social life all required enactment. A theater, for plays not operations, was one of the first buildings in the civic center of the colony: while the staff often directed, the players and the audience were lepers. It was not enough that they were represented as responsible patients or incipient citizens: they had to perform themselves as the subjects of civic narratives.[57]

Medical authorities expected lepers to work diligently in between their

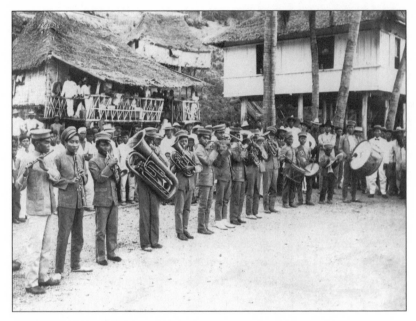

FIGURE 39. Leper brass band, Culion (RG 350-BS-1-4-177 [BS 995], NARA).

doses of chaulmoogra oil — indeed the treatment was supposed to enhance their industrial capacity. In front of each house, for instance, was a small flower garden, "and every effort is being made to instill a sufficient civic pride in the lepers to maintain them; but so far these efforts have not met with much success."[58] Some tried raising cattle or started "tiny sugar plantations." In order to produce the "conditions prevailing in ordinary communities," a store and, later, two bakeries and an ice cream parlor were opened to sell the lepers' manufactures. So that the money handled by lepers never reached the outside world, the authorities coined a special currency to serve as the medium of trade.[59] Many of the afflicted remained capable of carrying out simple domestic duties for a small salary: cooking, cleaning, dressmaking, taking care of streets, making repairs to buildings, and so on.[60] But Heiser lamented that "contractions of the limbs, destruction of tissue, losses of fingers and toes . . . and general debility" meant that only a few lepers performed sufficient manual labor to supply food for themselves. The bulk of the food was still prepared in a large kitchen by leper cooks. "Usually the leper is so depressed that he takes no interest in anything," Heiser reflected. "All he has to look forward to is the half-lingering hope that he may be among the very few who are to get well."[61] It seemed to him that most lepers remained "naturally apathetic" and dependent on government aid. Yet "the streets must be swept, the garbage cans emptied, assistance rendered at the hospital, and supplies carried."[62] When Heiser observed the neglect of civic responsibilities he "held a little meeting with the residents affected and asked them to attend to this matter, and they promised to do so."[63] The director of health expected a more meticulous and hopeful observance of the treatment regime in the future.

Even a carceral and probationary citizenship will provide a language of entitlement. As early as 1912, some of the less introspective lepers were writing to the Manila newspapers to complain about the neglect of their rights. The campaigning editors of *La Vanguardia* questioned Heiser's representation of the leper colony as "a model administration where men and women, more advanced than the rest of the archipelago, enjoy the fullest suffrage, voting as equals for the election of officials . . . [where] they have the best sanitary service, police, schools, gardens, walks, abundant and healthy food, and everything characteristic of modern life and comfort." Recent protests from the inmates had undermined the view that Culion was "a happy community in the full-exercise of self-government."[64] It seems that the food was poor, the housing was overcrowded, the police were oppressive, and the newspaper often censored. One leper lamented that he was "composed of lentils and salt up to the crown of [his] head." Others complained about forced labor on public works.[65] The lepers addressed the government in a language of civic entitlement, arguing that their corner of the archipelago, "abandoned by the hand of God but not the hand of Mr. Heiser," was apparently not the "earthly paradise" for lepers he had promised.[66] While Heiser and other Americans insisted on calling Culion the Island of Hope, Filipinos knew it as "la Isla del Dolor."

Hope was the theme of *Who Walk Alone*, Perry Burgess's popular account of the experiences of a solitary white American leper at Culion during this period. For Burgess, an advertising man trying to raise money for the leper colony, the island was a place of idealized aspiration, where abject embodiment might eventually be transcended. The story concerned "Ned Langford," a soldier in the Philippine-American War who had mixed too closely with an upper-class Filipino family, thus becoming an innocent and sympathetic victim of the disease. After abandoning his own family and changing his name, he admitted himself to Culion in order to get as far as possible from America. On his arrival, a tall, white doctor met him: it was Heiser, as "slender and lithe as an athlete." "Life appeared a continual frolic" to this physician, and optimistically he told Ned that recovery from the disease was now possible.

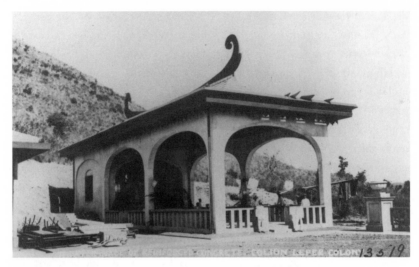

FIGURE 40. Culion theater, 1925. Courtesy of the Rockefeller Archive Center.

Heiser—or James Marshall, as Burgess called him—"liked Filipinos and he expected great things of them in the future." It seemed this "busy man with the welfare of millions in his hands, knew mankind as a whole."[67] Ned tried not to disappoint the director of health. Assigned a separate house, he installed a sink, a shower, and a septic tank. With other responsible lepers he took his treatments regularly: "I liked to study their faces, trying to guess what they were thinking as they winced under the thrust of the needle. Was it simple resignation? Or—was it hope?" Like Heiser, Ned realized how important it was to work; when lepers were "idle it was much more difficult not to lose hope."[68] Uninspired, they would stop taking their treatments.

Who Walk Alone becomes more exciting, though no less pious, with the arrival of Vicente, a "malcontent and political agitator" from Cebú. His advanced disease correlated with his "surly and critical" demeanor, and soon he fell in with "a gang averse to work."[69] Vicente began strutting about the colony shouting for independence and calling for the death of the physicians. With the help of Ned and other dutiful lepers, the miscreant was eventually arrested and imprisoned. Burgess then has Ned opine, "Lepers we were, but we were also citizens, not criminals deprived of our right to vote, but citizens."[70] Yet tragically, Ned died soon after his return to America, during his transfer to the Carville leprosarium, his disease uncured, and his rights not fully restored—what hope, then, for refractory Filipino lepers like Vicente? Despite the author's intentions, dolor still won out over promise at Culion.

Nevertheless, Culion became a model reformatory, influencing activities at Molokai and shaping the administrative apparatus of the new U.S. Federal Leprosarium at Carville, Louisiana. Although Hawaiian lepers had been exiled to the settlement at Kalaupapa, on the north side of Molokai, since 1866, it was only after the U.S. government assumed control in 1909 that inmates were disciplined and managed as at Culion. When Frederick Hoffman toured Molokai in 1915 he found a clean, hygienic town, with stores, churches, playgrounds, a baseball field, a music stand, and a movie theater. The six hundred or so lepers lived in small houses surrounded by pleasant gardens; they were supposed to work every day in the fields. Compared to Culion, research and treatment efforts were still meager, but in all other respects it now resembled the Philippine Island of Hope.[71] The impact of Culion on Carville was even more tangible. Since 1894 a run-down state leper home, Carville was transformed in 1917 into the Federal Leprosarium. Its establishment was in part a response to fears that returning soldiers and immigrants from places like the Philippines were bringing leprosy back into the United States — though the mainland had never been entirely free of the disease. Dr. Oswald E. Denny, the first director of Carville, had worked at Culion, and, according to Zachary Gussow, he re-created "an atmosphere of strict discipline" and a "quasi-military structure" in Louisiana.[72] For the next sixteen years, Denny strove to implant a new Culion in the bayou.

A COLONIAL OBSESSION

After Heiser resigned as director of health in 1915, he often returned to the archipelago, as director for the East of the International Health Division of the Rockefeller Foundation, and he continued to attempt to tinker with the health system. In the 1920s he became especially attentive to developments in the Philippines, advising and supporting his old friend and political ally Leonard Wood, M.D., who had been appointed governor-general. In particular, Heiser impressed on Wood the need for leprosy work. He was so persuasive that after 1922 more than one-third of the Philippines health budget was allocated to Culion, which then boasted six thousand residents in an archipelago of more than ten million people. Medical staffing improved at the colony, and treatment became more rigorous and sophisticated, allowing more paroles for inmates during this period.[73] As the number of "negatives" increased and few were prepared to go home, the population of the "negative barrio," later called *barrio* Osmeña, swelled, causing hardship and misery when the poor inland soils repeatedly yielded sparse harvests.[74]

During the 1920s, Wood became increasingly fascinated by the prospect of rehabilitating the inmates of Culion. He visited the island sixteen times as governor-general and immersed himself in the recent research on leprosy therapeutics. He hectored nationalist politicians, asserting that until they could take care of their lepers, Filipinos would not be fit for self-government.[75] But when members of the Philippine Senate visited Culion in 1922, they concluded it was a useless dissipation of funds, a peculiar American extravagance in a poor and needy archipelago. Manuel L. Quezon, the president of the Senate, was especially bitter. He compared the expense of reforming six thousand lepers with the pittance spent on the prevention of tuberculosis, a disease that killed some thirty thousand Filipinos each year. In 1923, Quezon told the annual meeting of the Philippine Islands Medical Association that the expenditure on the colony "for experimental purposes" was excessive. The medical results did not seem to justify the continued suffering and isolation of the lepers. Quezon was most concerned that tubercular patients were not separated from nontubercular lepers—he was stunned that even at Culion tuberculosis prevention and treatment were neglected.[76] Obsessed with leprosy, Americans appeared indifferent to "the tremendous ravages which this dreadful plague [of tuberculosis] is causing to the Philippine Islands." The nationalist politician regretted that there was "more interest here in doing things which promote immediate results, real or apparent, things that are so spectacular as to lend themselves to wide publicity calculated to invite universal commendation and to secure recognition as world achievements." The more tedious and unrewarding problems, such as tuberculosis prevention, elicited only Filipino commitment. "We have an army of doctors and nurses and well-paid experts in Culion . . . but what has been done by the Philippine Health Service to fight tuberculosis?"[77] The repeated hospitalization of Quezon during this period for bronchitis and other manifestations of tuberculosis, and his death from consumption at Saranac Lake, New York, in 1944, lend further poignancy to his pleas.[78]

Heiser and his colleagues would not allow the agitation of nationalist politicians to discompose them. Having staked his reputation on the rehabilitation of lepers, the former director of health made sure to monitor carefully developments at Culion. When he visited the colony in 1931, for example, he found the inmates "much more contented than formerly." They seemed to have settled down to the routines of therapy and hygiene. But he was saddened that so many of his efforts had been forgotten. Even worse, "the name of Mr. Worcester, who probably did more for leprosy than anyone else in the

Philippines, has been replaced with the name of Rizal on the plaza that was named after him."[79] The following year, however, when Heiser visited again, the entire colony turned out, and "several leper orators hailed our arrival in the most felicitous terms." Doctors still dispensed chaulmoogra oil, the hospital had been extended, and concrete barracks had largely replaced the nipa buildings. Heiser observed that many of those who became bacteriologically negative were still refusing to leave.[80]

During this period lepers also held several meetings demanding an end to segregation; they asserted that leprosy was not nearly as contagious as the health department had claimed, and they had a right to freedom of movement. Medical facts and social potential thus had become linked for doctors and patients alike. The attendant physicians were threatened, and a few inmates called for a strike.[81] In 1932, three hundred young men had forced their way into one of the female dormitories in protest against the reintroduction of restrictions on leper marriages: on this occasion, "the Culion police force was too small to disperse the ardent swains, who refused to pay attention to the law forces."[82] But the most popular forms of civic activism — or performance — were the petition and the public hearing. At Culion, in July 1935, the vice-governor-general Joseph Hayden listened to the fractious lepers as they presented their complaints. Ernesto S., invoking "individual rights and liberties of individuals," demanded that everyone receive a gratuity since they had all been brought to Culion against their will; Ciriaco S. P. protested against the reduced appropriation for the colony; Graciano A. directed attention to the dilapidated conditions of the school buildings; and Rufino M. noted that lepers "clean and cultivate" land without hope of owning it. In response, Hayden told the lepers he could now see that although they were still "afflicted," they "nevertheless, live in a well-ordered, well-directed, and well-operated community." He had been impressed by the review of scouts, pioneers, and police, and so he would consider their demands.[83]

BIOMEDICAL CITIZENSHIP AND THE DISTRIBUTION
OF AFFECT IN THE CARCERAL ARCHIPELAGO

In the Philippines leper colony, inmates were positioned as desiring and deserving treatment and civilizing. As the most needy and most malleable members of a marginal or disparaged population, they seemed the most eligible candidates for a coeval process of medicalization and civilization. Those most rejected from the society that Americans sought to reform appeared most amenable to the civilizing process. The iatrocratic disciplines of the leper colony were not supposed to reproduce the denigrated Filipino social body but rather were meant to normalize American ideals of civic responsibility, to attach recovering lepers to the colonial state and its agents. Accordingly, exile to Culion was represented not as the deprivation of liberty but as its creation. In the controlled environment of the microcolony — in that exemplary space — scientific experts watched over the disciplining, the bodily and moral reform, of those with "curable" yet chronic disease. Progressive intellectuals in the colonial and protonational state regarded the pathology of semicivilization as remediable, so long as those so afflicted were prepared to learn supposedly white ways of relating to the body, to family, and to authority. For Heiser and other medical officers, the most intimate activities of the body and the most intimate of human interactions were open to view and available for refashioning. The trajectory from "savage" (or leper) to citizen thus implied a reconfiguring of intimacies with one's own body and the bodies of others — a remaking of the private. It entailed at the same time a realignment of affect away from traditional family bonds and toward state abstractions like progress, modernity, and civilization.

Citizenship was linked symbiotically to corporeal metamorphosis, but the successful achievement of both was endlessly postponed. The result was a deferred and incomplete citizenship, as repressive as it was liberating: civic and medical responsibilities were always more salient at Culion than civil rights. As an exemplary part of the colonial process of modern subject formation, such carceral citizenship permitted no history beyond an individual's standardized medical history, and it sanctioned little public self-assertion: the leper-citizen was to become an individualized case record, oriented away from a messy past of illness and superstition toward a contained, therapeutic future. Citizenship at Culion thus was predicated on displacement, erasure, and transcendence of native embodiment in private and domestic life. Configured as moral reformation, medical protocol, and race elevation, this simulated citizenship would mostly be conferred as a discipline and only occasionally demanded as a right. Even those paroled from Culion required continued monitoring: they were in remission, not cured, and they were nationals, not full citizens. Their identities and relationships, their affective ties, were never as modern as hoped. The recovering lepers had, in effect, been left in nationalism's waiting room.[84]

Despite its flaws and disappointments, Culion remained the best model in the archipelago for "the making of men out of savages, the regeneration of a conquered people by the conquerors by teaching them the benefits of labor and industry."[85] Lepers would be "taught to speak, and to reason, and to . . . get their rights as citizens among those who have been so long their superiors."[86] It was the progressive colonial official's "work of civilization . . . of regeneration and instruction," organized through a multitude of individual medical careers.[87] In the microcolony, in the controlled laboratory of subject formation, the supposedly docile lepers might yet be enrolled in American modernity in advance of the nonleprous. To understand the American colonial project it was necessary to study Culion, for the leper colony had become an allegory of the prospects of the macrocolony. In the 1930s, as the Philippines moved toward self-government under U.S. guidance, the concentrating of lepers at Culion fell out of favor. Instead, new treatment stations scattered across the archipelago and a new leprosarium at Cebú allowed lepers to lead responsible, healthful lives while still integrated in their community.[88] Once expressively localized at Culion, the civilizing process was thus dispersed through the thickening carceral texture of the archipelago.[89]

Chapter Seven

LATE-COLONIAL PUBLIC HEALTH
AND FILIPINO "MIMICRY"

"But what an imitator the Filipino is!" wrote Victor G. Heiser, after visiting a hospital in Sulu, during an investigatory trip he conducted in 1916 for the International Health Board of the Rockefeller Foundation.[1] Just a year earlier Francis Burton Harrison, the new governor-general of the Philippines, had accepted Heiser's resignation from his post as director of health. Now the wily, authoritarian hygienist, supported by the Rockefeller Foundation, had an opportunity to return to the archipelago and make life difficult for those who sought, prematurely in his opinion, to "Filipinize" the American colonial bureaucracy.[2] In general, it was evident to him that health work had been degraded in his absence. The town of Legaspi, for example, had no latrines and was "filthy in the extreme." Heiser felt that Filipino infiltration of the public health service now meant that "politics seems to dominate everything for the worst."[3] In Manila, "the dead spirit seems to pervade everything."[4] All that remained was a corps of pathetic native imitators of American public health, carelessly supervising lower-class imitative natives in the *barrios*. "There is a great inefficiency," Heiser remarked, "and the machine is big and ponderous and the fuel does little more than oil the wheels, and progress is small, but this is to be expected with native control."[5] As they all went dutifully, slowly through the motions, producing unfaithful copies of the American originals, Heiser watched, gleefully reporting on their deficiencies. "In leaving Manila," he wrote, it was "a satisfaction to see the indestructible monuments of cement which I left on the landscape and which they will be unable to destroy."[6]

Wherever he went in the colonial Philippines, Heiser found imitation, theatricality, ornament, and politics. At times he was heartened by Filipino enthusiasm for his projects. "Hookworm treatment is very popular with the people," he reported on a later visit in 1925. They "have become greatly interested in its prevention; now that they understand how it is transmitted they are voluntarily building large numbers of latrines."[7] He was thrilled by local efforts to follow practices he regarded as typically American. But often these latrines would turn out to be quite different from what he had imagined: "The question of superstructure is left entirely to the householder's wish and it is amazing to see the numbers of directions into which this feature develops."[8] Nor were Filipinos seating themselves on their new toilets quite to his satisfaction. Heiser urged the local Rockefeller emissary, Dr. C. H. Yaeger, to modify the bowl design "to make it impossible to sit on except in the desired position."[9] Out in the field, boring holes for yet more latrines, Yaeger himself was never sure when locals were making fun of his hygiene enthusiasms or subverting his projects. In one town, they wanted to make a "wood carving of someone boring a latrine and suggested me. Well a joke is a joke and I didn't know if they were serious or not but took it in good spirit. What a reputation!"[10]

I return in this chapter to the colonial excremental vision not so much to indulge in toilet humor as to discuss imitation and difference in the new hygienic order, focusing on the role of mimicry in a colonial development project. In chapters 3 and 4 I described an American poetics of pollution in the colonial Philippines, a racializing of germ theories that conventionally contrasted a clean, ascetic American body with an open, polluting Filipino body. From the early twentieth century, public health officers argued that Filipinos, evolving with local pathogens, would surely have been fashioned as natural reservoirs of disease organisms, containers that racial customs and habits kept filled to the brim. Filipinos, then, were cast along with other local fauna as disease dealers — even apparently healthy Filipinos might secretly carry the invisible pathogens from which supposedly pure and cleanly bourgeois Americans were typically exempt and to which they seemed typically more vulnerable. Natives would thus appear as meretriciously healthy carriers and transmitters of local diseases, while those Americans who fastidiously restricted local contact were represented as innocent victims. As the American lower bodily stratum was erased or abstracted in tropical hygiene, the poorer class of Filipino, like other natives, became the chief source of contamination and danger. In other words, the new tropical hygiene developing at the end of the nineteenth century had led to an anthropomorphic mobilization of disease agency in the tropics as elsewhere, giving pathological depth and interiority to older racial and class stereotypes. I call this a poetics in order to emphasize the way in which colonial public health officers attempted to close the structure of medical metaphor and omit any relations of these imputative texts to political practice. The closed system of equivalence and opposition served to erase any historical or social context for disease patterns, substituting instead contrasting natural typologies, a poetics of purity and danger.[11]

The Manichean opposition in the medical text — the contrast of a white bourgeois American body, a formally expressive body, with a Filipino grotesque body — proved in practice excitingly assailable and perhaps necessarily unsustainable. American self-possession was always fragile, as we have seen, and no matter how repressed, a secret rottenness kept resurfacing in even the most apparently abstracted of bodies, disturbing and reconstituting American identity. American males repeatedly broke down in the tropics, going native or becoming neurasthenic or nostalgic. On the other hand, a few select Filipinos seemed ever more reformable, perhaps able through correct training to transcend their lower bodily stratum and thus eventually to become eligible for social citizenship. Positioned at the polluting pole of a binary typology, Filipinos were expected to confess their putrescence, to announce their desire for civilization or modernity, and to make themselves available for reformation. Medical and civic discourses were thus overlaid upon each other. The American civil authorities treated Filipinos as infants in need of, and capable of responding to, bodily training and guidance in proper behavior, that is, subject to a "benevolent assimilation" into a sort of American adulthood. In heeding the gospel of hygiene, some Filipinos, with lepers in the vanguard, might therefore be given limited civic rights, becoming probationary citizen-subjects. As President Woodrow Wilson remarked in relation to American duties in the Philippines, "Self-government is a form of character and it follows upon the discipline which gives a people self-possession, self-mastery, and the habit of order and peace. . . . No people can be 'given' the self-control of maturity. Only a long apprenticeship of obedience can secure them this precious possession."[12] Unlike most other colonial powers at the time, the American regime thus began to supplement a project of native homogenization with limited individuation and developmentalism—evidently, the copy was becoming as interesting as any typological construction of difference. The moral reform of the newly recognized individual was linked symbiotically to bodily reform, but the satisfactory achievement of both normalizations could, as Heiser attested, be endlessly deferred. Native imitations of American citizenship appealed to the narcissistic demands of colonial officials, but these performances usually appeared immature and unfaithful, that is, in need of further surveillance and discipline.[13]

I would like to extend this analysis and in this chapter consider further the role of mimesis in the colonial civilizing process.[14] I will focus on the Rockefeller campaign to prevent hookworm infection in the Philippines during the early 1930s, as this project demonstrates a medical effort to produce hybrid, imitative subject positions for Filipinos and indicates the ways in which "mimicry" sometimes might expose these constructions.[15] In the latrine business we can see the white man off-loading his burden, making hygienic subjects who participate in that subject-making, sometimes parodically. The story takes place during a period of rising nationalism and anti-Americanism in the Philippines, so the relations of colonial hygiene and citizenship become especially clear.

I have referred to this as a colonial civilizing project, for that is the goal to which American bureaucrats in the Philippines aspired, but in the 1940s this task would come to be called development. This chapter may therefore be read as an account of a colonial precursor of the development discourse that proliferated after World War II.[16] The early effort to produce and implement development knowledge would prove immensely influential, shaping later Rockefeller Foundation policies and stimulating other international agencies to conduct similar projects. Although development was soon taken up more widely by local elites and used as nationalist rhetoric, here it still appeared to offer, to Heiser and others, recolonizing possibilities. Indeed, one might argue that development never quite discarded the colonial legacy that pervades this story; it often seemed to repeat the older dichotomies of modernity and tradition, science and ignorance, global and local, purity and danger—only to characterize the subjects of development as arrested at stages in the traverse between these opposites. Much of development remained, at heart, a civilizing mission, disempowering local communities, demanding that the native or the underdeveloped person follow a single track toward a unique Western modernity, not really expecting that this distant prospect, the light on the hill, would ever be reached.

A NEW ORDER OF COLONIAL HYGIENE

In 1916, Victor Heiser, believing that the Filipinization of the colonial bureaucracy was premature, took special care to visit Sulu. The year before, the American health officer for the province, Dr. Ivan B. Hards, had approached a visiting U.S. congressman to tell him that since Heiser had left office, the Filipino civil authorities were grossly neglecting a cholera epidemic.[17] But when Governor Harrison investigated these allegations, Major L. A. I. Chapman, the commanding officer of the local barracks, reported that Hards, perhaps "more interested in maintaining a paid civil practice," had himself shown "but little interest in the cholera situation."[18] Hards now "emphatically" denied having suggested earlier that his Filipino superiors disliked him reporting the facts. "I have always been instructed by telegram and letters from my official superiors," he assured the authorities, "to report all cases of cholera occurring anywhere within the province."[19] Harrison regarded the accusation, now retracted, as typical of the attempts of Heiser and other health officers to "discredit and destroy the work of distinguished members of their own corps." "Among the most annoying and vexatious incidents in the establishment of the civil regime here," the governor-general wrote to Washington, D.C., "has been the effort of certain medical officers to discredit the newly appointed civil officers of the public health service." Hards resigned from his post late in 1915 and returned to the United States. Harrison replaced him with his deputy, Dr. Marcelino Gallardo. Unlike Hards, Gallardo was reputed to have "distinguished himself during the Sulu cholera epidemic" and displayed "a correct understanding of the fundamentals of combating cholera in accordance with the best modern practice."[20] Yet it was Gallardo who prompted Heiser, as he passed through Sulu, to exclaim, "What an imitator the Filipino is!"

Before 1914, Filipino physicians had generally occupied junior positions in medical institutions under the control of the Philippine government. All six senior officers of the Bureau of Health in 1913 were American; the only Filipino division chief was Dr. Manuel Gomez of the statistics department. At the Philippine General Hospital, Dr. Fernando Calderón was chief of the obstetrics section, but Americans managed the other five units. The senior officers of the bureau's inspection division were, with few exceptions, American physicians, but their assistants all were Filipino. Only two of the seven-

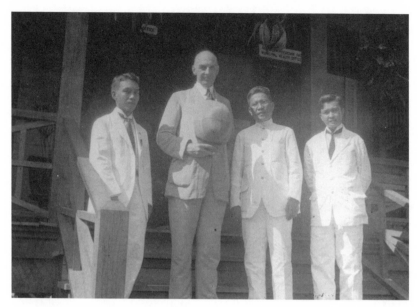

FIGURE 41. Dr. Luna, Dr. Heiser, Dr. Fajardo, Dr. Gallardo, Jolo Hospital, 1916.
Courtesy of the Rockefeller Archive Center.

teen inspectors in the field were Filipino, yet all of the nine junior inspectors
were locals. Of the twenty-seven district health officers, a lower-status job in
the medical service, no more than three were American.[21] All of the senior
instructors at the new Philippine medical school were foreigners. Similarly, at
the Bureau of Science, the senior researchers were American or European.
The first article by a Filipino published in the *Philippine Journal of Science* —
Calderón's discussion of obstetric practice in the archipelago — did not appear until 1908; the following year, Filipinos were junior authors of only
seven of the forty-seven papers presented in the journal. In 1913, Filipino
investigators contributed to no more than four of the journal's forty-one
medical articles.

During this period, Heiser and Dean C. Worcester repeatedly emphasized
the current incapacity of Filipino physicians for high office and their need for
unremitting supervision and tutelage.[22] American colonialists thought it possible that Filipinos, after learning the "whys and wherefores" of modern
hygiene and sanitation, would eventually develop the skills and the sense of
responsibility American physicians recognized in themselves, but that goal
still seemed far off.[23] Meanwhile Filipinos should occupy junior positions in
which they could observe and imitate the more accomplished foreigners.

Heiser took great pleasure in recalling a trip to the United States with Dr. Francisco Calderón — then "being groomed for an important administrative position" — whom he watched over "as though I was his keeper." According to Heiser, his charge was at a loss in modern society, unable "to conform to American notions of propriety."[24] "Things moved far too rapidly for him," and when Calderón addressed medical gatherings Heiser was convinced he "scarcely knew the meanings of the words."[25] Later, despite Heiser's misgivings, his *Rotpeter* became the dean of the Philippine medical school and president of the University of the Philippines.[26]

Heiser may have found support among some of the Filipino elite for his critical appraisal of their accomplishments. For example, T. H. Pardo de Tavera, the token Filipino physician on the Manila Board of Health and the Philippine Commission, had often thanked the Americans for promoting and institutionalizing the *ilustrado* anticlerical project. "America came to the Philippines to aid them, to sustain them and to give them the principles of liberty and free government," he wrote in 1902.[27] A founder of the Federal Party and editor of *La Democracia*, Pardo de Tavera hoped that one day the Philippines would be ready to become another state in the Union. According to Pardo de Tavera, Filipinos had not yet achieved the necessary "triumph over one's self" — they mostly remained "infected with the leprosy of superstition [*contagiodos con la lepra de la superstición*]." He argued that attainment of true self-government was not unlike the formation of "hygienic consciousness [*el sentimiento de la higiene*]." At first this sentiment had "existed in a latent state and we did not see, feel, or notice it because of lack of preparation." Gradually, Filipinos had come to clamor for more hygiene, but they had not yet reached American standards. In time, they would learn to imitate the "regime of liberty, industry, work and logical mentality [*mentalidad lógica*]."[28] Filipinos, Pardo de Tavera assured the graduates of the University of the Philippines in 1921, eventually would be "capable of following the infinite, progressive, and ascendant road of civilization," so long as they abandoned the "national type" and acquired American customs and habits. He urged the graduates to develop the qualities of "confidence in one's own self, of appreciation, respect and love for work, of hygiene and care of our body, of disregard for suffering." "Let us therefore lay aside sentimental patriotism," he declared, "and let us adopt scientific patriotism."[29] But after Pardo de Tavera's death in 1925, Heiser encountered few Filipinos who shared his disdain for their attainments, his sense of their unreadiness for self-government.

As governor-general, W. Cameron Forbes had demonstrated great reluctance to confer much responsibility on supposedly feckless Filipinos. In 1905, Forbes wrote to his old friend William James, wondering if the philosopher had ever "traveled around the world on a recently developed map and figured out how many countries there are in the torrid zone and in the neighborhood of the equator . . . and how many of them maintain self-government unsupported by men from the temperate zones."[30] Forbes was convinced Filipinos as yet were "without the sinews necessary to maintain a position among the nations of the world."[31] Although a committed anti-imperialist, James suspected this was indeed true, while he hoped the American emissary would at least nurture the soul of the Filipino. Occurring at a time when the United States was relying on a "collaborative compromise" with local elites to secure control of the islands, this exchange has a rather sad, detached, and self-serving tone. If he did not know in 1905, it must soon have become clear to Forbes that Filipinos continued to dominate commercial, professional, and political activities, even if they were excluded from the military, the American clubs, and the higher levels of the colonial bureaucracy. The local elites, even when they were not as complicit as Pardo de Tavera, proved capable of tolerating an American rhetoric of superiority, so long as they were allowed to get on with business.[32]

The enrollment of educated Filipinos in the institutions of American medicine, initially so gradual, accelerated greatly after 1914. The new U.S. president, Woodrow Wilson, had been elected on a platform that proposed early independence for the Philippines. Conventionally, Wilson argued that Americans should give Filipinos "a moral government which would moralize and sublimate their ideals"; having accepted the "compulsion of American character," locals might become true partners in government.[33] According to Wilson, the trajectory from savage to bureaucrat was already more or less accomplished, their apprenticeship was virtually over — an attainment that the Republican Forbes and his acolytes would still dispute. It came as no surprise, then, that soon after Harrison, a Democrat congressman from New York, replaced Forbes, he quickly announced his commitment to complete the Filipinization of the colonial bureaucracy. The reformist governor-general declared portentously that "a new era is dawning. We place within your reach the instruments of your redemption. The door of opportunity stands open and under Divine Providence the event is in your hands."[34] Harrison regarded the American colonial officials as a "stuffy body of restless, ambitious and adventurous young men," ill-suited to their self-appointed task as tutors of supposedly ignorant Filipinos. He suspected that "as the attractions of Philippine life grew upon American officials, so grew their willingness to believe in the incapacity of Filipinos for office."[35]

The number of American officials in the islands, including physicians and teachers, fell from 2,600 in 1913 to 614 in 1921.[36] The drop-off resulted in part from a deliberate policy of replacing Americans with Filipinos, but also was the consequence of Americans leaving to fight in the European war and of inveterate retentionists giving up in disgust at the drive toward independence. In 1916, the U.S. Congress passed the Jones Act, which extended the powers of the Philippine legislature, confirmed plans for early self-government, and disturbed those American colonial officials who doubted that Filipinos were ready to assume such responsibilities. When Heiser left the islands, he had been appalled that "many Filipinos were lifted into positions which they were not qualified to fill." His imitative subordinates had not yet got their act together. Heiser had been prepared to allow locals to "direct the lesser units of government and, as they showed fitness, to turn over to them the higher units," but Harrison seemed to believe that "the only way for people to learn how to govern was to let them do the governing as they wished."[37] Worcester, also isolated by the drift toward self-government, had resigned as secretary of the interior in 1913, "firmly convinced that Filipinos are where they are today only because they have been pushed into line, and if outside pressures were relaxed they would steadily and rapidly deteriorate." The task of "training physicians, surgeons and sanitarians so that the public health may be adequately protected" was not yet, he claimed, complete. "Shall they," he asked, "be left to stagger on alone, blind in their own conceit?"[38]

Worcester campaigned strongly against the Filipinization of the health service, and he enlisted expatriate friends and colleagues in the fight. The changes so incensed Dr. H. L. Kneedler, a physician who had worked as an insurance examiner in Manila since the American occupation and was an associate of Worcester, that he wrote to President Wilson, warning that the "weak puny bodies" of Filipinos would never be "transformed into a healthy vigorous race" if the "natives" were allowed to take over. When Kneedler first arrived, after the Philippine-American War, he had found the city's water grossly polluted; forty thousand or more died each year from smallpox; the lack of sewers meant that "noxious odors and gases were being constantly liberated"; five thousand lepers were at large; and malaria prevailed. "Those in charge of sanitation under these obstacles soon learned," Kneedler wrote, echoing Heiser, "that the passive resistance of the Oriental is a much more subtle and difficult force to overcome than the active opposition so frequently encountered among the inhabitants of the temperate zone." Nevertheless, a "system of sanitation" had been established, despite the "many efforts to avoid enforcement by the native Filipinos."[39] And now this apparently child-like race was taking over again.

Dissent from Harrison's Filipinization policy was expressed privately at the highest level. Charles H. Yeater, the vice governor and no friend of the chief executive, wrote to Daniel R. Williams, warning that the Bureau of Health "through the almost total elimination of American doctors, has already opened the way for the spread of epidemic and endemic diseases ever lurking for a foothold in the tropics." There were fewer than twelve American physicians in the whole archipelago. "Of the Bureau of Science," he went on, "which has done and was doing such wonderful work in original research, and discoveries relating to tropical diseases and their cure . . . now 'shot to pieces' and largely marking time." The basic problem was that the Malay race was incapable of forming nations — everyone knew this. Filipinos were generally "poor, ignorant, superstitious, and shiftless." "However much we might like to do so," Yeater reflected, "we cannot override ethnological truth nor hurdle the processes of evolution. The laws of nature are immutable. . . . If the Malay is to escape his inheritance it must be by the same road we have traveled, and history records that the journey was a slow and painful one."[40]

Heiser and most of his compatriots continued to find in the failures to enforce smallpox vaccination, the recurrences of cholera, and a rising death rate in the archipelago evidence of the unreadiness for office of the Filipinos they had trained. American papers unsympathetic to the Democratic administration declared that "the full harvest of the 'new era' is now in the reaping in the Philippines." "The Filipinization wind," warned the *New York Herald*, had caused the incidence of plague to "jump" in the islands.[41] Even the increasingly Filipinized health service conceded that in Manila the mortality rate for each one thousand inhabitants — 42.28 in 1903, at the end of the war, but as low as 24.48 in 1913 — had risen in 1918 to 46.33, and in 1919 was 27.55.[42] To Heiser this was a clear indictment of Filipino management. But Dr. Vicente de Jesús, the acting director of public health, had another explanation: the influenza pandemic in 1918 had exacted a heavy toll in lives and caused a "weakened organic resistance" to other diseases among the population.[43] New outbreaks of smallpox were the result of a wearing off of the immunity conferred in the general vaccination of 1905, the only truly thorough campaign the Americans ever carried out in the islands. Cholera had appeared again, as it usually did, for the archipelago had never been free of the disease. De Jesús was confident that 1920 would show some improvement in the Philippine death rate. Using the now-standard sanitary methods, cholera had been checked and smallpox was again under control. "Health conditions are returning to normal," he reported, "and with the increasing efficiency of this Service on the one hand, and on the other, with the population becoming better enlightened regarding hygiene and sanitation and readier therefore to respond to and cooperate with our efforts, the steady decrease in the death rate observed during the pre-grippal years will no doubt be recorded again."[44]

A few pro-Filipino American bureaucrats also defended the Filipinization of the health service. General Frank McIntyre, chief of the Bureau of Insular Affairs, noted that "unfortunately, cholera has visited the Philippine Islands every year since 1902." To charges of increased friction at the Philippine General Hospital, he replied that Heiser's earlier policies had probably caused the trouble, and currently care was as effective as ever, with no shortage of clinical material.[45] All things considered, "the great public health work in the Philippines is going on and it is being extended as rapidly as the resources of the government will permit."[46] Winfred T. Denison, the secretary of the interior, felt that the "venom" with which Heiser and Worcester "discussed the 'fitness' of the Filipinos, both here and at home, has been a dreadful misfortune to everyone concerned."[47] In 1914, Denison wrote to Teddy Roosevelt explaining that "what aroused my indignation was an apparent desire of the American colony to ride roughshod over the Filipinos in a tyrannical spirit, made unusually intense by racial difference." In fact, he continued, cholera had broken out when Heiser was still on duty, and unusual flooding had disseminated it: Colonel Edward L. Munson, M.D., later brought it under control, in cooperation with Filipino doctors. The health department had isolated cholera carriers for ten days in San Lazaro hospital — "you can imagine what a storm such a policy would arouse in New York City, and you undoubtedly remember the difficulties of Typhoid Mary's case."[48] After hearing that Richard P. Strong was telling people in Boston that the health service had been "wrecked," Denison wrote to David P. Barrows at the University of California to let him know that "the service is intact, and I believe in better shape than it ever has been, and it has also been put on the basis of better understanding with the legislature and Filipino physicians. They have been backing up sanitation in a very satisfactory way."[49]

Following the election of Warren Harding as president in 1920, Harrison was recalled, in 1921. The new U.S. administration appointed Forbes and

General Leonard Wood, M.D., both of them professed foes of rapid Filipiniza-tion, to report on conditions in the archipelago. Not surprisingly, they con-cluded that "the orderly process of promotion of proved efficiency from the less important positions was changed to a hurried Filipinization, placing Fili-pinos in nearly all of the higher positions." The report condemned the lack of hospitals and dispensaries, inadequate appropriation for sanitary work, and a shortage of properly trained doctors, nurses, and sanitary workers. It added that the "excellent health service which previously existed has become largely inert; much of the personnel remained, but it has lost the zeal and vigor which formerly characterized it."[50]

Heiser liked to think that the "Harrison bonfire which had blazed so merrily for many years and round which the Filipinos had danced so blithely, finally flickered and went out, leaving only dead ashes." Having attached himself to the Wood–Forbes mission, Heiser took pleasure in visiting the islands again, once more "in harness at the old job of hauling the Filipinos out of the slough." He felt warmly welcomed in Manila by his "prize cholera fighter," De Jesús, who "seemed overjoyed at my return to share his respon-sibilities." "He had already had a desk placed beside his," Heiser recalled, "and offered to retire temporarily while I was there. I was never more touched than by this demonstration of trust."[51] But despite the Wood–Forbes mis-sion's criticisms of Filipinization and Heiser's immense capacity to patronize local colleagues, the process continued even after General Wood was ap-pointed as governor-general. By 1925, only 1.5 percent of the civil service (not including teachers) was American.[52] It was about this time Heiser began organizing the Rockefeller hookworm campaign in the Philippines, a scheme that would become a means of recolonizing health work in the archipelago, of reintroducing American discipline and American role models. For Heiser and many other American bureaucrats there was only one right way to manage the colony and only one way to inhabit it with propriety; Filipinos necessarily were unfaithful or inadequate imitators of this model.

Rizal and others among the first generation of *ilustrados* had linked sci-ence and medicine to militant nationalism: for them, to be scientific repre-sented an authentic affiliation with modernity, and it indicated the capacity for independence of mind and therefore of polity. But the following genera-tion, which included De Jesús and the Calderón brothers, had largely un-coupled science and militancy: they were more likely to regard themselves as bureaucratic functionaries, efficiently managing the colonial state. Science was a matter of state and rarely excited thoughts of the nation any longer. For

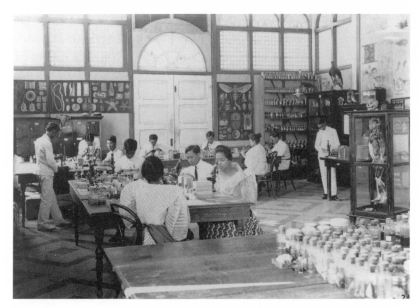

FIGURE 42. Class in biology, Manila. Courtesy of the Rockefeller Archive Center.

Rizal, medicine had radical political implications; for De Jesús, it meant hygiene reform of the masses.[53] But even though medicine came to be shorn of nationalist significance, Filipino public health officials resisted imagining themselves as mere mimics of Americans. Rather, they believed they could normalize state medicine in the Philippines in a way foreign colonizers could never achieve. In a sense, they had identified American colonial public health officers, not themselves, as the profane copy. They wanted to administer mundane state medicine, not colonial medicine; they wanted to be ordinary scientific professionals, not scientific radicals.

Many Filipino medical bureaucrats thus resisted following U.S. prescriptions, but without drawing radical nationalist lessons from this refusal. It was still the opinion of many Americans, including Heiser, that Filipinos could not yet evade fully their unhygienic racial habits: thus any Filipino, until proved otherwise, would remain a contributor to tropical pathology. Educating out such ingrained habits would, it seemed, take generations; in the meantime only the strictest regulation would control them. But this made little sense to De Jesús and other members of the Filipino elite. For them, disease stigma more properly belonged not to race but to social class. Thus while Heiser continued to look askance at *Filipino* customs and habits, De Jesús argued for the "unsanitary habits of the *masses* as the largest factor in the transmission of cholera and other intestinal diseases, such as eating with the fingers, care-lessness in the disposal of excreta." The bad behavior was the same, the ideal techniques of surveillance, persuasion, and enforcement altered little, but a simple racial understanding of tropical disease transmission dropped out of most Filipino epidemiological theory. It had become "the masses," not the race, "as yet untouched by either example or precept."[54] When Dr. Eu-genio Hernando rehearsed the dogma of the "new public health" in 1919, the racial concerns that had pervaded earlier tropical accounts of the subject were absent: he confined his remarks to the individual (of any race) and contact with infective discharges.[55] Thus if cholera continued to be spread in the provinces, it seemed to the urban Filipino elite that this was because "the poorer classes"—and not their educated compatriots—continued to drink water contaminated by others of their low social stratum.[56] When infant mortality was finally recognized as a problem in the 1920s, Fernando Cal-derón blamed it on the superstitious and faulty maternity practices of the lower classes.[57]

The natural resistance to hygiene reform that Heiser took to be racial and illicit was, for many Filipino physicians, at once social and comprehensible. De Jesús, for example, repeatedly urged that the sanitary code "be given a certain flexibility, so that the application of certain regulations would be left to the discretion and sound sense of the district health officer."[58] But sanitary regulations might, on other occasions, still be enforced severely. In 1914, De Jesús had thought that the only effective way to eradicate cholera in the provinces was "through a trained central force sent from Manila and operat-ing under direct supervision of the Bureau of Health in cooperation with the Constabulary."[59] But if an apparent sanitary crisis could still elicit a military style of prevention, Filipino medical officers were more commonly claiming an increased sensitivity to local social values. A senior health official in 1929 observed that the conquest of disease "is so closely bound up with the eco-nomic condition and personal habits of the people that improvement must necessarily come gradually with sympathetic guidance and education." He incensed the great interventionist Heiser when he continued, "Few things arouse greater resistance and antipathy than efforts to enforce changes in the daily lives of people and the conditions that surround them, and it is but natural that they should resist measures which, so far as they can see, are devised solely to make them unhappy and uncomfortable."[60] Such remarks prompted Heiser to reflect yet again on what poor imitators the Filipino physicians had proven to be.

Under the American civil regime, the biological laboratory of the Bureau of Science assiduously examined specimens taken from the new tropical territory and from the bodies that inhabited it. Each day, scientists assayed more than 100 samples of body fluids and excretions, mapping the pathological terrain of the archipelago, identifying the racial salients of disease. In 1909 alone, the scientists examined 701 specimens of blood, over 900 urine specimens, and more than 7,000 fecal specimens.[61] When the influx of Filipino material had indicated a widespread, and often asymptomatic, pathogen carriage, the scientists attributed this condition to inherently racial "customs and habits," not to social disadvantage. The search for occult germ carriage became an obsession of the biological laboratory. It prompted C. L. Cole in 1907 to survey the "natives of the Philippine Islands" for the presence of the hookworm, *Necator americanus*; P. E. Garrison organized a more orderly study of the "animal parasites of man"; J. M. Phalen and H. J. Nichols reported on the distribution of *Filaria nocturna* among the local inhabitants; R. E. Hoyt presented the results of 300 examinations of feces "with reference to the presence of amoebae"; Garrison and Llamas described the intestinal worms of 385 Filipino women and children in Manila; and E. R. Stitt studied the intestinal parasites of Cavite province.[62] At Heiser's request, Dr. David Willets went to the Cagayan valley, where he made nearly 7,700 fecal examinations.[63] But even as many of these studies demonstrated widespread hookworm carriage in the archipelago, Heiser, while director of health, would do little to prevent it.

American doctors in Puerto Rico were treating hookworm infestation far more seriously. A year or so after the American occupation of the island, Dr. Bailey K. Ashford had identified hookworm as the cause of the anemia that prevailed there. Ashford knew of the work of Charles Wardell Stiles, who claimed he had found hookworm in the stools of poor whites in the southern United States in the 1890s.[64] The pattern of behavior of this novel pathogen was soon established. Entering humans through the skin, usually through bare feet, the parasite eventually reaches the intestines by way of the trachea, esophagus, and stomach. Once in the duodenum, worms fix themselves to the intestinal walls and feed from the bloodstream, in time causing a marked anemia. Blood loss might produce the symptoms of pallor, tiredness, and fatigue — thus hookworm became popularly "the germ of laziness." The infected person, unknowingly, excretes thousands of ova each day, and if deposited on warm, moist soil, the eggs generate infective larvae that seek another host. While Stiles thought he had found *Anchylostoma duodenale* in the southern United States, Ashford's worm was a new type, later called *Necator americanus*. Returning to Puerto Rico in 1902, Ashford, together with Dr. W. W. King, set aside two wards of the Ponce hospital for hookworm patients; the following year, the governor, William H. Hunt, allocated five thousand dollars for hookworm prevention and treatment (an unpleasant, nauseating thymol mixture). "An intelligent combination of educational and prohibitory measures," the program expanded further in 1904, resulting in the establishment of the Hookworm Commission of Puerto Rico, which used mobile field hospitals and clinics to distribute information and provide treatment.[65] When Ashford returned to the United States in 1906, the commission continued its work, led by Puerto Rican physicians, and by 1910 more than 250,000 people had been treated in an effort to eliminate the germ that was sapping their industry and efficiency.[66]

In the United States, Stiles had been talking to Frederick T. Gates, the advisor of John D. Rockefeller, about the frightening prevalence of the germ of laziness in southern regions. Rockefeller, eager to promote health and industry, decided in 1909 to fund a Sanitary Commission for the Eradication of Hookworm Disease, appointing Stiles as scientific secretary and Wickliffe Rose as administrative secretary. Hearing of Ashford's work in Puerto Rico, Rose visited the colony in 1910, hoping to use the hookworm commission as a model for health work in the southern United States. He was impressed with the Puerto Rican program, which combined educational and dispensary activities. During the next few years, the Rockefeller Commission set up similar organizations in each southern state. Led by a director of sanitation, who reported to the state board of health and to the commission, a corps of inspectors, microscopists, and laboratory technicians engaged in educational campaigns, diagnostic investigations, and the dispensing of thymol. Working mostly through newspapers, fairs, and the public schools, they produced articles, pamphlets, cartoons, and circulars and delivered stirring lectures. They traveled from town to town, putting up exhibits of the hookworm, displaying models of sanitary houses and latrines, and exhorting the public to avoid the germ of laziness — it was a form of hygienic evangelism that often echoed the tent revival meetings.[67] The local sanitary officers tended to racialize the message, though their more extreme opinions rarely received endorsement from the commission. Dr. Charles T. Nesbitt, for example, pointed to the African origin of the parasite and suggested a likely affinity between it and

African-Americans: "The hookworms, so common in Africa, which are carried in the American Negroes' intestines with relatively slight discomfort, were almost entirely responsible for the terrible plight of the southern white. It is impossible to estimate the damage that has been done to the white peoples of the South by the diseases brought by this alien race."[68] Nesbitt interpreted such racial susceptibilities as evidence of the need to separate vulnerable, valuable whites from the bowels of African-Americans. Stiles, in contrast, suggested that this ecological détente meant that "the white man owes it to his own race that he lend a helping hand to improve the sanitary surroundings of the Negro."[69]

Although the campaign followed, in broad outline, earlier work in Puerto Rico, significant deviations soon became evident, especially in its relations with southern whites. The promoters of the "gospel of hygiene" in the United States took special care to enroll local medical doctors and to appoint sanitary officers who already claimed the respect of their white communities. Such sensitivity to local concerns had been rare in the colonial setting when American officers were program managers. Moreover, Rose and others in the South chose to emphasize dispensary work more than sanitary reform: they recognized the need for behavioral reform and a privy construction program but conceded that social changes among white citizens would have to be voluntary, not compulsory, as in the colony. The sanitation and treatment of African-Americans, however, were frequently forced and blatantly colonial in style.

By 1914, Gates was satisfied that the sanitary commission had alerted white southerners to the microbial peril. As the hookworm campaign stimulated the growth of a network of state and local public health agencies, his attention shifted to global health work. The new International Health Commission (later Board) of the Rockefeller Foundation needed a means of entry into the colonial tropics, and hookworm seemed to offer ready access, just as it had in the southern United States. The hookworm campaign might prove to be a tool permitting ingress to a colony, or a new state, and a means of enabling the Rockefeller Foundation to build, or rebuild, a broader health program. Rose soon became the head of an international hookworm program, setting up campaigns first in Egypt and then northern Australia, both modeled on the sanitary commission's work in the United States. When passing through Manila in 1914, Rose recruited Victor Heiser, the disaffected director of health, and made him director for the East of the International Health Board. Rose reported that Heiser's "demonstration that the super-

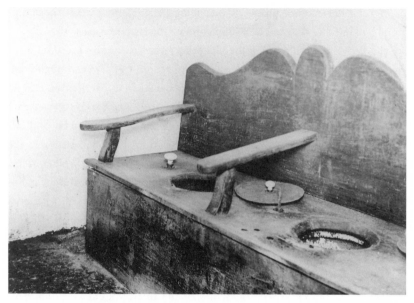

FIGURE 43. "An old Spanish type of toilet." Courtesy of the Rockefeller Archive Center.

stitious and fixed customs of Asiatic natives can be transformed" was "one of the very best things he accomplished."[70] Heiser, who had paid little attention to hookworm until then, would soon demonstrate that he could also become an indefatigable warrior in the sanitary battle against the germ of oriental laziness.

When Heiser's successor, Dr. J. D. Long, compiled the annual report of the Philippine Health Service for 1915, he scarcely mentioned hookworm, but he did include a lengthy consideration of persistent "soil pollution" in the archipelago. While climate and terrain had been exonerated as causes of ill health in the tropics, as elsewhere, it seemed native customs and habits might yet pollute and render dangerous the otherwise salubrious soil. As noted in chapter 4, Health officers feared that Filipino "promiscuous defecation" would spread the germs of typhoid and cholera—hookworm no doubt figured in their concerns, but they rarely focused on it. Attempts to install a pail system of toilets in the Philippines had failed, since it was difficult to "secure personnel for the repulsive work of collecting, dumping, and cleaning the pails, and any part of the system from the pail closet to the pit where final disposal is made, may easily become a nuisance if there is the slightest relaxation of sanitary precautions or lack of intelligent supervision."[71] The sophisticated privies favored by the Rockefeller Sanitary Commission in the United States would be far too expensive for an impoverished colony. Health authorities in the Philippines had initially resorted to a simple pit in which body wastes were deposited and covered with earth or lime, but this rapidly became a breeding place for flies. The new Antipolo closet was cheap and more effective, though Long feared the typical Filipino excretory system would soon overload it, and he warned against its use in public buildings. The director of health believed that the providing of better toilets would eventually be "far reaching beyond calculation in the education of the rising generation, who will continue the sanitary habits inculcated during their period of school life. . . . When this has come about, the nightmare of waterborne epidemics and the economic inefficiency due to intestinal parasites will have disappeared."[72]

Soon after leaving office in the Philippines, Heiser announced that "effort should be continued to control intestinal parasites, to extend malaria control work as rapidly as the field studies warrant, to encourage the use of latrines, and other campaigns to make friends for the health department."[73] Under his direction, the Philippines activities of the International Health Board, through to the early 1930s, would concentrate on medical and nursing education, hookworm eradication, and malaria control. Heiser thought these projects would prove the most effective means to "promote self-help and prosperity in a needy, (I must admit it!) exasperating, and hitherto irreconcilable people."[74] In 1922, the foundation loaned Dr. William S. Carter to the medical school at the University of the Philippines, where he acerbically evaluated and supervised the training of Filipino doctors. Later that year, the first field experiments in malaria control began, initially managed by W. D. Tiedeman and then by J. J. Mieldazis and Paul F. Russell. They would develop a malaria program that involved surveys, field research, control demonstrations, and the training of medical and subordinate personnel.[75]

In particular, the Rockefeller Foundation thought it could do better at toilet training refractory Filipinos than the increasingly Filipinized health service, with its "imitative" Filipino doctors—allegedly less fastidious and vigilant than Americans—who now were largely in charge of the civilizing mission. A hookworm survey conducted in 1922 indicated that infection had increased during the previous ten years; Filipinos apparently were still polluting the soil and avoiding latrines, especially in rural areas. Heiser lamented,"The habits of the people are such that the control of intestinal borne diseases is extremely difficult."[76] When Dr. Charles N. Leach visited Cebú in 1923, on behalf of the International Health Board, he reported that almost 80 percent of the inhabitants harbored hookworm; and yet, during the past few years, twenty-six thousand people had received treatment with carbon tetrachloride, an effective vermifuge, though sometimes toxic to the liver.[77] Leach advocated the "frequent instruction of school children residing in infected areas regarding the dangers of soil pollution and the methods by which hookworm disease can be avoided." He hoped, too, for more mass treatment with carbon tetrachloride.[78]

Traveling through the southern islands in 1922, Munson, the aging military hygienist, reported that "some of the sanitary inspectors are unquestionably inert and incompetent." They were permitting widespread soil pollution and did little to encourage latrine construction.[79] Heiser also thought the problem was not a lack of money, but the failure of Filipinos to offer "intelligent and forceful direction." There were too many councils, committees, and advisors and not enough American know-how and efficiency.[80] It seemed to Heiser that the Rockefeller Foundation might make available a better model of health work, just as his old health service had once served as an exemplar of proper conduct. At the medical school, Carter was finding it "discouraging to try to do something for people who will not do anything for themselves, and I am free to say that the inertia of these people passeth all understanding."[81] He regretted that "these people are so blinded by their mistaken ideas of patriotism that they cannot see things in the light of efficiency."[82] That the Filipino was a mere perfunctory imitator of American medical ideals became a Rockefeller litany. Of course, this was exactly what Heiser wanted to hear. In 1927, Dr. E. B. McKinlay, a representative of the International Health Board, confirmed that "it is most difficult to stimulate the native worker to do more than his daily routine work. . . . The scientific tone is in general very low." "All will agree that the mass of Filipinos represent an inferior race," he wrote to Heiser. "They are not in a position to know what's best for them."[83]

It was not until the late 1920s that the Rockefeller Foundation began to sponsor rural health demonstrations and sanitation studies in the islands. In 1928, Dr. C. F. Moriarty first suggested to Heiser the establishment of a demonstration unit for rural sanitation in Cavite province, a poor, malarious region accessible from Manila. A model system, it would make available clean water, a sanitary excreta disposal system, antilarval methods of malaria control, dispensaries, immunization programs, education, and propaganda. "The Filipino is not usually capable of independent judgment due to his environment and relative lack of culture," warned Moriarty. "He must have a routine program and should be taught only one method for each task."[84] The

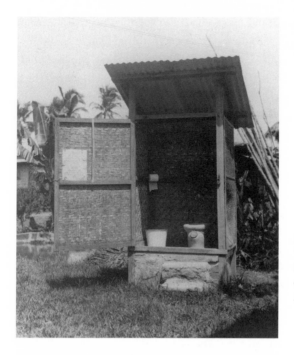

FIGURE 44.
"Build a bored-hole
latrine." Courtesy
of the Rockefeller
Archive Center.

following year, the town of Calauan, in Laguna province, was chosen as the
site for the first demonstration unit, in part because it had a death rate of
sixty-four for every thousand people, compared with twenty-six to twenty-
eight per thousand in other rural areas. The pioneer primary health care
project would improve the water supplies, investigate the suitability of various sanitary latrines, replace the sanitary inspectors with public health nurses,
develop the school health program, enforce immunization, and ensure better
mother and baby care. Heiser specifically instructed Yaeger to get rid of the
male Filipino sanitary inspectors and have the more pliant nurses conduct
"repeated intensive house-to-house public health education."[85] He hoped
that the Laguna unit would soon be "coming to grips by intimate personal
contact with health problems."[86] By the end of the year, Yaeger could report
that police were dealing with unsanitary nuisances and nurses were promoting personal and domestic hygiene, giving "special emphasis to the importance of using latrines." He was in charge of a special "boring squad" and was
delighted to point out that, thanks to the Rockefeller Foundation, "now
latrines are being built every day."[87]

Yaeger set up another demonstration unit at Navotas, in Rizal province, in
1931, where he concentrated again on ousting feckless sanitary inspectors

and boring holes for latrines. A few years earlier, when Yaeger had investigated health work at Daet, he found that the local sanitary officers spent a lot of time on "general inspection," which meant "loafing if we judge by results."[88] Both he and Heiser wanted to remove them, but they met considerable opposition. " 'Replacement by nurses,' " he wrote to an insistent Heiser, "I suppose I would dream that if latrines didn't interfere. I have had all kinds of verbal promises and suave agreements, and even letters and resolutions on the sanitary inspector problem, but excuses come in persistently."[89] Heiser became more impatient and demanded some clear evidence of success. Yaeger simply asserted that substituting public health nurses had already led to excellent results. "This is as we expected," Heiser replied. "Nurses are so much better trained, have superior access to the family, and do not have to serve as assistants to the doctors."[90] But Paul Russell pointed out there was great resentment of nurses "for enforcing the regulations regarding sanitary toilets" and ignoring local sensitivities.[91] One of these nurses has described how she went about her duties. Ignacia Limjuco promoted the importance of cleanliness and correct eating; she warned against overcrowding and poor ventilation; she was dedicated to the propagation of school hygiene and the "proper disposal of excreta." As a nurse she demanded assent to modern science, to the knowledge that an individual was "an arsenal of germs" and that the mouth was nothing more than "the gateway of infection."[92] In 1933, though, the provincial council stopped its part of the funding of nurses like Limjuco and spent the savings on the carnival. "They evidently preferred carnival exhibits," lamented Yaeger, "to saving babies and other public health work."[93] According to the Rockefeller emissaries, male Filipinos remained disobedient, willful, and childlike, fond of entertainment, decoration, and political gambits. They still did not know what was best for them.

"Politics, personal opinions, the retrenchment policy of government," explained Yaeger, "seemed to come up daily, and without any official power on my part made the work seem almost hopeless."[94] Indifference and opposition meant he was far from his goal of one hundred thousand bored holes. At times Yaeger was optimistic: "The spectacle of boring and particularly of blasting is one which appeals strongly to the people. . . . This appeal to the imagination is an important aid in attempting to persuade a community to install a large number of latrines. There is nothing dramatic about the old pit latrine."[95] But more often he was disappointed. "In one instance," he reported, "too much insistence on latrine installation resulted in an anonymous letter threatening the life of the district health officer."[96] Just before it closed

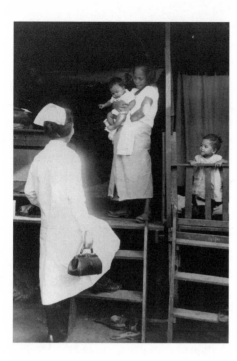

FIGURE 45. "Sanitary nurse."
Courtesy of the Rockefeller
Archive Center.

in 1934, Yaeger admitted that the Rizal health unit had been nothing but "a little volcano."[97]

In 1930, Heiser had met with Dr. Jacobo Fajardo, the new director of health in the Philippines, and tried to impress on him that "the ultimate success of health work in the Philippines would depend upon the degree of education of the masses and that the best hope there lies in a sound school health program."[98] The need for education and reform was a truism of progressive public health, and Filipinos were already well aware of its importance. A few years earlier, Dr. Agerico B. M. Sison had urged the state to teach proper care of the body and fastidious behavior in the public schools. "The masses need to be informed of the rudiments of hygiene and public health," he wrote. It was crucial that more effort be made to "inculcate the principles of hygiene and sanitation in the more plastic minds of the school-children."[99] As Fajardo announced in the commencement address at the nursing school in 1931, "Many of our major health problems now, such as infant mortality, tuberculosis and respiratory diseases, can only be satisfactorily solved with the aid of personal hygiene, which means an alteration in daily habits of the individual, and such alteration can be accomplished by one means — education." Fajardo wanted each nurse to become "exemplary as a good citizen, interested always in the best solution of public questions, social and health problems, and in everything that pertains to the community."[100] But Filipino doctors, nurses, teachers, and the subjects they were supposed to be molding would find that the achievement of self-government, of corporeal and social citizenship, was difficult to validate: for Americans like Heiser it was never quite satisfactory, always immature, and poorly imitative.

As Americans registered the performance of hygienic citizenship as inadequate or partial or perfunctory, they took it to imply that continued surveillance and discipline were required in the colony. For example, as Yaeger observed, most of the teachers whose responsibility it was to educate children about latrines themselves lived in houses without privies. "It is almost unbelievable," he wrote to Heiser, "to think that the very teachers who are following health education department instructions can keep talking latrines to the students and not make an attempt to live in houses with latrines themselves." The idea of privy-deficient teachers pretending to preach sanitation disturbed and unsettled him. They did not seem to take the message seriously. He could see no excuse "for a single teacher being allowed to teach without having a latrine."[101] Toward the end of his stay in the archipelago, Yaeger reported he was "very much disappointed in the results among the people in general of public health education. Perhaps I expect too much."[102] The Rockefeller health advisor did not believe most Filipinos were ready for self-government, whether of the body or the polity. "Level-headed persons in general," he mused, "see only a gloomy future if the present provisions for independence are not changed."[103] In 1933, after dinner in Manila, Heiser too found himself "rather exhausted this evening after a full day of struggling with the Malay mind."[104] As the archipelago moved toward independence in 1935, the Rockefeller Foundation decided to cut its losses and close down its programs.

"I was none too well impressed with the zeal or the manner in which our activities were conducted," Heiser reported in 1931 to Colonel F. F. Russell, the director of the International Health Board. "I suppose the tropics have a tendency to promote apathy."[105] Privately, Heiser noted that "our own work lacked logical planning, initiative and punch. . . . [Paul] Russell was more interested in traveling somewhere than thinking of practical malaria control. Yaeger, while doing brilliant things in the mechanics of boring holes, lacked perspective in spreading the work on an island-wide basis."[106] Yaeger had never bothered to establish the baseline for the rural health programs, so it was impossible to ascertain their effectiveness. Heiser criticized his junior

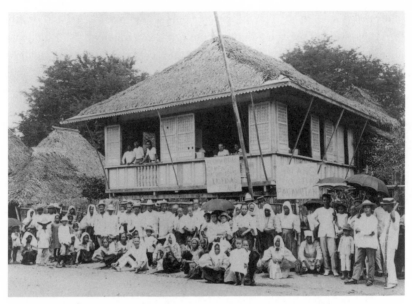

FIGURE 46. Hookworm dispensary, Las Piñas, Rizal. Courtesy of the Rockefeller Archive Center.

colleague's "inability properly to set forth his work on paper."[107] The Americans had themselves been shown up as illogical and lacking in initiative and perspective; Yaeger was demonstrating a childish fascination with boring holes everywhere. Filipino imitations of American hygiene had drawn attention to the inadequacy of the American models—were perhaps the Rockefeller emissaries themselves mimics? After all, elite Filipinos were fond of saying that the Americans were no more than flawed copies, crude imitators, of Europeans.

Americans were anxious about revealing any affiliation with the practices they regarded as typically Filipino. Paul Russell had frequently complained that "local doctors will not get their feet muddy except in cases of urgent personal necessity, as when being chased by beast or potent superior officer."[108] But his criticisms of others often turned on himself. Heiser remarked wryly that "the itinerary of your southern trip includes many of the Islands' best fishing places, at all of which there seems to be a dearth of malaria-transmitting *Anopheles*."[109] Neither Yaeger nor Russell would leave anything of value behind in the Philippines. Others fared much worse, breaking down or "going native." Moriarty, according to Heiser, "did nothing the first five or six months except consume alcohol." He refused to go out on field trips and

indicated he would like a job in India, where, it was suspected, "if no results followed the blame could be put on religion, caste, and superstition."[110]
Heiser interviewed him in Manila. "After a long diatribe against Filipino inefficiency and unreliability, and the impossibility of obtaining results," Heiser
reported, "I asked [Moriarty] point blank how much his drinking habit had
interfered with his work."[111] Moriarty resigned on the spot. But eventually
Heiser too would suffer from his interactions with the poor Filipino imitators.
His disparaging of their political activities and ceaseless self-promotion drew
attention to his own intrigues and egotism. In 1934, F. F. Russell forced him to
resign, having tired of his irritability, his scheming, his resentment of rivals,
and his claims, as a *cacique* of tropical hygiene, to own the Orient.[112] Who,
then, was imitating whom? Who was not imitative?

UNCANNY HYGIENE

Nancy Tomes has argued that in the United States during this period "notions
of public health citizenship . . . offered a seemingly neutral ground for building consensus, for purposes of both inclusion and exclusion."[113] Heiser had
dreamed of fabricating such self-possessed hygienic citizens in the Philippines,
and he had promised that, in the indefinite future, needy natives would be
transformed into a respectable proletariat. But it was hardly a neutral ground,
and frequently it seemed to him that Filipinos were subverting his designs,
that they remained incomplete, unfinished; he was fond of representing local
inhabitants as unstable hybrids, dressed natives, childish imitators. No longer simply the polar opposites of bourgeois Americans in civic decorum,
Filipinos allegedly were becoming flawed or profane copies.[114] Repeatedly
Heiser imagined hybrid Filipinos seductively attesting to their unreadiness for
self-government. In order to reveal more clearly their poor mimesis of American hygiene, Heiser tried to create islands of good conduct and rigorous
discipline in the archipelago, supervised by American doctors. The health
demonstration units in Rizal province were utopian medical microcolonies
designed, like the Culion leper colony, to produce, in the distant future, citizens who avoided promiscuous contact and forswore irresponsible habits. As
usual, Heiser expected, and indeed hoped, that American supervision and discipline would have to go on for generations before such a goal was achieved.
The medical marking of mimicry, the insistence on it as a sign of developmental delay, thus functioned still to limit boundary crossing in the Philippines
and worked to defer the entry of Filipinos into civic modernity. If Filipinos,
even Filipino doctors, were so obviously and so poorly imitative, then they

had not yet developed a fully adult American subjectivity, and could not yet be counted as authentic citizens.

"Infantile mentality is that of the men who demand for their people their immediate, complete and absolute independence!" The nationalist politician Claro M. Recto was addressing the Philippine Senate in 1933. "Maturity of judgment that of those who favor the law of colonialism! What thoughts are these?"[115] When Recto spoke to the graduating class of the University of the Philippines, some thirty years after Tavera had offered a homily on the danger of *ignorantismo*, he condemned his compatriots for "parroting the slogans and mimicking the gestures of American foreign policy."[116] He also lamented that "many of our countrymen have assiduously cultivated a servile mentality." But "those of us who pretend to be Americans risk only the ridicule and laughter of their so-called brothers behind their backs."[117]

At the same time, a critical awareness of mimicry, of the uncanny sense of the copy, could also challenge the boundaries of citizenship in the colony. Supposedly mimetic performance might serve, at this deeper level, to reveal the artificiality, the play, of conventional distinctions between native and other, to illuminate and make strange the "cultured self" of colonized and colonialist—in the case of the latter, to disturb a narcissistic overvaluation of his own mental processes, to eat away at his sense of authenticity and control. There were moments when the whole project of colonial hygiene and bodily reform came to appear a little silly, and self-proclaimed models of fastidious conduct realized that they looked foolish, inadequate, and self-deceiving. Surrounded by perceived imitation, the constructedness of their own identity was, on occasion, revealed to colonial officials and Rockefeller emissaries in the Philippines. In imagining profane copies of themselves, they would experience an uncanny doubling. In 1919, Sigmund Freud had described the uncanny as the secretly familiar that has been repressed and then returns in a distorted form.[118] In particular, the figure of the Filipino imitator of hygiene was revealing what ought to have remained hidden, that which Americans had sought to overcome or repress in themselves: their own supposedly infantile or primitive or underdeveloped elements, the abject that returns repeatedly to disturb identity.

Chapter Eight

MALARIA BETWEEN RACE AND ECOLOGY

As early as the 1920s, ideas of racial difference were losing some of their explanatory power in Philippine medical science. For most Filipino physicians, hookworm had become a disease of poverty, not the manifestation of Filipinos' innate incapacity for hygiene—not, therefore, a sign of racial inferiority. Leprosy seemed ever more curable, and soon individual lepers might assume their rights as citizens beyond the confines of Culion. Self-government of body and polity was increasingly related to educational and economic improvement. The latrine had joined the ballot box as a domestic possibility. As the old racial impediments to progress began to dissolve, some medicos gained confidence in the capacity of Filipinos—even the masses—to inhabit the archipelago with propriety. There was less reason than ever to assert that the race would be permanently arrested somewhere on the imagined trajectory from native to citizen. At the same time, white mentality could seem just as generic and mundanely conflicted as any other: tropical neurasthenia was dwindling into Freudian neurosis. Moreover, whites were not the only people capable of elaborate brain-work; not all natives were entirely slaves to their id. Of course, many experts were still resisting any such decline in the valence of race. The changes in scientific reasoning were gradual, at times scarcely perceptible. American discussions of hygiene, in particular, still regularly invoked allegedly racial customs and habits and biological limits to reform. But social, economic, and ecological explanations of disease, and indeed of civilizational achievement, did nonetheless gain some ground during the 1920s, and not only in the Philippines.

In the late 1920s, even Victor G. Heiser could on occasion be diverted from the familiar comforts of racial prejudice. In conversations with Filipino physicians, he too began occasionally to identify the masses, not the race, as the focal point of hygiene education.[1] During the Depression, the old race warrior told Theodore Roosevelt, Jr., then governor-general of the islands, that "lifting the economic level . . . would probably do more for the health of the Philippines than any other measure."[2] Improved nutrition would reduce beriberi directly and moderate the impact of other diseases. According to Heiser, the International Health Board of the Rockefeller Foundation had avoided efforts to involve the Philippines government in a tuberculosis campaign "on account of its great cost and the probability of poor results so long as the economic standards of the Islands are so low."[3] But more commonly, Heiser still clung to theories that postulated inherent racial limits to Filipino accomplishment in hygiene. Social and economic explanations had begun to infiltrate his etiological reasoning and to contaminate his health advice, yet they never entirely displaced the racial disparagement so commonplace in his work. In his accounts of the civic status of lepers, the toilet habits of all Filipinos, and the attainments of local physicians, race would keep reasserting its prominence well into the 1930s.

The response to malaria — never a major interest of Heiser's — perhaps illustrates best the more general and gradual displacement of race and the rising enthusiasm for ecological investigation and technical intervention. In the early twentieth century, the racial factor had still dominated explanations of malaria outbreaks: control of the disease was predicated on the identification and treatment of native carriers of the causative plasmodium. Thus Major Charles Woodruff, as we have seen, warned in 1903 that asymptomatic Filipino soldiers were the main "source of fatal infection to white men" in the Philippines, since the foreigners lacked their racial immunity.[4] Others pointed to the dangers posed by apparently healthy Filipino children, most of them loaded with malaria parasites. When Dr. Charles Craig investigated an outbreak of malaria at Fort William McKinley, he concluded that "the greatest source of danger to the white man in a malarial locality lies in the native population, especially in the native children." Therefore, it would be futile to attempt to "rid any locality of malaria so long as the native element in the question is neglected."[5] If Camp Stotsenberg was always malarious, it must have been because the local, apparently healthy inhabitants constituted a persistent reservoir of plasmodia upon which the *Anopheles* mosquito might draw. But by the 1920s, the contribution of this "native element" had virtually disappeared from the etiological calculus. Instead, malariologists, mostly from the Rockefeller Foundation, were focusing on mosquito distribution and behavior and on the influence of agricultural development on vector population and patterns. They were testing new larvicides, such as Paris Green, and manipulating the environment in order to control, or even eradicate, mosquitoes. Technological enthusiasm was displacing racialist anthropology as the chief determinant of what might be achieved. Dosing reluctant races with quinine was not forgotten, but mosquito control usually came to take priority.

Race was not so much deconstructed and abandoned as put aside in favor of the exploration of local ecologies. The human factor, whether defined as race, population, or community, had simply come to seem a less important part of the malaria equation. This hardly represented an explicit critique of the idea of race. Indeed, as we have seen in previous chapters, where hygiene and human development were concerned race could remain very much in play. Ecological and technical approaches thus came to supplement, not to substitute for, racialist assumptions in international health and development before World War II. Nowhere is this odd symbiosis more evident than in the tensions between the Rockefeller Foundation's efforts to control hookworm *racially* and malaria *ecologically* in the colonial Philippines.

RACE OR ECOLOGY?

The relative merits of quinine and vector control had been disputed since the 1890s. It had become clear by then that quinine, used as a general febrifuge since the seventeenth century, was also a specific toxin for the malaria parasites, or plasmodia, which Alphonse Laveran identified in 1880. Patrick Manson soon suggested a role for mosquitoes in the transmission of plasmodia, modeled on his mosquito-vector theory of filariasis, but he continued to believe that humans ingested the parasites only after mosquitoes deposited them in water. In 1897, however, Ronald Ross reported from India that he had found malaria parasites in the bellies of *Anopheles*, and the next year he determined that the mosquitoes could transmit them directly to birds.[6] These discoveries implied two key measures that might reduce the spread of malaria: dosing of affected or vulnerable populations with quinine; and the control or eradication of *Anopheles*. More of a naturalist than most physicians, Ross advocated further investigation of the mode of life of mosquitoes, which would inform efforts to destroy them.[7] But it took some time before this ecological advice was heeded in the colonial Philippines: malaria control in the archipelago initially tended to follow racial contours, tracing familiar lines of human isolation and selective dosing with quinine.

Malaria was endemic in the Philippines, causing significant mortality and much more widespread morbidity. On occasion, war, famine, or development could whip it up into major epidemics: in 1903, after the Philippine-American War, more than one hundred thousand people died of malaria — even in the 1930s, though, more than ten thousand were succumbing to the disease each year.[8] The parasite was primarily *vivax*, though *falciparum* was well represented too. The mosquitoes that carried plasmodia evidently preferred the foothills, where mountain streams emerge from the jungles, for there malaria was most prevalent. Unlike many other mosquito vectors, they avoided swamps and marshes, so drainage never made any impact on the disease's incidence. It seems unlikely that Manila, a low-lying metropolis, was ever malarious, though it felt as though it should be, and there were always cases in the city's hospitals.

From the beginning of the occupation, the U.S. Army recommended mosquito netting for its soldiers and on rare occasions prophylactic quinine for those stationed in especially malarious places. At the Lucena Barracks men were court-martialed for not using their mosquito nets properly.[9] But the mosquito bars proved difficult to set up in field tents, and in any case their mesh was often too wide and their coverage inadequate. Weston Chamberlain complained that on some mornings he caught as many as forty engorged mosquitoes within these course, short nets.[10] Not surprisingly, then, attention turned to the nearby meretriciously healthy native hosts of the malaria parasite. In 1904, Major W. D Crosby, M.D., reported from Camp Stotsenberg, "There are a few cases of malaria, which will appear at this post which it is apparently impracticable to prevent, and these are the cases in which the men are infected in the native barrios in the evening. The barrios are situated on running water and the malaria mosquitoes are very numerous, and these are mostly infected mosquitoes, from the fact that most of the natives are full of malaria."[11] Crosby's accurate identification of the mosquito's habitat was prescient, but like his colleagues he believed that vector control was impractical. Instead, he recommended the separation of troops from infected Filipinos and regular dosing of the whole *barrio* with quinine.

When a new battalion arrived at Camp Stotsenberg in 1906, the soldiers, like others before them, soon found their mosquito bars were ineffective; and before long, more than 150 troops came down with malaria. The authorities decided to move the men into hastily constructed bamboo quarters, but evidently the new buildings "harbored mosquitoes and permitted them to breed in bamboo joints." As more men contracted the disease, the post commander finally decided to issue prophylactic quinine, and within days the outbreak was controlled.[12] At the same time, sanitary officers filled in or oiled stagnant pools and covered or screened receptacles for drinking water. In order to eliminate malaria from the camp, the investigating surgeon thought "the removal of all native barrios existing within the reservation" would eventually be necessary.[13] During this period, Craig, in a series of papers, established — or rather, reconfirmed — the menace to the soldier of the native carrier of malaria.[14] Around Camp Stotsenberg, for example, 50 percent of the Filipino children and 60 percent of adults had latent malarial infection.[15] The army would therefore continue to insist on mosquito netting in the barracks and a *cordon sanitaire* around its bases; and when this policy failed, it demanded the treatment or removal of any Filipinos in the vicinity of soldiers.

Unlike the army, the Bureau of Health initially expressed little concern at the prevalence of malaria in the islands. In part, this complacency reflected the relative rarity of clinical malaria in the capital; and in part it indicated the gravity of the threat from other diseases, such as cholera, smallpox, leprosy, and dysentery. Still, some perfunctory, and perhaps misdirected, efforts eventually were taken to reduce malaria transmission. In 1905 the bureau reported extensive oiling of mosquito breeding places in Manila. It recommended, too, that the fetid moat around Intramuros be filled to reduce the chances of malaria infection — at the time it seemed a typical site for the breeding of malarial mosquitoes.[16] Yet malaria was not transmitted in Manila. After 1906, the bureau decided instead to distribute free quinine to Filipinos across the archipelago in the hope this would reduce the incidence of the disease. More than two million doses of quinine were distributed during 1910 just in the provinces of Albay and Ambos Camarines. The schools began a vigorous educational campaign, emphasizing the danger of mosquitoes and the need for netting at night. No one, though, was sure if these projects had any impact on the death rate; few seemed to care. In general, Heiser did not regard malaria as a disease of spectacular importance, or its possible control as offering any enhancement of his reputation. He was more concerned with leprosy.

Around 1910, a few of the health officers and scientists in the Philippines began to investigate mosquito control more seriously. C. S. Ludlow gradually elucidated the character of the Philippines *Culicidae*, differentiating the various species, while others attempted to determine which of them transmitted malaria. When outbreaks occurred, more emphasis now was placed on mosquito reduction than on quinine treatment or prophylaxis. At the Olongapo naval base, one man in ten was unfit for service because of malaria during the year 1910. The narrow mosquito nets gave imperfect protection. But once breeding places were filled and cleared and quarters thoroughly screened, the admission rate for malaria plummeted.[17] A year later, inspectors from the Bureau of Health reported that San José, Mindoro, suffered a 40 percent morbidity from malaria. Long known as "the white man's grave," Mindoro had for three hundred years resisted the efforts of Europeans and Americans to exploit its exceptionally fertile soil. The health officers proposed control measures that mostly targeted mosquitoes, including drainage, clearing of vegetation, screening of doors and windows, and oiling of stagnant water — though quinine prophylaxis still had a place. Of all these measures, effective screening was probably responsible for the subsequent (evanescent) dip in malaria mortality.[18] A later investigating team did reassert the importance of the "systematic treatment of all persons (compulsory if necessary) harboring the malaria parasite" and the prevention of reinfection by "the importation of malaria-free laborers and by restricting the intercourse between inhabitants of the protected zone and infected persons in nearby territory." But quarantine and compulsory treatment seemed too difficult to organize. Instead, the Mindoro plantation companies took up the more practical recommendations for the reduction of anopheline mosquitoes, which the investigators had suggested would finally break the chain between the infected and the "non-immune" person.[19]

After 1912, the Bureau of Health conducted successive campaigns to reduce mosquito numbers in Manila, fining householders who allowed any stagnant water to collect or any rank vegetation to grow. A bulletin from the bureau, issued in 1913, urged all residents to destroy the breeding places of mosquitoes: no water should be left standing for more than forty-eight hours before it was drained or oiled. The bureau also recommended that houses be fumigated regularly with sulfur, or else smudge fires might be lit to smoke out the insects. But "since it is a difficult matter to eradicate mosquitoes entirely," residents were still advised to consider taking prophylactic quinine. Above all, anyone sick with malaria must always be kept under nets and screens, away from any surviving mosquitoes.[20] That same year, the bureau proudly announced the arrival in the archipelago of mosquito-eating fish from Hono-lulu.[21] By 1914, health authorities had come to the conclusion that "at best, of course, quinine distribution can only be palliative and the problem resolves itself into preventing the breeding of mosquitoes that carry malaria."[22]

Also in 1914, E. L. Walker and M. A. Barber described experiments that had determined the susceptibility of four Philippine *Anopheles* to malaria infection. They found that the *minimus-flavirostris* subgroup (which they called *febrifer*) was by far the most prone to midgut infections with plasmodia.[23] This mosquito was abundant in the shaded brooks of Laguna, though it also frequented irrigation ditches with overhanging banks. It liked to breed in fresh, flowing water in ditches, brooks, and rivers and enjoyed resting at the banks of streams and the edges of islets of grass. The investigators regarded as futile, therefore, older efforts to combat the mosquitoes who favored stagnant pools and rice fields: these were not the malarial culprits. Barber and his colleagues recommended that "antimalarial measures should be based upon a thorough anopheles and malaria survey, and those measures should be employed which will best meet the conditions. The best single measure is the destruction of the larvae of malaria carriers, and in this work the breeding places of the stream-breeder should receive first attention."[24] Even so, for the following decade most medical officers did not heed this advice, preferring to resort conventionally to the drainage of swamps, marshes, and still water in order to reduce mosquito numbers — or, simply, to quinine.

The equivocation between mosquito control and quininization was hardly unique to the Philippines. Most colonial health officers in the early twentieth century were prepared to try many different measures to reduce malaria, but they were often constrained by ecological ignorance or financial pressures. Metropolitan theorists could afford to be more abstract and absolute, usually demanding either mosquito control or quinine and segregation.[25] Robert Koch, who led a German malaria expedition to East Africa and New Guinea in 1898–99, had been the leading advocate of systematic mass prophylaxis with quinine. He firmly believed that partially immune native children represented a reservoir of infection for nearby white men and urged colonial authorities to dose them thoroughly with quinine. A trial at Stephansort, New Guinea, in 1900 proved successful, although too expensive to become routine. British malariologists, often with Indian experience, continued to heed Koch's advice, in part because it resonated with long-standing racial assumption, clinical interest, and enclavist practice. Thus J. W. W. Stephens, a lecturer in tropical medicine at Liverpool, warned that malaria is a contagious disease.

Moreover, "the source of the contagion . . . lies in the fact that in the tropics the native population, especially the child population, carries malarial parasites in its blood; that it does so often while presenting not the least outward sign of sickness. It is this apparently healthy but actually highly infected population which is the greatest source of malarial parasites, and hence of danger to the European." Stephens disputed the practicality and value of mosquito control, urging instead the use of netting, limited quinine prophylaxis, and segregation, especially the "removal of native bazaars with their infected population from the vicinity of European barracks."[26]

Ronald Ross, in contrast, was an untiring advocate of mosquito control measures. He could cite the moderately successful experiment in Freetown, Sierra Leone, in 1901 in which the number of mosquitoes diminished and malaria incidence seemed to fall for a time. But he was dismayed when his opponents pointed to the attempt, in 1902, to reduce mosquitoes at Mian Mir, in India — the enterprise appeared to him halfhearted, and more mosquitoes soon displaced the few eliminated. "Work like this at Mian Mir only tends to arrest enthusiasm in the cause without really adding anything definite to our knowledge," he claimed.[27] More than twenty-five years later he was still lamenting that "it was probably the worst type of country for a test case." According to Ross, "doctors to the right of me, doctors to the left of me, laughed at the mere notion of reducing mosquitoes."[28] More inspiring was Malcolm Watson's somewhat quixotic attack on Malayan mosquitoes. In 1901, as government surgeon in Klang District, Selangor, Watson decided it was unrealistic to expect feckless Chinese to take quinine regularly, so he embarked upon a campaign of drainage and filling. It proved a "fortunate choice" and soon rendered the adjacent town of Port Swettenham far less malarious. A few years later, Watson associated his success with the more celebrated efforts to eradicate mosquitoes from the Panama Canal Zone — which were "without question the most brilliant achievement in Preventive Medicine which the tropics, and for that matter the whole world, has seen."[29] Ross, in reflecting on Watson's work, also endorsed his view of the importance of Panama as an example. It suggested to him that colonial administration was changing: "We are passing away from the older period of incessant wars and great military or civil dictatorships into one of more minute and scientific administration."[30]

Few medical officers in the Philippines would have followed closely the debates over mosquito control and quininization; but they all knew about William Gorgas's campaign to eradicate mosquitoes from Panama.[31] As chief sanitary officer of Havana, Cuba, at the end of Spanish-American War, Major Gorgas had based his campaign against yellow fever on the recent confirmation — by Walter Reed, James Carroll, and Jesse Lazear of the U.S. Army and Aristides Agramonte — of Carlos Finlay's theory that the mosquito *Culex fasciatis* (later *Aedes aegypti*) was the transmitter of the disease.[32] Gorgas therefore put yellow fever patients in screened rooms, removed water receptacles, and burned pyrethrum in the houses — soon Havana was free of yellow jack and also far less malarious. In charge of sanitary work in the Panama Canal Zone, Gorgas continued his fight against the mosquito. When Ross visited Gorgas in 1904, he found a "spare, resolute man of the best type," a progressive sanitary officer committed to eliminating the vector of malaria.[33] Gorgas insisted on draining marshes and swamps, cutting brush and grass, oiling still water, spreading soluble larvicide, screening quarters, and swatting adult mosquitoes. The measures proved effective, reducing malaria and allowing the construction of a canal, though too expensive for regular use. Here, nonetheless, was a model of successful disease control through ecological intervention — decades later, Paul F. Russell recalled the "tremendous impression that Gorgas made by his sanitary victories in Havana and Panama."[34]

While the British (apart from Ross and Watson) still tended to regard malaria as a racial disease, Americans after 1910 were becoming more interested in its ecological character. No doubt the American tendency derived in part from the shining example of Gorgas; but experience in the Philippines was also confirming their predilection for technical intervention into the patterns of life of the relevant mosquitoes. Of course, in practice, local health officers would continue to try both quinine and vector control — and anything else that seemed worthwhile at the time — in order to subdue malaria. There were no methodological purists in the field. Still, as Lewis Hackett, from the International Health Board, recollected, the British leaned toward mitigation and Americans increasingly came to push for mosquito eradication.[35]

ROCKEFELLER EXPERTISE

Like hookworm, malaria was a familiar disease in the southern parts of the United States. Although its range and incidence had diminished during the late nineteenth century, malaria still killed thousands of Americans each year. From 1912, Henry R. Carter, who had served in Panama with Gorgas, and R. H. von Ezdorf, both from the U.S. Public Health Service, began planning experiments in malaria control in the South. They established a malaria headquarters at Mobile, Alabama, and organized pilot programs at Roanoke Rapids, North Carolina, and Electric Mills, Mississippi, using the conventional, pragmatic combination of drainage, screening, and quinine. By 1915, Wickliffe Rose, the director of the International Health Commission of the Rockefeller Foundation, was expressing interest in developing more rigorous field trials of mosquito control and quininization in the South. Malaria, like hookworm, appeared to offer the foundation a means of seeding state health activity in the poorer parts of the country.[36]

Rose emphasized the importance and practicality of prevention either "by protecting people from being bitten by mosquitoes, or by destroying the parasite in the blood of the human carrier."[37] In 1916, a field experiment at Crossett, a low-lying lumber town in southern Arkansas, concentrated on *Anopheles* reduction, through drainage of breeding places and removal of undergrowth and vegetation. "A serious menace to health and working efficiency," malaria accounted for almost 60 percent of medical attendances in the county. The first effect of the vector control measures was the virtual elimination of mosquitoes as a pest; and within six months it was evident that malaria incidence had declined by more than 70 percent. The Rockefeller Foundation reproduced this field trial in other Arkansas towns over the following two years and found a similar alleviation of morbidity. Rose concluded that "malaria control in such communities, considered merely as a business proposition, pays."[38] It cost far less to reduce mosquito numbers than to pay doctors' bills, which were just a small part of the total cost of malaria. Outside the towns, however, mosquito control was less cost-effective. Screening, along with occasional quinine, appeared more practical. Rose reported on a field trial of screening at a group of cotton plantations near Lake Village, Arkansas, a region with high malaria incidence. The cabins on the plantations were ramshackle and difficult to protect against mosquitoes, but carpenters managed to cover most of the holes with galvanized wire cloth. Within a year, the infection rate had dropped from 12 percent to 4 percent, at little cost to the plantation owner.[39]

Inevitably, the Rockefeller Foundation became entangled in the racial politics of malaria in the South. As in the Philippines, the idea of the typical malaria carrier had racial intonations; like Filipinos, African-Americans came to be represented as a biological type that favored plasmodial carriage. Many physicians in the South were more interested in the elimination of human carriers than in apparently expensive and perhaps futile mosquito control.[40] At the urging of Dr. C. C. Bass, a New Orleans physician, the Rockefeller Foundation therefore began in 1916 a field trial of quininization in Bolivar

County and later in Sunflower County, Mississippi. A survey of thirty thousand Bolivar residents revealed that malaria carriers were common: evidently treatment of acute attacks with quinine or "chill tonics" had not sterilized the blood of most victims. The project leaders ensured that carriers received adequate quinine dosages for eight weeks to destroy the parasites. In Sunflower County, a patchwork of sluggish streams, bayous, and swamps, blacks outnumbered whites by four to one, and the predominant industry was cotton. Malaria was endemic, some 70 percent of all sickness disability on the plantations being attributed to this disease alone. A Rockefeller survey in 1918 indicated that more than 40 percent of tenant farmers suffered from clinical malaria within the previous twelve months, and a further 20 percent carried plasmodia. All those who had contracted malaria or who carried the disease parasite received eight weeks of supervised treatment. A marked decline soon occurred in malaria cases, but the demonstration proved too expensive and difficult to sustain. The investigators despaired that blacks were not intelligent enough to take medicine without instruction.[41] Rose, however, maintained high hopes for further field investigations of various strategies of malaria control in the South and perhaps in the Philippines.

When Heiser amplified Rockefeller Foundation involvement in the Philippines in the 1920s, after the installation of Leonard Wood as governor-general, malaria control was among the programs he developed. The Philippine experiments in mosquito suppression thus paralleled — and sometimes anticipated — the more celebrated Rockefeller work in Italy. Heiser assigned W. D. Tiedemann, a sanitary engineer, to malaria control in the Philippines in 1922, two years before the establishment of the Stazione Sperimentale per la Lotta Antimalarica in Italy. By 1928, Rockefeller activities in the archipelago were coalescing into the new School of Sanitation and Public Health in Manila, whereas the Italian Instituto di Sanità Pubblica did not open until 1934. Darwin H. Stapleton has argued that the attempt to eradicate *Anopheles* from Sardinia in the 1940s "became a source of standards by which eradication efforts throughout the world were measured."[42] One of the leaders of the Sardinian efforts was Paul F. Russell, who learned his skills in the Philippines years earlier. The standards he enforced in the Mediterranean were hard-won Philippine lessons. Heiser had made sure that the International Health Board of the Rockefeller Foundation used the Philippines, his old stamping ground, as a test bed for many of its international health projects, whether in racial development (as in hookworm prevention) or ecological intervention (as in malaria control).[43]

On arriving in the archipelago, Tiedemann set about establishing a laboratory in Los Baños and conducting malaria and mosquito surveys in nearby towns. The survey was always the initial technology of malaria control, just as the census had been the first tool of the health service and intelligence the necessary primary activity of an advancing army. In surveying the Del Carmen section of Pampanga province, Tiedemann found plentiful *Anopheles*, widespread malaria, and inadequate treatment facilities. Two freshwater species, *A. minimus* and *A. ludlowii*, seemed the most dangerous vectors of the malaria parasite. Tiedemann experimented with various methods of larval destruction, including poisons, top minnows (*Dermogenes*), and cannibalistic mosquito larvae (*Lutzia fuscana*)—but only the new Paris Green seemed to have any effect.[44] He discounted the extensive use of quinine as a prophylactic measure, since he believed it would require military discipline for it to be taken regularly, and that now appeared unlikely.[45] Tiedemann's successor, J. J. Mieldazis, another sanitary engineer, also endorsed the use of Paris Green in vector control. In 1924, Mieldazis and his staff of sixteen, including a field director, a microscopist, inspectors, and sanitary engineers, began to expand the malaria control demonstration in the Del Carmen area. They collected *Anopheles*, studying the mosquitoes' habitat and characteristics, and confirmed the effectiveness of Paris Green. In surveys of Mindoro, Bataan, Culion, and Laguna, Mieldazis found plenty of malaria, especially along the rivers and streams favored by *A. minimus*.[46] "I am convinced," he wrote in 1928, "that control of malaria here means control of the *A. minimus* breeding places only. We can now determine whether a community is malarious simply by the presence of *minimus*."[47]

On the surface, it was a meritorious scheme: *A. minimus* larval control with Paris Green and minor drainage, and, secondarily, carrier elimination with targeted use of quinine or plasmodin. But when Heiser visited the control demonstrations in Pampanga, he privately expressed skepticism and frustration: the projects seemed too costly, and their efficacy was not proven. "It was," he wrote, "difficult to judge the value of control work owing to the constantly shifting population."[48] In particular, it proved impossible to determine how many deaths there were from malaria, as few autopsies were performed. Moreover, "the doctors do not care to do field work, and laborers and inspectors become lax and control measures are not dependable."[49] Laborers, struggling with the blower, were not fastidious in spraying Paris Green, and probably fewer than 15 percent of those given quinine actually took it.[50] While the incidence of the disease fell where larval control was attempted, so too was it falling elsewhere without any intervention. In a

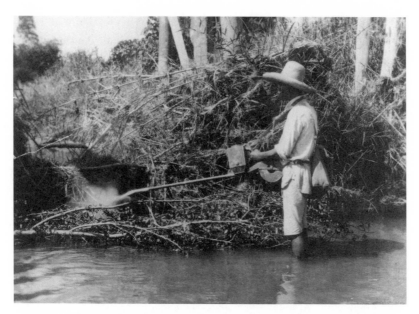

FIGURE 47. Spraying Paris Green, 1926. Courtesy of the Rockefeller Archive Center.

statistical review of the project at the Rockefeller Foundation, Persis Putnam declared that the reports from Mieldazis and C. F. Moriarty, his field director, were "more unsatisfactory than any I have attempted to work with," and she condemned their "lack of system." The accuracy of the figures was dubious, and no one had provided an adequate control site.[51] In response, Heiser weakly defended Mieldazis, arguing that he had accomplished "more important work than the reports indicate."[52] But in 1929, when C. H. Yaeger interrupted his latrine boring to act as a temporary replacement for Mieldazis, he complained that even after a thorough review of the data he could not "draw any conclusions as to why malaria has increased or decreased in any area."[53] Publicly, Yaeger put a positive veneer on the shambles: "Malaria control work during the past couple of years has been done for the purpose of demonstrating practical control measures, and not as a detailed scientific study of the malaria problem. These early demonstrations led the way to increased activity to control the disease throughout the Philippines." In an attempt to justify the lack of complete records and controls, he claimed that "the fact was that people were suffering from malaria and we wanted to give them relief."[54]

Cost was always a special concern for Heiser. Typically, he calculated that if the malaria control measures came to encompass the archipelago it would cost over seventeen cents per capita, when the total expenditure on health work was currently twenty-seven cents per capita.[55] He later concluded there was "a very general feeling that much money has now been spent . . . on studies and so little accomplished in controlling the disease. The great outstanding obstacle to control is its cost."[56] While the present expense of vector control schemes appeared to rule out their broad application, Heiser believed they might still prove useful in specific government projects, private *haciendas*, and commercial enterprises.

"We are coming to the conclusion," Heiser wrote in 1927 to Jacobo Fajardo, the director of health, "that after the method of control has once been thoroughly established it should be carried out by the regular health service and not by a specially organized malaria squad."[57] Evidently, Heiser was eager to off-load the malaria control project and to limit his staff in the Philippines to occasional field surveys and the training of local physicians, nurses, and inspectors. The Philippine Health Service, with Rockefeller support, obligingly established a new malaria control section, with Dr. C. Manalang as director. It took over the troubled demonstration units and set up others at Calauan, Laguna; San José, Mindoro; Zamboanga, Mindanao; and Novaliches, Rizal. These units continued to concentrate on mosquito surveys and spraying the habitat of *A. minimus* with Paris Green. But it was tedious, expensive, and unrewarding work. Manalang was never sure if a fall in malaria incidence was the result of natural fluctuations, quinine, or Paris Green. The rates normally increased again soon afterward anyhow.[58] The U.S. Army was having more success with vector eradication. After thoroughly applying Paris Green to Camp Stotsenberg — and after thirty years of futile intervention — the number of malaria admissions to the hospital finally had fallen dramatically, from four hundred each year to fewer than twenty.[59]

PAUL RUSSELL AND THE ECOLOGY OF CONTROL

Paul Russell arrived in Manila late in 1929, with instructions to replace E. B. McKinley as the Rockefeller Foundation's "laboratory man" at the ailing Bureau of Science and to find time to conduct experiments on malaria control. Heiser and other Rockefeller emissaries liked to deplore the decline in scientific standards at the bureau since Filipinos came to dominate it. In particular, during the Depression they worried that it was turning into a merely practical institution, driven by industrial needs. Russell confirmed that there was in the archipelago "no longer any government laboratory in which pure research in theoretical science may be pursued." The Bureau of Science had degenerated into "a fourth-rate museum, a testing and measuring labora-tory, an uninspired manufactory of germs and vaccines, and a place where men will play at industrial research."[60] In contrast, he was supposed to repre-sent the exemplary white American scientist. As Selskar M. Gunn, at the Rockefeller Foundation, put it, "Through excessive Philipinization [*sic*] of the staff and weak direction, it [the Bureau of Science] has deteriorated enor-mously and its future as a research institute seems to me very dubious."[61] Only Americans like Russell, an "activator of research," according to Heiser, might salvage it.[62] Indeed, regardless of the obstacles, Russell soon began investigations into the transmission of malaria among birds, the model Ross had used thirty years before.

Russell initially sought to distance himself from the sloppy fieldwork of the Rockefeller demonstration units, now under the authority of the Philippines Health Service. "The records of past work," he wrote to Heiser, "are a hope-less mess from which it is practically impossible to ascertain anything at all." Even though he felt sure that "the previous work here has had a very benefi-cial and stimulating effect on malaria control," it was not an effect that would ever prove scientifically demonstrable.[63] Before long, though, Russell was taking more interest in malaria control projects. He agreed with Governor Roosevelt that "malaria control as an activity of the Health Service should follow soil sanitation and anti-tuberculosis (including nutritional) endeavors. But malaria control requires a great deal of attention, nevertheless." Russell soon recommended a new, more localized scheme, one with greater commu-nity participation. To Paris Green he would add more effective treatment with quinine, the use of netting, and educational efforts. "The present centralized unit control system," he told Heiser, "has proved to be a total failure."[64] Sending out a special control unit from the central government paralyzed local initiative — "or if by some miracle it does reduce the malaria there is a prompt recurrence when the unit leaves a year or two later." Instead, Russell wanted to engage community leaders, not lazy, fee-obsessed Filipino medicos, and develop a corps of "unimaginative laborers under lay supervision." "I feel strongly that control work must be locally desired and locally carried out," the young malariologist concluded. "The work of a central malaria control division should be advisory, experimental and instructive."[65]

Despite his professed disdain for previous demonstration projects, Russell soon embarked on his own control program. But the project at the Iwahig Prison Colony, on Palawan, necessarily would lack the community involve-ment he had earlier stipulated. Nonetheless, just as the nearby microcolony at

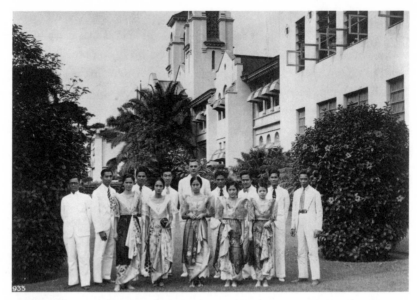

FIGURE 48. Dr. Paul F. Russell and local personnel, Manila 1933. Courtesy of the Rockefeller Archive Center.

Culion had proven to be an exemplary site for the "recovery" of lepers, so the microcolony at Iwahig might demonstrate the technics of malaria control—only without genuine local initiative and leadership. The great advantage of Iwahig was that the prisoners did not move about much and were easily controlled. The Spanish had settled there long ago, but intermittent fever eventually caused them to abandon the site. After the prison colony was established in 1904, it was never free of malaria, despite the health services' regular efforts to control the disease with prophylactic quinine and drainage works.[66] Russell had noticed Iwahig in 1933 while touring the southern islands, fishing and collecting mosquitoes. Heiser urged him to try out his new control scheme at the prison colony: "Unless malaria can be controlled at Iwahig, where the personnel is under discipline, the prospects for doing it elsewhere in the Philippines are not very encouraging."[67] Russell had access to decades of medical records at Iwahig and a docile population to work on, so he could make sure his demonstration project produced valid results. He organized the prison authorities to spray Paris Green, dosed the inmates with Atebrin, a new antimalaria drug, told them about the role of mosquitoes in transmitting disease, introduced netting, and continued drainage operations. By early 1935, when the project was abandoned, the incidence of malaria had fallen greatly.[68]

At the time, Russell believed it was pointless to administer quinine outside the disciplined conditions of an institution like Iwahig. "All available evidence," he wrote, "indicates that drug control of malaria is impossible from a practical standpoint in the Philippines as elsewhere."[69] According to Russell, "The difficulties of getting a large group of civilians to take anti-malarial drugs systematically are as insurmountable in these Islands as elsewhere."[70] He disagreed with Manalang, who now favored quininization, believing the masses would adhere to a drug regimen if it was explained to them; Paris Green, in contrast, Manalang thought either ineffective or too costly.[71] Russell, in response, argued that the demonstration projects had proven the value of larval control—or "species sanitation," as it was now called—and bitter experience indicated that Filipinos could not be trusted with quinine. "There is no evidence that without larval control malaria rates can be lowered much below their present level in these Islands," Russell concluded. "Control in decades rather than years should be expected." Moreover, in the tropics, "no more permanence may be anticipated in malaria control than in road repairs or water sterilization."[72] In a dig at his Filipino colleagues in the health service, Russell insisted that such long-term control must be carried out by engineers and entomologists, "and not by physicians, who in the Eastern Tropics, at least, show little aptitude for such work." Echoing Heiser, the Rockefeller emissary remarked, "The average physician, whether or not he is called a health officer, dislikes to get his hands, his feet, or his white collar muddy and he is rarely qualified for anti-mosquito supervision."[73]

When the International Health Division began to withdraw from the Philippines in 1934, Russell took the unexpended funds with him to Madras, India, where he continued his experiments in malaria control. Initially, he was dismayed that "dogma and superstition" prevailed in India even more than in the Philippines. But he praised incipient efforts to eliminate mosquito breeding places across the subcontinent. Although the "so-called 'lesson' of Mian Mir" had delayed larval destruction in India, health authorities were slowly coming to recognize its value. In contrast, the attempt to use quinine to control malaria was an abject failure. Since 1933, at Memari in the Bengal Presidency, a treatment experiment had struggled along. "As in all other control-by-treatment experiments thus far recorded, so in Memari, such adverse factors as the opposition of quacks and some physicians, expense and practical difficulties of distribution, and the usual public aversion to repeated dosage with any drug, however freely offered, have combined to curtail sharply the results theoretically possible." Instead, Russell planned to set up a trial of mosquito control, using "naturalistic methods" adapted to the local ecology, just as he had in the Philippines.[74] At Kasangadu, in the Madras Presidency, Russell and Fred W. Knipe began to spray with a pyrethrum mixture in order to kill the adult vector species, which preferred houses and outhouses for daytime rest. Human infection rates soon fell from 68 percent to 24 percent, but it seemed that the cost, while modest, still was more than most South Indian villages could sustain.[75]

NEW "DANGEROUS RACES," NEW WARS

"An outstanding need in the Tropics today," Russell wrote in 1933, "is an automatic or biological weapon, with which to attack malaria-carrying mosquitoes."[76] Throughout his career, Russell would use towns, villages, and rural areas as field laboratories in which to test such putative biological weapons, whether Paris Green or, later, dichloro-diphenyl-trichloroethane (DDT). He sought, above all, a technological fix, an intervention into the local microbial ecology which visiting experts, like himself, might engineer and monitor. Despite his claims, community participation was usually less salient in these plans than technical skill and data security. In the multitude of mosquito-control laboratories scattered across the tropics, Russell and his colleagues from the emerging international health services would try to alter the intimate relations of malaria parasite and vector, frequently discounting or even abandoning intervention into resistant local cultures.[77] Thus neglect of the "human factor" in malaria transmission perpetuated earlier disparagement of native races: it was predicated on a deep pessimism about the capacity of natives to behave responsibly or to follow instructions. Despite some differences with Heiser, Russell shared his superior's disdain for native competence and trustworthiness. Heiser, however, persisted in perfunctory and often showy efforts to reform supposedly inadequate and refractory race cultures; Russell instead was more likely to circumvent them altogether, turning to ecological explanation, which decentered humans, and to techniques of modern biological warfare, targeting insects.[78] It was not until the development of medical anthropology in the 1960s that a nonracialized method of accounting for the human factor was added to the calculus of malaria control.

The war against mosquitoes therefore was distinct from the older pacification and attraction strategies that Heiser and other hygienists had waged since the later stages of the Philippine-American War. The new war did not require the laying down of sedimentary strata of disciplinary institutions across occupied territory; it did not demand the surveillance and reformation of local customs and habits. Above all, it was not a technique of human population management: it did not try to change people. Rather, the new campaign drew on models of continental warfare, as experienced in World War I, with their emphasis on the maintenance of fixed positions, acquisition of territory, and defeat or extermination of enemy forces. The attraction and assimilation of humans was less important than the killing of mosquitoes. During the 1920s and 1930s, then, these more traditional military metaphors, strategies, and tactics came to supplement in international health work those derived from combat with guerilla forces, from small wars doctrine. Methods of hygiene administration and population management, or race development, persisted, as we have seen, in hookworm campaigns, and in the delivery of child and maternal health services. But the fight against malaria, yellow fever, and dengue increasingly resembled a pitched battle against mosquitoes.[79]

Russell's experiences in the Philippines and India could be duplicated elsewhere. From 1924, L. W. Hackett had directed the Rockefeller Malaria Experiment Station in Italy, where he too set up "practical experiments in prevention." It was not long before the "use of larvicides became the measure on which most reliance was placed." Malaria in Sardinia and Calabria was not "driven back" before 1926, when "the almost miraculous efficiency of Paris Green . . . saved the day." To the health officer, Hackett expounded, "the malaria problem presents itself as a sort of nocturnal traffic in gametocytes and sporozoites. . . . The physician seeks a drug to cure the disease, the health officer a means to suppress transmission."[80] Elsewhere, Hackett observed that the "presence of malaria had nothing to do with latitude or standard of living, or any other social or physical character," only with the density of the "dangerous races" of *Anopheles*.[81] Therefore, it was against these dangerous races — insect, no longer human — that the war must now be fought. After the introduction in the 1940s of DDT, an amazingly effective residual insecticide and larvicide, Hackett and Russell realized they now possessed the "biological weapon" they were seeking. Along with Fred L. Soper, who had led Rockefeller efforts to eradicate *A. gambiae* from Brazil, Hackett and Russell initiated a trial of DDT in Sardinia after World War II. Although the mosquito persisted in small numbers, malaria was eliminated from the island.[82] By the 1950s, afire with enthusiasm for their new technology, malariologists were confidently forecasting the global eradication of the disease.[83] Russell, like many other disease ecologists, then began to warn of the dangers of human overpopulation and urge the regulation of reproduction in the tropics — thus concern for the quality and quantity of native populations kept resurfacing.[84]

In the new war on nature, the previously homogeneous tropical environment was disaggregated and reconnected in unconventional ways. Russell, for example, could point to a hitherto unsuspected ecological affinity between Assam and the Philippines, as both were places where *minimus* was the vector of the malaria parasite. Sardinia had become comparable with Malaya, Mississippi with Kenya. Accordingly, general, abstract concepts such as climate were fragmenting into a series of specific microenvironments, engendering new distinctions and associations. "Local malaria problems," Russell insisted, "must be solved largely on the basis of local data. It is rarely safe to assume that the variables in one area will behave in the same way as they do in another area, however closely the two regions may seem to resemble each other in topography and climate."[85] In these emerging, multiform networks of correspondence and difference, generic classifications like "the tropics" became less meaningful than ever. "Everything about malaria," Hackett cautioned, "is so molded and altered by local conditions that it becomes a thousand different diseases and epidemiological puzzles. Like chess, it is played with a few pieces, but is capable of an infinite variety of solutions."[86] To explain malaria, and many other so-called tropical diseases, the environment had been reintroduced as a factor in the etiological equation, but it was now a far more animated and piecemeal concept than the older notions of place and milieu that had prevailed in medical geography.

In 1935, Richard P. Strong, by then professor of tropical medicine at Harvard, observed that diseases like malaria, dengue, and yellow fever were compelling fresh attention to local ecologies, to competing and commensal populations of micro- and macroparasites. Multiple, particular environments appeared more than ever to exert *indirect* influences on disease, furnishing "unsanitary conditions, and especially, the parasites which cause and the insects which transmit infectious disease."[87] As F. Macfarlane Burnet argued in 1940, "The necessity for the ecological outlook on disease is probably more clearly evident in relation to . . . insect-borne diseases than elsewhere." Medical geography in the early twentieth century had largely been subsumed into the racial pathology that prevailed in the colonial Philippines; now notions of race were themselves being partially displaced in favor of a more complex and realistic ecology. "Native populations," as Burnet put it, "remain the passive objects of a vast ecological experiment," an experiment that only visiting experts could identify, monitor, and regulate.[88]

CONCLUSION

D uring the 1930s, under the direction first of Dr. Jacobo Fajardo and then Dr. José Fabella, the Philippine Health Service concentrated on social welfare, tuberculosis control, mental hygiene, maternal and infant health, and the education of "the masses." Spurred on by enthusiasm for the doctrines of social medicine — which recognized socioeconomic causes of disease — Filipino physicians departed from the straight path of racial hygiene to which Dr. Victor G. Heiser had pointed and from the narrower ecological route that Dr. Paul F. Russell was taking.[1] Theirs was predominantly a program of state medicine or national hygiene, similar to those undertaken in postcolonial settler societies such as the United States itself and Australia to the south.[2] Gone was the simple, though mobile, dichotomy of white American and Filipino; instead, class structure joined finer, generally unspoken internal gradations of ancestry and color to frame public health intervention. Of course, many continuities also were evident: colonial methods and practices had come to haunt national health services. The emphasis on personal and domestic hygiene persisted, along with an assumption that medical facts determined civic potential. Civilized or hygienic behavior, control of bodily functions, limits on social contact, all still indicated eligibility for social citizenship — only now, being Filipino did not necessarily imply natural faultiness or deficiency in these qualities. That depended much more on class position, though disparagement of people in the hills and on the southern islands lingered. With the election in 1935 of Manuel L. Quezon as the first president of the Philippines Commonwealth, under U.S. sovereignty, this normalization of state medicine gained pace in the archipelago. Expenditure on public health more than doubled within a few years, and services extended further into rural areas. It comes as no surprise that the new government boasted that it had constructed more than one hundred thousand latrines: by the 1930s, the privy was nowhere more firmly affixed to the nation.[3]

After the Japanese invaded in January 1942, the health service, hospitals, and medical schools initially maintained their activities. Claro M. Recto, that staunch opponent of U.S. imperialism, became the commissioner of education, health, and public welfare, while Dr. Eusebio D. Aguilar continued as director of health, until he died at the hands of the Japanese in 1945. It was not long, however, before the health services and other resources were harnessed to the needs of the invading forces. The commandeering of the means of communication and transport gravely hindered centralized public health work. Waste disposal was not strictly monitored, and latrine building was abandoned. Tuberculosis, malaria, and dysentery became rife. The lepers at Culion, quarantined and neglected, soon were starving, and hundreds died. As food became scarce across the archipelago, many medical students, nurses, and doctors drifted from the cities to the country to live off the land with their relatives. Then, when Allied forces returned to the Philippines early in 1945, fierce fighting destroyed many hospitals and other facilities. Under the command of General Douglas MacArthur, the U.S. Army restored public health control across the archipelago, as it had more than forty years before under the command of his father. Each division contained a Philippine Civil Affairs Unit, directed by a civil affairs officer and a medical officer. The Civil Affairs Units reestablished hospitals and health offices and brought Atebrin, penicillin, pentothal sodium (an anesthetic), and blood substitutes to the ravaged islands. Doctors and nurses moved back to the cities and resumed their work. After the Philippines achieved formal independence in 1946, the U.S. Public Health Service invested heavily in hospitals and rural health centers throughout the archipelago, rebuilding much of the infrastructure lost in the war. But the weakness, decentralization, and corruption of the postwar Philippine state would always greatly hamper public health activities.[4] The prestige of public health work plummeted, and few doctors chose to join the poorly supported bureaucracy—another example, perhaps, of the "normalization" of state medicine.

And yet, even in the United States, such normal, or national, public health still could demonstrate colonial features and inspiration.[5] Urban health services in America that targeted immigrants and minorities were, in part, legacies of empire. Colonial influences had been symbolic and direct. After 1910, few health departments in the United States could resist referring to American sanitary achievements in Panama and aligning their own efforts with those of Colonel William C. Gorgas, M.D., and other heroes of tropical medicine. As late as 1918, the director of the Illinois Department of Public Health was repeating Hermann Biggs's truism that "public health is purchasable," a fact that "can be illustrated no better than in the construction of the Panama canal."[6]

In the early twentieth century, the logic of some medical careers connected American metropolitan health much more directly with colonial engagements. Military surgeons in the Spanish-American War, once demobilized, often found they had developed a taste for preventive medicine and applied their energies and new skills to public health, rather than to the retail aspects of the profession. A decade or so later, many colonial bureaucrats, repatriated as the result of Filipinization, moved into senior positions in city and state health departments. In 1912, the U.S. Public Health Service chose Dr. Rupert Blue as surgeon general in preference to Heiser, but within a few years the colonial reject had the satisfaction of refusing an offer to direct the New York City Department of Public Health. Instead, his old friend Dr. Haven Emerson set about reforming administrative procedures in New York, having to endure Heiser's insistent advice and reiteration of Philippine lessons.[7] Dr. William E. Musgrave, the director of the Philippines General Hospital, fled to San Francisco in 1917 after some disaffected nurses tried to poison him, and he became a leading hospital administrator and professor of tropical medicine at the University of California—he, too, constantly proffered advice to local health authorities.[8] In the Milwaukee public health department from 1913 to 1914, Dr. Louis Schapiro applied lessons from his time in Bontoc to improve further the personal hygiene and vaccination rates of the inhabitants of "the healthiest city." But he longed for the tropics and soon left Wisconsin for Costa Rica, where he directed the Rockefeller hookworm campaigns.[9] Such examples of professional mobility could be multiplied further. Many American public health officers during this period were pragmatic cosmopolitans: they roamed the Pacific and the Western Hemisphere, translating and adapting models of modern preventive medicine, and with them the mixed predicates of race and class, their careers building an intricate web, an informal and converging network, of colonial and national health services.

The influence of the colonial Philippines on the new public health in the United States varied considerably across the country: it might be negligible, as in Chicago; filtered and mediated but still detectable, as in San Francisco; or profound, as in Boston.[10] In general, the medical experience of empire served to amplify or channel existing features of domestic public health work, to reshape or extend structures and policies already in place, rather than introducing wholly new procedures and goals. In particular, colonial experience tended to focus more attention on the fault lines of race and force recognition of the need to intervene more vigorously to reform the personal and domestic hygiene of those on the margins of society, to propel them into civic and medical trajectories.

The career of Dr. Allan J. McLaughlin epitomizes the metropolitan reach of the colonial bureaucrat. As deputy director of health in the Philippines, McLaughlin had demonstrated the importance of cholera carriers in spreading the disease and warned against promiscuous defecation by inferior races. After his appointment as commissioner of health for Massachusetts in 1914, this evangelist of personal hygiene "set the pace and direction for reorganization" of the public health department.[11] Proving himself a "physician skilled in sanitary science and experienced in public health administration," McLaughlin recruited full-time district health officers, created a new division of hygiene, and improved operational efficiency and transparency.[12] He wanted the public health department to run like a "well-regulated business," as it had, unimpeded, in the Philippines, and to ensure this he introduced formal administrative procedures and organizational charts. His colonial experiences had made him aware of the need for a "wider application of the principles of personal hygiene by the individual citizen himself" and sensitive to opportunities to carry sanitary instruction into the home, especially those of immigrants and minorities.[13] McLaughlin appointed visiting nurses and arranged for a physical and mental survey of every schoolchild in the state. The hygiene division delivered health lectures, set up exhibitions, and published educational pamphlets: its first, revealingly, was on mosquitoes and malaria — the insect was a summer nuisance, but the disease was rare in New England. By 1918, when he resigned to take up the position of an assistant surgeon general of the U.S. Public Health Service, McLaughlin had more or less adapted the Philippine Health Service to Massachusetts. To be sure, class mattered more than it had in the colony, and the main target of preventive medicine was now the urban white child. But whether in Manila or Boston, McLaughlin tried earnestly to convince all his charges, Filipino, American-born, and immigrant, that "there is more romance in the achievements of right living than in all the other episodes of glamorous lives."[14]

Public health, military medicine, and industrial hygiene all could be, at least in part, surrogates of colonial health services in the United States. Despite the efforts of Dr. Richard P. Strong and Dr. Andrew W. Sellards at Harvard and Colonel Charles F. Craig, M.D., at Tulane, tropical medicine itself did not flourish in North America.[15] The military legacy, of course, is not surprising: as we have seen, the links between the army and colonial medicine were lasting, intense, and multiform. Military medical officers readily traversed the health services of empire and returned to army or navy posts. For example, Craig and Weston P. Chamberlain became commandants of the Army Medical School after their colonial rotation; Edward L. Munson alternated instruction in military hygiene at the Army Service Schools in Fort Leavenworth with advice to the Philippine government and ended his career as commandant of the Medical Field Service School at Carlisle Barracks; P. C. Fauntleroy taught hygiene at the Army Medical School; P. E. Garrison directed the Naval Medical School. The training camp and the colony had come to resemble each other; raw recruits and natives displayed a striking affinity, even if they were credited with disparate capacities for discipline and improvement. Military hygiene had become a transferable skill and a widely available mechanism of modern government.

The logic of the colonial medical officer's career could also bridge fields that now seem much more distinct and separate than military and colonial medicine. Struggling to make a living in tropical medicine back in the United States, some repatriated physicians instead contributed to the further development of the new specialty of industrial hygiene. Munson had drawn attention to military hygiene as a resource for managing the domestic workforce, and many former colonial bureaucrats, once in the United States, recognized the sense of his precepts. Dr. John R. McDill, the first president of the Philippine Islands Medical Association, became professor of surgery at the Medical College of Wisconsin, but by the 1920s was advising the Federal Board for Vocational Education in Washington, D.C. More strikingly, in 1938, the National Association of Manufacturers (N.A.M.) made Heiser its consultant on "healthful working conditions." After his forced retirement from the International Health Division of the Rockefeller Foundation, Heiser had written *An American Doctor's Odyssey*, which proved immensely popular, selling half a million copies and breathing new life into the genre of medical tales from the tropics.[16] As a celebrity physician, Heiser urged workers to take personal responsibility for preventing injury and sickness in American industry. On behalf of the N.A.M., he organized clinics for local manufacturers' groups at which he extolled the benefits of vitamin supplementation, regular exercise, and personal hygiene. Accidents, he argued, were usually the result of worker carelessness, fatigue, and malnutrition. Heiser's goal was to help management use its personnel to greatest advantage in production. He believed that the physician's mission in the factory was "as bold and as adventurous as in any of nature's jungles."[17] Later, during World War II, the aging colonial medico turned his attention to improving stamina on the home front, addressing radio audiences and writing pamphlets, urging white Americans to enhance their diets and "toughen up" to meet the Nazi challenge.[18] Throughout this period he continued to express disdain for African-American capacities.[19]

The repatriation of white American physicians after 1910 anticipated by a decade the mass immigration of Filipino workers to the United States. As nationals, Filipinos could not legally be excluded, so during the 1920s they flocked to California's shores. Historians of migration have observed a racialization of Filipinos and Mexicans during this period — in particular, the disparagement of the foreigners' hygiene, along with warnings of their innate propensity to spread diseases that would threaten white communities.[20] But American health officers had fabricated this stigma long before in the colony, and later exported it back to the United States, where it might be applied to all immigrants. Filipinos, in particular, arrived already medicalized and racialized. Whereas in the colonial Philippines such stereotypes had prompted hygiene education and race improvement — the civilizing project — in the continental United States they more often elicited calls for exclusion and repatriation, which perhaps indicates the limits of influence of the liberal colonial model and of ideals of republican virtue more generally. But then, even the most reformist of physicians always recognized that there was little return on the disciplining of some human material: enforcing the hygiene of allegedly inferior races often seemed a frustrating and thankless task, to be undertaken only when no alternative presented itself. After the passage of the Tyddings McDuffie Act of 1934, which created the Philippines Commonwealth, Filipinos were reclassified as aliens, and their entry to the United States was restricted. But the postwar exchange visitor program and the relaxation of immigration criteria in the 1960s permitted the influx of thousands of Filipino nurses and a few physicians. By the end of the twentieth century, American nursing care was becoming markedly Filipinized.[21]

The focus on Pacific crossings — from the United States to the Philippines and vice versa — should not obscure widespread efforts to translate American colonial medical practices elsewhere in Asia and the Western Hemisphere. A complex circulation and repatterning of practices of public health emerged, flexibly coupled with ideas of race and development, and as these models passed from place to place they would be readjusted before moving on. Out of this play of assertion and caution came alterations in the style and form of the hygienic management of populations and in the manipulation of the environment as well as in the self-fashioning that public health work engendered. While director for the East of the Rockefeller International Health Board, Heiser attempted to reshape health services in more than forty countries, supporting more efficient and interventionist bureaucracies, directing attention to racial hygiene and health instruction, and developing medical and nursing education. Other Philippines medical officers followed his example. After working in Manila and at Culion, Dr. John E. Snodgrass took over the Rockefeller hookworm scheme in Ceylon, seeking through latrine building and hygiene reform to improve the productivity of plantation laborers.[22] Dr. John D. Long, Heiser's successor as director of health in the Philippines, shuffled between Manila and San Francisco, where he repeatedly led the Public Health Service's response to disease outbreaks, before joining the Pan-American Sanitary Bureau in the 1920s. Making analogies between colonial discipline and urban health in Asia and the Americas, he drafted the Pan-American Sanitary Code in 1923–24 and later wrote national health codes for Chile, Panama, and Uruguay, based on a Philippines model.[23] Dr. Paul F. Russell, as we have seen, turned away from the frustrations of "race development" and concentrated on manipulating the nonhuman elements of disease ecology, on fighting mosquitoes. His Philippine experiences directed him toward specific disease eradication campaigns, which necessarily became global in scope, abrogating colonial and national boundaries.

Thus the international health services, as they came to be known after World War II, derived in part from various Philippine models and approaches. A mosaic of influences gave rise to a mosaic of responses to disease threats, global and local. Such were the multiple sequels of Philippines colonial public health: in the archipelago, social medicine and national hygiene; in the United States, urban health services, industrial hygiene, and military medicine; and in Asia and Latin America, national and international health services, ecological intervention, and racialized development regimes.

Abbreviations

AMA	American Medical Association
APA	American Philosophical Society
BMJ	*British Medical Journal*
IHB	International Health Board
JAMA	*Journal of the American Medical Association*
JAMS	*Journal of the Association of Military Surgeons*
JMSI	*Journal of the Military Service Institution of the United States*
NARA	United States National Archives and Records Administration
NLM	National Library of Medicine
PHS	Public Health Service
PJS	*Philippine Journal of Science*
PMA	Philippine Medical Association
RAC	Rockefeller Archive Center
RF	Rockefeller Foundation
RFA	Rockefeller Foundation Archives
RG	Record Group
TAMS	*Transactions of the Association of Military Surgeons*

Note on citations: Citations to records in NARA are generally in the following form: record group-(subgroup)-series-folder.

Notes

INTRODUCTION

1. Rudyard Kipling to W. Cameron Forbes, August 21, 1913, Forbes papers, bMS Am 1364, Houghton Library, Harvard University. Kipling was an active promoter of U.S. intervention in the Philippines: see his "The White Man's Burden."

2. Heiser, "Unsolved Health Problems," 177. My focus here is on colonial hygiene and health education; I pay relatively little attention to clinical medicine and psychiatry and less to other healing traditions in the Philippines.

3. Rosenberg, "Framing Disease." On the social body, see Poovey, *Making a Social Body*. For other accounts of the racializing of pathology, see Gilman, *Difference and Pathology*; O'Connor, *Raw Material*; Craddock, *City of Plagues*; and Shah, *Contagious Divides*.

4. Stoler and Cooper, "Tensions of Empire"; Dirks, ed., *Colonialism and Culture*; Thomas, *Colonialism's Culture*. Also Arnold, *Colonizing the Body*; Packard, *White Plague, Black Labor*; Vaughan, *Curing Their Ills*; and Comaroff and Comaroff, *Ethnography and the Historical Imagination*.

5. Importantly, the model is not the concentration camp, described hyperbolically in Agamben, *Homo Sacer*. That is, I am describing the biopolitics of colonial subject formation, not a thanatopolitics.

6. Ileto, "Outlines of a Non-linear Emplotment," 110.

7. On the "civilizing process," see Elias, *The Civilizing Process*. Adas finds in the colonial Philippines "the fullest elaboration of America's civilizing mission ideology" but disassociates it from ideas of race (*Machines as the Measure of Men*, 406; and "Improving on the Civilizing Mission?"). On the colonial inculcation of civic virtue, see Conklin, *A Mission to Civilize*. Fieldhouse briefly alludes to the United States attempting "to fit her colonies into a republican framework" (*The Colonial Empires*, 343). Cannell suggests that "Americans demanded from their colony the evidence of the growth of a 'democratic' civic sensibility of a certain kind" (*Power and Intimacy*, 203). On the persistence of the rhetoric of republican civic virtue in American culture, see Furner, "The Republican Tradition"; Pickens, "The Turner Thesis and Republicanism"; and Cohen, *The Reconstruction of American Liberalism*. It is important to recognize the overlap, or mutual reinforcement, of republicanism, corporate liberalism, and Christian social gospel in the United States during this period: see Hofstadter, "Cuba, the Philippines and Manifest Destiny." Anti-imperialists (such as William Jennings Bryan) and imperialists (such as Theodore Roosevelt) debated whether an empire would endanger American republicanism or reinvigorate it (at least forestall its corruption) as continental expansion once had — see chapter 2. Of

course, the practice of republicanism in the Philippines was necessarily limited by the various racialist frameworks into which it was fitted.

8. Public health officers homogenized "the Filipino" in this period, ignoring Chinese or Spanish ancestry, contrasting the emerging type with the homogeneous white American type. The so-called non-Christian tribes were regarded as irredeemable and therefore the province of anthropology, not medicine. My usage of *triage* differs somewhat from Visvanathan's in "On the Annals of the Laboratory State," 272.

9. On discipline, see Foucault, *Discipline and Punish*; on governmentality, see Foucault, *The History of Sexuality. Volume 1*, and "Governmentality." See also Scott, "Colonial Governmentality."

10. Anderson, "Leprosy and Citizenship." For other uses of the concept, see Porter, *Health, Civilization and the State*, chapter 12; Ong, "Making the Biopolitical Subject"; Briggs with Mantini-Briggs, *Stories in a Time of Cholera*. In *Life Exposed*, Petryna also explores the entwining of identity, rights, and diagnosis but argues that those who suffered most from the nuclear disaster at Chernobyl gained most social capital.

11. Smith-Rosenberg and Rosenberg, "The Female Animal"; Pateman, *The Sexual Contract*; Young, "Polity and Group Difference"; and Scott, *Only Paradoxes to Offer*. On the continuing "partial citizenship" of migrant Filipina domestic workers, see Perreñas, "Transgressing the Nation-State."

12. Stepan, "Race, Gender, Science and Citizenship," 65. See also Mohanty, "Under Western Eyes"; and Spivak, *In Other Worlds*.

13. On the tendency to produce Manichean dichotomies in colonial discourse, see Fanon, *Black Skin, White Masks*; and Said, *Orientalism*.

14. On European historicism as a means of saying "not yet" to the colonized, see Chakrabarty, *Provincializing Europe*. On liberal strategies of exclusion, see Mehta, "Liberal Strategies of Exclusion"; and Parekh, "Liberalism and Colonialism." Mehta observes that the "liberal theorist in the broad structure of his or her theoretical enterprise works in a way quite akin to the modern doctor," in that the prescription is adjusted to "the minimally constitutive features of the human body" (82n).

15. Stoler, *Carnal Knowledge and Imperial Power*, 138. Indeed, Stoler sees increasing segregation and exclusion during the 1920s and 1930s (77, 111).

16. Arnold, *Colonizing the Body*, 280. Prakash, in contrast, describes the "unbridgeable gap" between the colonial state and its subjects in India during this period (*Another Reason*, 157).

17. Cooper, "Modernizing Bureaucrats, Backward Africans, and the Development Concept." Cooper has also observed that "the idea of empire as a transformative mechanism is indeed available, but one has to be careful about how one locates it" ("Modernizing Colonialism," 8). See also Packard, "Visions of Postwar Health and Development."

18. In this sense, the American colonial state in the Philippines was "late" from the outset: see Darwin, "What Was the Late-Colonial State?" For an account of Filipino nationalist developmentalism during the late-Spanish period, see Ileto, "Outlines of a Non-linear Emplotment."

19. Studies of colonial intimacy and affect and of the framing of the private usually emphasize the biopolitics of transgressive sex: here I am suggesting that we recognize that the care of the body, medical examination, and personal and domestic hygiene all reconfigure intimacy, affect, and privacy. See Stoler, "Tense and Tender Ties."

20. This may also explain the relatively relaxed legal attitude toward interracial sex in the Philippines, compared to many other colonial locales and to many of the U.S. states. See Stoler, *Carnal Knowledge and Imperial Power.*

21. Bhabha, "Of Mimicry and Man," 158. As Bhabha also puts it, "Almost the same but not white" (156).

22. Ileto, *Pasyon and Revolution*; Rafael, *White Love.*

23. Salman, "The United States and the End of Slavery in the Philippines, 1898–1914"; Kramer, "The Pragmatic Empire" and "Making Concessions"; Go and Foster, eds., *The American Colonial State in the Philippines*; and McFerson, ed., *Mixed Blessing.* See also the chapter on the Spanish-American War in Jacobson, *Whiteness of a Different Color;* and Hoganson, *Fighting for American Manhood.*

24. "Sensationalized racial contrast" is from Kramer, "Making Concessions," 96. Most of these works also focus on lowland Christian Filipinos, especially Tagalogs, and not Moros, hill tribes, or the substantial Chinese community.

25. Taussig, *Mimesis and Alterity,* 156.

26. Latour, "Give Me a Laboratory and I Will Raise the World"; and *Pandora's Hope.* See also Cunningham and Williams, eds., *The Laboratory Revolution in Medicine.*

27. The laboratory metaphor still has some appeal: see Visvanathan, "Lineages of the Laboratory State"; Rabinow, *French Modern,* 117, 289; and Wright, *The Politics of Design in French Colonial Urbanism,* 306. According to Prakash, the colonies were "underfunded and overextended laboratories of modernity" (*Another Reason,* 13). Conklin argues, though, that the "colonies were never just laboratories, they were sites, however unequal, of conflict and negotiation between colonizer and colonized" (*Mission to Civilize,* 5). On the related idea of the colony as "an object of experimentation," see Mbembe, *On the Postcolony,* 2.

28. Stoler, *Race and the Education of Desire;* and Anderson, *The Cultivation of Whiteness.* As McClintock suggests, "The invention of whiteness . . . is not the invisible norm but the problem to be investigated" (*Imperial Leather,* 8). In the Philippines after the first few years of occupation, *white,* or simply *American,* was the preferred self-designation, not *Anglo-Saxon,* which seems predominantly to have been a U.S. metropolitan political discourse during this period, though occasionally an ironic counterdiscourse among elite Filipinos. See Martellone, "In the Name of Anglo-Saxondom"; and Kramer, "Empires, Exceptions, and Anglo-Saxons."

29. On progressivism and the efficiency movement in the United States, see Haber, *Efficiency and Uplift;* Wiebe, *The Search for Order;* Galambos, "The Emerging Organizational Synthesis" and "Technology, Political Economy and Professionalization"; Skowronek, *Building a New American State;* and Rodgers, "In Search of Progressivism." On the development of an increasingly instrumentalist and scientific bureaucracy in Washington, D.C., and its links to republicanism and progressivism, see Lacey, "The World of the Bureaus." Abinales argues that "nothing in the existing

work on American colonialism examines the effect of the Progressive Movement on the colonial state" ("Progressive-Machine Conflict," 157). But see, for education policy, May, *Social Engineering in the Philippines*.

30. On the "prosthetic Gods" of modernity, see Freud, *Civilization and Its Discontents*, 28–29.

31. This is, then, a story of the successes and failures of *techne* in the tropics and the ineluctable presence of *pathos*—the *techne* and *pathos* of the colonized and the colonialist. See Heidegger, *The Question Concerning Technology*.

32. Thomas has criticized the use of "colonial discourse" as a "global and transhistorical logic of denigration" and called for "an understanding of a pluralized field of colonial narratives, which are seen less as signs than as practices" (*Colonialism's Culture*, 3, 8). See also Anderson, "The 'Third-World' Body" and "Postcolonial Histories of Medicine."

33. On the absence of empire in American historiography, see Williams, "The Frontier Thesis and American Foreign Policy." Kaplan has also observed that "the study of American culture has traditionally been cut off from the study of foreign relations" ("Left Alone with America," 11). Desmond and Domínguez have urged us to "chart the integral international flow of cultural products, material goods, and people across United States borders as a constitutive element of United States history and national identities" ("Resituating American Studies," 487).

34. Saldivar, "Looking Awry at 1898," 388. See also Adelman and Aron, "From Borderlands to Borders."

35. Julian Go urges us to study "how imperial or cross-colonial connections shaped the efforts and self-fashioning of U.S. colonial agents" ("Introduction," 25).

36. Rogaski, *Hygienic Modernity*, 3.

I. AMERICAN MILITARY MEDICINE FACES WEST

1. Capt. S. Chase de Krafft to Chief Surgeon, Manila, June 13, 1900, RG 112-E26-75139, NARA.

2. George S. Sternberg, Surgeon General, to Adjutant General, April 2, 1900, p. 6, RG 94-318183, NARA. The mean strength in this period was 27,712. The annual death rate from disease was therefore 17.1 for each 1,000 of strength, compared to 39.38 in Puerto Rico, and 61.15 in Cuba. In the first eighteen months of the Civil War, the annual death rate from disease was 52.27 (p. 7).

3. While quinine was catching on as a specific for malaria in the 1890s, it was still used more generally as a stimulant and febrifuge, as it had been for a century or more.

4. De Bevoise, *Agents of Apocalypse*, 11, 13. De Bevoise attributes the high annual death rate since 1860 to a combination of social disruption, changing agricultural patterns, and improvements in transport, giving rise to epidemics of cholera, malaria, smallpox, and rinderpest (a cattle disease). Any epidemiological review of the Spanish period is difficult because records are so scarce and unreliable—as a result, comparisons between Spanish and American colonial public health tend to favor the former. For local epidemiological reconstructions of the war years, see May, *Battle for Batangas*; and Smallman-Raynor and Cliff, "The Epidemiological Legacy of War."

5. Ashburn, *A History of the Medical Department of the United States Army*; Gillett, *The Army Medical Department, 1865–1917*; and Cirillo, *Bullets and Bacilli*.

6. Woodruff, "Military Medical Problems," 227. Woodruff identifies a significant trend, but, as usual, he overstates the point. Even during the U.S. Civil War, sanitation was not unimportant. See, for example, Woodward, *Outline of the Chief Camp Diseases*; and Hammond, *A Treatise on Hygiene*.

7. Smart, "Medical Department of the Army," 193.

8. See Horsman, *Race and Manifest Destiny*; and Jacobson, *Whiteness of a Different Color*. On the impact of colonial cultures on the structuring of bourgeois white masculinity more generally, see Stoler, *Race and the Education of Desire*. I discuss black American soldiers in the Philippines in chapter 3.

9. Hobsbawm has written that military service became a mechanism more generally for "inculcating proper civic behavior, and, not least, for turning the inhabitant of a village into the patriotic citizen of a nation" (*The Age of Empire*, 304–05).

10. LeRoy, *The Americans in the Philippines*; Hofstadter, "Manifest Destiny and the Philippines"; Cosmas, *An Army for Empire*; Gates, *Schoolbooks and Krags*; Trask, *The War with Spain*; Miller, *"Benevolent Assimilation"*; Linn, *The United States Army and Counter-Insurgency* and *The Philippines War*. In June 1898, the Philippine Expeditionary Force became the Eighth Army Corps. A corps consisted of three divisions plus artillery and cavalry, and each division consisted of three brigades, a brigade being three regiments. Initially only one-quarter of the force was regular army, the rest having volunteered. In the spring of 1899, the volunteers of '98 were mustered out and replaced by thirty-five thousand men of the new volunteer regiments. By autumn '99 there were still sixty-five thousand troops in the Philippines, more than thirty thousand of them volunteer. In March 1900 the Department of the Pacific became the Division of the Philippines, with four geographical departments, each divided into military districts. Even in late 1901 more than forty-five thousand U.S. soldiers remained in the archipelago.

11. This is the way it was characterized in Washburn, "The Relation Between Climate and Health." A medical doctor, Washburn became chairman of the Philippine Civil Service Board.

12. Anderson, *The Spectre of Comparisons*, 227.

13. Water from the Marikina River was pumped into a reservoir at San Juan and then piped into the city, to public water taps and residences (only 1,825 by 1902). See D. F. Doeppers, "Water, Milk, and *Chocolate* versus Coffee," unpublished ms., 2003. Sanitary engineering was more advanced in the United States, but it should be noted that three-quarters of the urban population of New England was served by public waterworks. In 1890, only 1.5 percent of the American urban population was supplied with filtered water, 40 percent by 1914 (Rosen, *Preventive Medicine in the United States*, 46).

14. Bantug, *A Short History of Medicine in the Philippines*, 64–77; and Marcelo C. Angeles, "History of the Public Health System in the Philippines," c. 1967, 1–4, Archives Section, Department of Health, Republic of the Philippines.

15. Lopes-Rizal, *Annual Report of the National Research Council*, 159.

16. LeRoy, "The Philippines, 1860–1898." Under the Spanish regime, *mestizo* meant a

person of mixed Spanish–local ancestry or mixed Chinese–local ancestry; *penin-sulares* were Spaniards from Spain; *criollos* were persons of Spanish ancestry born in the Philippines; and *indios* were descendants of the original inhabitants. There were, in addition, mountain peoples — Igorots, for example — and Moros, the Islamic peoples of the south. For a revealing account of Spanish colonial racial classifications, which were becoming more stringent and influential toward the end of the century, see Comisión Central de Manila, *Memoria complementaria de la sección 2 del pro-grama*. This was produced for the Philippine Islands Exposition in Madrid — in it, *indios* are treated as degenerate or inferior but not inherently pathogenic.

17. Schumacher, *The Propaganda Movement*; and Ileto, *Pasyon and Revolution*.

18. LeRoy, *Philippine Life in Town and Country*, 98.

19. LeRoy, "Philippines, 1860–1898." See also Agoncillo, *The Revolt of the Masses*; and Zaide, *The Philippine Revolution*.

20. Rizal, *El Filibusterismo*, 141. I have altered the quotation slightly in accordance with the original text. On Rizal and other leading nationalist physicians, see Guerra, *El Médico Político*, chapter 6.

21. Schumacher, "Philippine Higher Education."

22. Bantug, "Rizal and the Progress of the Natural Sciences."

23. Schumacher, "Rizal and Blumentritt."

24. Billings, "The Military Medical Officer," 350, 353. Billings established the collection that became the basis of the National Library of Medicine and later was the founding director of the New York Public Library. See Garrison, *John Shaw Billings*; and Chapman, *Order Out of Chaos*.

25. Sternberg, "Presidential Address," 15. Sternberg, who briefly trained with Koch in 1886, had been surgeon general since 1893: see Sternberg, *George Miller Sternberg*; and Gibson, *Soldier in White*. Although Sternberg is chiefly remembered for his promotion of laboratory science and discovery of the pneumococcus, he was equally concerned with improving training in medico-military administration. In 1898 he wrote that "physicians and surgeons from civil life, however well qualified profes-sionally, as a rule, are not prepared to assume the responsibilities of medical officers charged with administrative duties and the sanitary supervision of camps" (quoted in Sternberg, *George Miller Sternberg*, 200–201). The Association of Military Sur-geons of the United States was established in 1891; the *Transactions* of its meetings later became *JAMS* and then *Military Surgeon*.

26. The army surgeon in the past had often depended on chance to find shelter for the wounded, though Tilton had built hospital huts at Valley Forge and Erwin used tents as a field expedient at Shiloh in 1862.

27. Halley, "First-aid to the Wounded."

28. Ibid., 131.

29. Woodruff, "Military Medical Problems," 231.

30. Boekmann, "Some Remarks about Asepsis," 229.

31. Ibid., 230.

32. Smart, "Medical Department of the Army," 193. On late-nineteenth-century im-provements in colonial military hygiene and their epidemiological consequences, see Curtin, *Death by Migration*.

33. Munson, *The Theory and Practice of Military Hygiene*, 115. The other important guides to American military hygiene in this period — both indebted to Munson — were Ashburn, *The Elements of Military Hygiene*, and Havard, *Manual of Military Hygiene*.

34. Notter, "On the Sanitary Methods," 113, 112.

35. The most influential of the nineteenth-century medical geographers was undoubtedly Hirsch, especially the revised, expanded, and much-translated second edition of his *Handbuch der Historisch-Geographischen Pathologie*. On medical geography in general, see Grmek, "Géographie médicale"; Ackerknecht, *History and Geography of the Most Important Diseases*; Valenčius, "Histories of Medical Geography"; and Barrett, *Disease and Geography*.

36. Hirsch suggested that some geographically distributed diseases might be biologically mediated, that is, arise from associated plant or animal life. In the early twentieth century, Clemow claimed that most had proven to be mediated, in *The Geography of Disease*, esp. 5. In the interval between these publications, the great discoveries of the microbial causes and insect transmission of many diseases were made: for example, Robert Koch had identified the cholera bacillus in 1882 and the tubercle bacillus in 1883; Alphonse Laveran had discovered the plasmodium of malaria in 1880, and Ronald Ross identified *Anopheles* as its vector in 1897. Patrick Manson had found filariae in *Aedes* in 1882, but filarial transmission was still thought to be diffusedly environmental until the 1890s. See Worboys, *Spreading Germs*.

37. But for an effort to explain the techniques of bacteriology, see Woodruff, "The Military Uses of Bacteriology."

38. Munson, *Theory and Practice of Military Hygiene*, 336, 338, 339.

39. Woodward, "The Sanitation of Camps," 144.

40. Notter, "On Sanitary Methods," 116, 116–17, 117.

41. Bache, "The Location of Sites," 415, 416.

42. Ibid., 417, 416.

43. Ibid., 419, 420.

44. See Munson, *Theory and Practice of Military Hygiene*, esp. chapter 17. Munson noted that "venereal infection, especially that of a syphilitic nature, appears to take place more certainly, and to assume a much more severe character, when relations are entered into between individuals of different racial characteristics" (828). He recommended the regulation of prostitution and the frequent inspection of soldiers, measures he introduced into Philippines. More generally see Levine, "Venereal Disease, Prostitution and the Politics of Empire."

45. Bache, "Location of sites," 429. Some examination of recruits had occurred earlier, but it was not systematic and rigorous until the late nineteenth century. See, for example, Henderson, *Hints on the Medical Examination*.

46. Burrill, "Is It Expedient to Have a Physical Examination?" 137.

47. Munson, *Theory and Practice of Military Hygiene*, 1, 3.

48. Greenleaf, *An Epitome of Tripler's Manual*, 7. Greenleaf asserted that "the recruit must be effective, able-bodied, sober, free from disease, and of good character and habits" (9). As assistant surgeon general during the 1890s, Greenleaf had reorganized record keeping, the entry examinations, and the table of medical supplies (see

his file, RG 94-521ACP90, NARA). On his assistance to John van Rensselaer Hoff in the organizing of the hospital corps in 1887, see Henry S. Greenleaf, "The Medical Corps U.S. Army: A History of its Establishment. Excerpts from the Correspondence of Brig. General Charles R. Greenleaf," in C. R. Greenleaf papers, MS C91, History of Medicine Division, NLM.

49. Munson, *Theory and Practice of Military Hygiene*, 1.

50. Ibid., 33, 71, 72.

51. See Notter, "On Sanitary Methods," 113; and Munson, *Theory and Practice of Military Hygiene*, chapters 5 and 6.

52. Munson, *Theory and Practice of Military Hygiene*, 384, 393, 400.

53. Ibid., 589, 590.

54. Greenleaf, "Practical Duties of an Army Surgeon."

55. The other members were Major E. O. Shakespeare, M.D., and Dr. Victor C. Vaughan: see Reed, Vaughan, and Shakespeare, *Abstract of the Report of the Origin and Spread of Typhoid Fever*; and Vaughan, "Typhoid Fever Among the American Soldiers." Reed later became celebrated for his work with the Yellow Fever Commission in Cuba, which associated transmission of the disease with a particular mosquito. On the typhoid outbreak, see Cosmas, *An Army for Empire*, chapter 8. The initial response to the epidemic was generally condemned: almost twenty-one thousand soldiers contracted the disease, and about fifteen hundred died (Reed, Vaughan and Shakespeare, *Abstract of Report*, 185–86, 190–92).

56. Vaughan, "Typhoid Fever," 85, 85–86.

57. As Sternberg pointed out, "It was not the site [of the camp] but the manner of its occupation which must be held accountable for the general spread of disease among the troops" (*Report of the Surgeon-General of the Army*, 110). Reed and Sternberg also took the opportunity to insist on command responsibility for health and education of line officers in hygiene (introduced at West Point in 1904–05).

58. Smart, "Medical Department of the Army," 200. See also Traub, "Military Hygiene."

59. Alden, "The Special Training of the Medical Officer," 676, 683. Defects in training, revealed in the winter of 1890–91 in the campaign against the Sioux, had led to the establishment of a school for the training of sanitary corps at Fort Riley, Kansas. In 1892, a system for the examination of assistant surgeons was introduced. The Prussian military medical school had been founded in 1795 (reformed 1818); the French military medical school at Val de Grâce dates from 1852; and the British Army Medical School, the model for the U.S. school, was established in 1860, after the disaster of the Crimean War. John Farley observes that the U.S. Army Medical School gave more time to bacteriology and hygiene and less to parasitology and helminthology than the Liverpool and London schools of tropical medicine, both founded in 1899 (*Bilharzia*, chapter 2). Considering the known disease distribution in the temperate part of the United States, which it also served, this is not surprising. On the U.S. Army Medical School, see Craig, "The Army Medical Service"; Lull, "The Days Gone By"; and Nichols, "Notes on the History of the Laboratories of the Army Medical School." Most of the regular army surgeons in 1898 would not have attended the Army Medical School, and only a few National Guard medical officers had trained there.

60. Hoff, "Sanitary Organization in the United States Army." See also his "Scheme of Military Sanitary Organization."

61. Woodruff, "Military Medical Problems," 221. From the 1880s, army regulations had required the post or line commanding officer to forward medical reports on the health of command without amendment, though comment was permitted. This considerably enhanced the influence of the medical officer.

62. Hoff, "Some Steps in the Organization," 112, 114.

63. Griffith, "Hospital Experience in the War with Spain," 161. One of the few articles in *TAMS* to deal with tropical disease before 1898 was Foster, "Notes by a Medical Officer in the East." Foster concentrates on antiquated British methods of surgical antisepsis, but he does observe that "all over the tropics fever is a matter of course," and it appalls him that "east of Cairo water closets become very rare; I do not believe there are a dozen in all of India" (367, 365).

64. Hoyt, *Frontier Doctor*, 322. See also Hoyt, "Observations Upon and Reasons for a More Complete Physical Examination." During this period, occupational medicine and military medicine were emerging in parallel as specialties, and some physicians, like Hoyt, worked in both.

65. Hoyt, *Frontier Doctor*, 323.

66. Ibid., 333, 335.

67. Ibid., 346. For more on Flexner and Barker, see chapter 3.

68. Ibid., 353. From Corregidor Hoyt wrote, "I don't seem to recuperate in this climate and I know that I will if I go to the States" (Hoyt to Adjutant General, August 6, 1899, RG 94-272956, NARA). A few years later, Hoyt returned with his family and stayed at Nueva Caceres (now Naga City) until his son was badly burned, and the family had to go back to the States.

69. Kemp, "Field Work in the Philippines," 73, 74.

70. Ibid., 75.

71. Ibid., 78, 77, 80. The use of Chinese bearers was banned in 1900, as they were deemed a deterrent to the employment of Filipino workers.

72. Ibid., 80.

73. Ibid., 81. In such conditions, the consumption of contaminated water often led to illness.

74. Lippincott, "Report of Lt.-Col. Henry Lippincott," 263. He also observed, "The Spaniards have given little attention to sanitary matters, so that coming from our country to this, one is reminded of the advantages our people have in the United States" (264).

75. Lippincott, "Reminiscences of the Expedition," 172–73. See also Lippincott, "Medical and Sanitary History of the 8th Army Corps," January 31, 1899, RG 112-E26-39109-182, NARA; and Gillett, "Medical Care and Evacuation During the Philippine Insurrection."

76. Lippincott, "Reminiscences of the Expedition," 170, 171.

77. A. A. Woodhull to Sternberg, May 24, 1899, RG 112-E26-57592-E, NARA. Greenleaf, Lippincott, and Woodhull had all served in the medical corps since the Civil War. Lippincott had distinguished himself with Custer's forces against Black Kettle's Cheyennes at the battle of Washita. Woodhull relieved Lippincott, who was sick

from dysentery and malaria, on April 18, 1899 (RG 94-4414ACP72, NARA). According to William H. Welch, Woodhull was "something of stickler for forms and ceremonies in military matters" but "a thoroughly good man" (Welch to Simon Flexner, March 17, 1899, Welch papers, folder 12, box 16, Alan Mason Chesney Archives, Johns Hopkins Medical School; on Woodhull's career, see RG 94-5620 ACP1876, NARA). By August 1899 there were 1,682 men in the First Reserve and 35 vacant beds (Woodhull to Sternberg, August 28, 1899, RG 112-E26-57592-5, NARA). In September, nipa huts in the Manila suburbs accommodated a further 2,000 sick (Major-General Elwell S. Otis to Adjutant General, September 6, 1899, RG 112-E26-57592-4, NARA). By April 1900 there were fewer demands on the hospitals: in Manila the hospitals accommodated 1,460 patients, with 760 vacant beds; and in the country there were approximately 3,500 patients with 500 vacant beds (C. R. Greenleaf to Sternberg, April 23, 1900, RG 112-E26-57592-107, NARA).

78. Woodhull to Sternberg, June 4, 1899, RG 112-E26-57592-C2, NARA.

79. Woodhull to Adjutant General, May 23, 1899, RG 112-E26-57592-8, NARA.

80. Woodhull to Sternberg, October 25, 1899, RG 112-E26-57592-45, NARA.

81. Lanza to Adjutant General, June 20, 1899, RG 112-E26-57592-8, NARA.

82. Mary E. Sloper, "Arraignment of the Medical Department in the Philippines," January 31, 1899, RG 112-E26-56797-J, NARA.

83. Woodhull to Sternberg, May 24, 1899, RG 112-E26-57592-C, NARA. By November 1899 a hospital of bamboo and nipa was erected at Corregidor, but it still lacked a kitchen and mess hall (Woodhull to Sternberg, November 16, 1899, RG 112-E26-57592-56, NARA).

84. Letter, January 25, 1900, in Spanish-American War Survey — U.S. Hospital Corps, W 1149, U.S. Army Military History Institute, Carlisle Barracks, Penn. Soon though, Fleming fell apart: "The dyarrhaea has been running or was running up till the time the dysentary broak out about 2 months on me" (July 27, 1900).

85. Hoyt to Sternberg, March 1, 1899, RG 112-E26-57592-O, NARA; and Lawton to Adjutant General, July 1, 1899, RG 112-E26-57592-J, NARA. See also Henry I. Raymond to Adjutant General August 29, 1899, RG 112-E26-57592-20, NARA.

86. Woodhull to Sternberg, June 19, 1899, RG 112-E26-57592-S, NARA. For the surgeon general's responses, see Sternberg to Woodhull, July 19, 1899, RG 112-E26-57592-C, and August 7, 1899, RG 112-E26-57592-S, NARA.

87. Woodhull to Sternberg, August 15, 1899, RG 112-E26-57592-14, NARA. In February 1900, 28 medical officers were on sick report, and Greenleaf, the chief surgeon of the troops in the field, asked for a further 40 surgeons (Greenleaf to Sternberg, February 10, 1900, RG 112-E26-57592-85, NARA). At the time, the number of military surgeons in the Philippines was 191; by April 1900, the number was 239, approximately 4 for each 1,000 of strength (Surgeon General to Adjutant General, July 26, 1900, RG 112-E26-57592-86, NARA).

88. Woodhull to Sternberg, September 28, 1899, RG 112-E26–57592-31, NARA.

89. Woodhull to Sternberg, November 28, 1899, RG 112-E26-57592-63, NARA.

90. Woodhull to Sternberg, January 30, 1900, p. 34, RG 112-E26-57592-76, NARA.

91. P. C. Fauntleroy to Sternberg, January 1, 1900, RG 112-E26-57592-78, NARA. For

another detailed account of the First Reserve, see Kulp, "A Manila Military Hospital," esp. 228–31.

92. Lippincott, "Reminiscences of the Expedition," 171–72.

93. Lippincott to Sternberg, January 30, 1900, p. 5, RG 112-E26-57592-76, NARA.

94. Lippincott, "Reminiscences of the Expedition," 172.

95. Lippincott to Sternberg, January 30, 1900, pp. 15, 26–27, RG 112-E26-57592-76, NARA. In 1898, there were 1,902 admissions to sick report for every 1,000 of strength in the Philippines, 1,777 by disease and 138 by injury—the overall sick rate and mortality rate (24/1,000) were much lower than in Cuba (where the Fifth Army Corps had initially been disorganized, and yellow fever and a more lethal form of malaria prevailed). In the Philippines, malaria and diarrhea contributed most to the sick report, but typhoid caused most deaths. In 1899, the sick rate in the Philippines rose to 2,396/1,000: 2,206 from disease and 241 from injury. The increase was primarily due to more diarrheal disease and malaria. The mortality rate rose to 31/1,000 but the contribution of disease to this rate fell, since there was considerably less typhoid (Sternberg, *Report of the Surgeon-General of the Army*, 1900, 86). Between 1898 and 1902, 3,693 U.S. soldiers died of disease, and 449,918 were admitted to the sick list ("Statistics from the Office of the Surgeon General," RG 112-E26-10086-M, NARA).

96. Notter, "On Sanitary Methods," 118.

97. J. J. Curry, "The Diseases of the Philippine Islands: Report to the Surgeon General," c. 1900, p. 31, RG 112-E26-68075-G, NARA.

98. Hoyt, "Appendix," 262.

99. Mason, "Notes from the Experiences of a Medical Officer," p. 309.

100. Sternberg to Adjutant General, April 2, 1900, p. 11, RG 94-318183, NARA.

101. Notter, "On Sanitary Methods," 118, 112.

102. Greenleaf to Sternberg, January 30, 1900, pp. 13, 14, RG 112-E26-57592-76, NARA. In this report, Greenleaf pointed out that "direct heat to the lower back of the head, and the spine, means increased susceptibility to illness, even when actual illness does not result" (p. 31). His observations were probably influenced by the long-standing military interest in sunstroke in temperate regions: see Brown, "The Effects and Treatment of Heat and Sunstroke."

103. Greenleaf to Sternberg, January 30, 1900, pp. 14–15, RG 112-E26-57592-76, NARA. Lt. Col. Parker confirmed the climatic problems: "The air lacks vitality; undue exertion exhausts the men and takes the heart out of them. . . . A march of 12 or 15 miles in this country is a *forced* march" ("Some Random Notes on the Fighting in the Philippines," 319).

104. Charles F. Mason, "Observations upon Diseases in the Tropics," p. 1, RG 112-E26-77851, NARA.

105. Palmer, "Notes on Luzon," 228–29. For a critique of theories of a climatic "death trap," see L. M. Maus, "Military Sanitary Problems in the Philippine Islands," September 1, 1908, p. 1, RG 112-E26-18668-27, NARA.

106. Guthrie, "Some Observations While in the Philippines," 143.

107. Munson, *Theory and Practice of Military Hygiene*, 860, 908. There was perhaps

one subject that soldiers still concentrated on: Munson noted that "the genital function" seemed to increase in the tropics, but that "excesses in venery are especially trying to the unacclimated" (910).

108. Greenleaf to Sternberg, January 30, 1900, p. 18, RG 112-E26-57592-76, NARA.

109. L. M. Maus, "Military Sanitary Problems in the Philippine Islands," September 1, 1908, p. 16, RG 112-E26-18668-27, NARA. Mason also observed malignant nostalgia: "Men became morbid and homesick. When they did get sick they thought of nothing but home, and if the disease proved intractable and they had set their hearts on going home, it was death not to send them ("Medical Officer in the Tropics," 310). Sternberg reported, "Home sickness prevailed to a considerable extent in some of the regiments, causing depression of spirits and aggravating trivial ailments" (Sternberg to Adjutant General, April 2, 1900, p. 4, RG 94-318183, NARA). These must have been among the last examples of the medical diagnosis of nostalgia: see Rosen, "Nostalgia." On the cognate problem of "shell shock" during World War I, see Stone, "Shellshock and the Psychologists."

110. Anon., "Insane Soldiers Coming," *Evening Star*, February 13, 1900, clipping in RG 112-E26-57592-143, NARA. Nurse Alice Burrell was worried that on the steamer home there were "several insane soldiers on board. Result of disease and exposure in the P.I.'s" (Diary, June 8, 1900, ms. 81–1, UCSF Archives). In fact, in the six months to June 30, only 101 "insane soldiers" went home (Greenleaf to Surgeon General, July 13, 1900, p. 2, RG 112-E26-57592-143, NARA).

111. Munson, *Theory and Practice of Military Hygiene*, 854, 858, 860, 861.

112. Birch, "Influences of Warm Climates on the Constitution," 4, 19. See Livingstone, "Human Acclimatisation: Perspectives on a Contested Field," "Climate's Moral Economy," and "Tropical Climate and Moral Hygiene"; Kennedy, "The Perils of the Midday Sun"; and Harrison, *Climates and Constitutions*.

113. Kidd, *The Control of the Tropics*, 48, 54.

114. Mason, "Medical Officer in the Tropics," 309.

115. Stelle, "Some Notes on the Clothing," 17. See also Birmingham, "Some Practical Suggestions of Tropical Hygiene."

116. Mason, "Medical Officer in the Tropics," 312–13. See also Renbourn, "Life and Death of the Solar Topi."

117. Stelle, "Some Notes on the Clothing," p. 22. See also Renbourn, "The Spine Pad." I am grateful to Robert Joy for directing me to this reference (and many others).

118. Guthrie, "Observations in the Philippines," 148.

119. Philippine Commission, *Report of the Philippine Commission to the President, 1900*, 161.

120. Woodruff, "Hygiene in the Tropics," 297. Woodruff, a military surgeon since 1887, was considered clever but troublesome. At Missoula, a senior officer concluded, "He is not fit to command the hospital detachment, nor does he know his duties as a subordinate" (Wesley Merritt to Major Schwan, September 21, 1891, RG 94-1946APC 87, NARA). In 1901, his commander at Fort Riley, Kansas, admonished him. See chapter 5.

121. Munson, *Theory and Practice of Military Hygiene*, 878. See also Munson, "The Ideal Ration."

122. Stone, "Our Troops in the Tropics," 367.

123. Greenleaf to Sternberg, January 30, 1900, pp. 35–36, RG 112-E26-57592-76, NARA. See also Birmingham, "Some Practical Suggestions"; and Seaman, "Observations in China and the Tropics."

124. Woodruff, "Tropical Hygiene," 298. Greenleaf wryly observed, "The soldier craves and gets, some way or other, the food he has been accustomed to eat at home, and he eats plenty of it; he wants meat twice or three times a day and he eats bacon or uses it in some form or other in his cooking whenever he can get it. He will not eat rice" (Greenleaf to Sternberg, July 13, 1900, p. 4, RG 112-E26-57592-143, NARA).

125. For another aspect of the relations between the Philippine war and American manliness on the home front, see Hoganson, *Fighting for American Manhood*. More generally, see Mrozek, "The Habit of Victory." I discuss American manliness in the Philippines in more detail in chapter 5.

126. Turner, "The Significance of the Frontier in American History." See also Coleman, "Science and Symbol in the Turner Frontier Hypothesis."

2. THE MILITARY BASIS OF COLONIAL PUBLIC HEALTH

1. Von Clausewitz, *On War*, 603. Foucault inverted another of Clausewitz's aphorisms when he wrote that "politics is the continuation of war by other means" (*"Society Must be Defended,"* 15). Foucault went on to argue that war is a "matrix for techniques of domination" (46).

2. Ileto has described the sanitary response to the cholera epidemic of 1902 in Manila as war by other means, in "Cholera and the Origins of the American Sanitary Order." In his comments on Ileto's paper, Arnold notes, "The involvement of the military in the medical interventionism of the imperial period is one of its most striking features" ("Introduction: Disease, Medicine and Empire," 19). According to Arnold, in South Asia during this period, "the institutional connections between the military and state medicine were close and enduring," and the army and jails provided models for "the wider colonization of Indian society by Western medicine." These were, he writes, "exemplary sites, perceived as models of how Western medical and sanitary practices might — in theory at least — be deployed in the wider society" (*Colonizing the Body*, 62, 61, 114). And yet, Feierman has observed that "the most important stream of early colonial biomedicine is one to which scholars have paid little attention: military medicine" ("Struggles for Control," 120).

3. Gottman, "Bugeaud, Galliéni, Lyautey," 235, 246. Rabinow discusses the influence of colonial warfare on French modernity and urbanism in *French Modern*. It is striking the extent to which the doctrine of colonial warfare appears to anticipate Foucault's *Discipline and Punish*.

4. Lyautey, "Du rôle coloniale de l'armée." See also Lyautey, "Du rôle social de l'officier"; Galliéni, *La Pacification de Madagascar*; and Callwell, *Small Wars*. For the development of U.S. tactics, see Utley, *Frontier Regulars*; Jamison, *Crossing the Deadly Ground*; and Bickel, *Mars Learning*.

5. More generally, Lawrence has argued that disciplines of hygiene in the Royal Navy helped to shape medicine's "governmental" involvement ("Disciplining Disease").

Cooter has identified the (very different) model of the Prussian military, with its tight efficiency and hierarchical control, as a model for orthopedic surgery at the end of the nineteenth century (*Surgery and Society in Peace and War*). See also Sturdy, "From the Trenches to the Hospitals at Home"; and Harrison, "The Medicalization of War."

6. Gates, *Schoolbooks and Krags*; May, "Filipino Resistance to American Occupation"; Filiberti, "The Roots of U.S. Counterinsurgency Doctrine"; Linn, *The U.S. Army and Counterinsurgency in the Philippine War*; and Birtle, "The U.S. Army's Pacification of Marinduque." Ironically, after the Philippine-American War there was no systematic effort by the U.S. Army to develop formal small wars doctrine, and it resumed an obsession with continental warfare. But see Hamilton, "Jungle Tactics"; Bullard, "Small Maneuvers"; and Bickel, *Mars Learning*. More generally, see Linn, *Guardians of Empire*. The legacy of colonial warfare in the Philippines was therefore primarily medical, not military.

7. Munson, "The Civil Sanitary Function of the Army Medical Department."

8. Guthrie, "Some Observations While in the Philippines," 142.

9. Quoted in Young, *The General's General*, 265. MacArthur had translated Isobelo de los Reyes's *Guerilla Tactics: Surprises, Ambuscades, and Attacks on Convoys* in 1899.

10. Sternberg, *Report of the Surgeon-General of the Army, 1900*, 94.

11. Ibid., 98.

12. Maus, "Report of Major L. M. Maus," 123.

13. Meacham, "Report of Major Franklin A. Meacham," 139.

14. Woodhull, *Notes on Military Hygiene for Officers of the Line*, 315.

15. Munson, "Civil Sanitary Function of the Army Medical Department," 274, 290.

16. Smith, "Edward L. Munson, M.D." The "Munson last" was the army's official boot from 1912 to 1942. In 1914, Munson declined a permanent appointment as director of health in the Philippines, saying he would rather go to Alaska than stay longer in the tropics (RG 94-2115ACPI893, NARA). But he returned for three years in the 1920s. After retirement in 1932, Munson became professor of preventive medicine at the University of California Medical School.

17. Munson, *The Management of Men*, 735, 36, 70.

18. Board of Health, *Manual of the Board of Health*. See also Greenleaf, "A Brief Statement of the Sanitary Work Accomplished"; Fales, "The American Physician in the Philippine Civil Service"; and Gillett, "U.S. Army Medical Officers and Public Health in the Philippines."

19. Greenleaf to Adjutant-General, Division of the Philippines, May 21, 1900, in Sternberg, *Report of the Surgeon-General of the Army, 1900*, 99.

20. Worcester, *The Philippines Past and Present*, 333. Bourns, who had accompanied Worcester on his zoological expeditions to the Philippines in the early 1890s, proved much more amenable to his friend's plans than most of the other medical officers. Worcester, a zoologist from the University of Michigan, was secretary of the interior from 1901 until 1913: see Sullivan, *Exemplar of Americanism*; and Stanley, " 'The Voice of Worcester Is the Voice of God.' "

21. Munson, *Theory and Practice of Military Hygiene*, 944, 946.
22. *Report of the Secretary of the Interior to the Philippine Commission for the Year ending August 31, 1902* (Manila: Bureau of Public Printing, 1902), 6–7.
23. Ileto has argued that in practice "the new colonial order, in fact, merely reproduced the classic Philippine pattern of principalia-dominated, sanitary towns, whose outskirts faded into a world of 'uncontrollable,' 'disorderly' or 'subversive' elements" ("Cholera and the Origins of the American Sanitary Order," 142).
24. On November 1, 1905, the Board of Health would become the Bureau of Health (Act 1407). Over the following year district health officers were substituted for the provincial boards of health, thus permitting the director of health a more effective personal control over local actions (Act 1487, May 16, 1906). This act gave the director of health power "to revoke, or modify any order, regulation or bylaw, or ordinance of a local board of health or of any municipality, except in the City of Manila, concerning any matter which in his judgment affects the public health." In a general reorganization of the colonial administration, the Bureau of Health in turn became the Philippine Health Service (PHS) on July 1, 1915 (Act 2468). The PHS, like its precursors, exercised administrative supervision over hygiene and sanitation in the islands through its divisions of general inspection, sanitation, hospitals, statistics, district nursing, and publicity and hygiene.
25. Maus was thus head of the Board of Health. The other members were H. D. Osgood, sanitary engineer; Dr Franklin A. Meacham, chief sanitary inspector; Dr Paul C. Freer, superintendent of government laboratories; and Manuel Gomez, secretary. The Manila Board of Health was established by Act No. 157, Philippine Commission, July 1, 1901 (RG 350-3465-0, NARA). Act No. 187, on August 5, 1901, transferred the staff of the Manila board to the Board of Health for the Philippine Islands (RG 350-3465-1, NARA). Maus, a graduate of the University of Maryland, had joined the medical department in 1874 and served in the Dakota and Arizona territories before becoming chief surgeon of the 7th Army Corps in Havana and then chief surgeon of the department of northern Luzon and commissioner of public health (June 1900–August 1902). He was again chief surgeon for the army in the Philippines from 1907 till 1909. Notorious for his bad temper, Maus was also a vigorous campaigner for prohibition and eugenic sterilization. According to Brigadier General George H. Torney, the surgeon general, Maus was "one of the most disgruntled members of the medical corps and . . . a selfish, self-seeking officer. . . . He is constantly seeking favors for himself, and I have been informed by medical officers that when serving in the Philippines he persecuted officers who were not in accord with his views" (Memorandum, 1913, RG 112-E26-18668, NARA). Maus regarded Torney as a deliberate and malicious liar (Maus to Adjutant General, January 12, 1914, RG 112-E26-476ACP82, NARA).
26. Charles Greenleaf, 1900, quoted in Robert D. Gorodetzer, "A Concise Biography of Col. Louis M. Maus," p. 9, box 2, Halstead-Maus family papers, Archives of the U.S. Army Military History Institute, Carlisle Barracks, Penn.
27. Maus organized examinations and mandatory treatment in isolation hospitals for prostitutes. His allowance of a "tolerance zone" for prostitution antagonized mis-

sionaries, who prevented the issuing of certificates, though the examinations continued. See Maus, "Venereal Diseases in the United States Army"; and Dery, "Prostitution in Colonial Manila."

28. Worcester to W. H. Taft, governor, September 6, 1902, and June 26, 1903, RG 112-E26-476ACP82, NARA.

29. Maus to Adjutant General, October 29, 1903, RG 112-E26-476ACP82, NARA. Maus reflected that "anyone serving under Mr. Worcester could not fail to note his vindictive and overbearing spirit, or his personal prejudices, and on account of his general manner and personal bearing, I have never heard anyone speak favorably of him" (Maus, Sworn Statement, November 26, 1906, p. 9, RG 112-E26-476ACP82, NARA).

30. According to Sternberg's "efficiency report" in 1901, Carter was a "very zealous and competent officer"; see Carter's personnel file, RG 94-5059ACP86, NARA. Carter, a graduate of the University of Virginia and a courteous man of military bearing, arrived in the Philippines on July 29, 1902, and would stay until 1905, when his health broke down (W. H. Taft to Carter, March 31, 1905, RG 94-5059ACP86, NARA). In 1882 he had been a surgeon with the Chihuahua campaign, and in 1885–86 he accompanied an expedition into Mexico in search of hostile Apaches.

31. Carter, "Sanitary Conditions," 544.

32. Ibid., 544–45. Similarly, the director of the census of 1903 was Major General J. P. Sanger.

33. Root, "Report for 1902," 261. In 1901, Surgeon J. O. Skinner had written to Root, reporting on conditions in the Philippines: "The natives appear to me to be utterly incapable of self-government in any proper form. . . . I do not believe the present generation can ever appreciate much less absorb and assimilate American ideas and institutions. . . . While a very few of them have been able to memorize and repeat, parrot-like, the wording of our Constitution and Declaration of Independence, neither they nor their followers have, in my opinion, the proper conception of the provisions and purposes, the privileges and penalties of these instruments" (RG 350-59-26, NARA).

34. Roosevelt, "Message of the President of the U.S., Communicated to the Two Houses of Congress at the Beginning of the First Session of the 57th Congress," 590. For Roosevelt's complex views on race, see Dyer, *Theodore Roosevelt and the Idea of Race*; Bederman, *Manliness and Civilization*; and Gerstle, *American Crucible*. On Roosevelt and the Philippines, see Alfonso, *Theodore Roosevelt and the Philippines*.

35. Roosevelt, "At Arlington, Memorial Day, May 30, 1902," 59, 65.

36. Roosevelt, "At the Banquet Tendered for Gen. Luke E. Wright, at Memphis, Tennessee, Nov. 19, 1902," 206.

37. Roosevelt, "Message of the President of the U.S., Communicated to the Two Houses of Congress at the Beginning of the Second Session of the 57th Congress," 628. As Ashburn put it, "Military officers were made governors general of countries, governors of provinces and towns, and it is interesting to note that there was a general parallelism between their success in their jobs and their ability to visualize, grasp, and control the sanitary evils which afflicted the countries" (*A History of the Medical Department of the United States Army*, 227).

38. Appleby, *Liberalism and Republicanism in the Historical Imagination*; Brugger, *Re-*

publican Theory in Political Thought; and Cohen, *The Reconstruction of American Liberalism*.

39. Pickens, "The Turner Thesis and Republicanism."

40. Bryan, *Bryan on Imperialism*, 55. See also Schurz, *For American Principles and American Honor*; Stillman, *Republic or Empire?*; and Smith, *Commonwealth or Empire?* See also Lasch, "The Anti-imperialists, the Philippines and the Rights of Man"; Beisner, *Twelve Against Empire*; Shirmer, *Republic or Empire?*; and Welch, *Response to Imperialism*.

41. On the policy of "attraction," see Stanley, *A Nation in the Making*; and Owen, ed., *Compadre Colonialism*.

42. Roosevelt, "At the Coliseum," 95.

43. Roosevelt, "Message of the President of the U.S., Communicated to the Two Houses of Congress at the Beginning of the First Session of the 57th Congress," 570.

44. Roosevelt, "At the Coliseum," 95.

45. *Affairs in the Philippine Islands: Hearings before the Committee on the Philippines of the United States Senate*. Senate Document 331, 1st Session, 57th Congress, 1902. 3 vols. (Washington D.C.: Government Printing Office, 1902), 1:270–71. The Taft commission, which included Worcester, Wright, Henry C. Ide, and Bernard Moses, arrived in June 1900, although the full transfer of power did not occur until July 1901. Taft was governor from June 1900 until December 1903. He was later president (1908–12) and then chief justice of the United States. See Pringle, *The Life and Times of William H. Taft*. His successors, Wright (1903–05), Ide (1906), James F. Smith (1906–09), and W. Cameron Forbes (1909–13), largely endorsed Taft's assessment of Filipino character—as did most other Americans in the archipelago. Peter Stanley quotes the editor of the (Manila) *Cablenews*, August 8, 1907, on this point: "If a race, through ignorance or perverseness, will not heed the advice of civilized nations about, it must be cared for as a child by its step-mother or a wild beast by the keeper who cages it but treats it humanely" (*A Nation in the Making*, 107–8).

46. *Affairs in the Philippine Islands*, 1:61, 322, 343.

47. Taft, "The Work of the United States in the Philippines," 243, 240. Even in 1921, colonial officials like Frank Carpenter, the executive secretary of the insular government, were still recommending "the political reconstruction of Asia upon the basis of our institutions, the saving of the world to Occidental civilization and thereby, we may hope, the survival of our race" (Carpenter to General Leonard Wood, July 30, 1921, quoted in Stanley, *A Nation in the Making*, 107).

48. Moses, "Education of a Stranger" (address at Berkeley, August 28, 1903), Moses papers, c-b 994, Bancroft Library, University of California-Berkeley.

49. Moses, "Control of Dependencies," 87. Moses claimed that distinctively liberal American colonialism "recognizes racial differences, but at the same time it finds in the less developed races other sentiments than fear to which it may successfully appeal" (95).

50. Moses, "American Control of the Philippines" (ms., c. 1913), Moses papers, c-b 994, Bancroft Library, University of California-Berkeley.

51. Beveridge, "Our Philippine Policy," 65, 71. Moses felt that "Senator Beveridge is

undoubtedly a bright but superficial person, but his conceit as manifested at times was oppressive" (Diaries, vol. 5, September 1, 1901, Moses papers, C-B 994, Bancroft Library, University of California-Berkeley). On Beveridge, see Braeman, *Albert J. Beveridge*. One of the major awards offered by the American Historical Association honors Beveridge.

52. Beveridge, "Our Philippine Policy," 73, 85.

53. Beveridge, "March of the Flag," 49, 50.

54. Taft, "Progress of the Negro," 320, 328.

55. Roosevelt, "Message of the President of the U.S., Communicated to the Two Houses of Congress at the Beginning of the Second Session of the 57th Congress," 639.

56. See Hoxie, *A Final Promise*; and Berkhofer, *The White Man's Indian*. Hoxie points to the influence of Henry Lewis Morgan's ideas of social evolution and his postulated trajectory from savagery to barbarism to civilization.

57. Roosevelt, *A Book Lover's Holidays in the Open*, 51. During his presidency Roosevelt was also interested in immigration restriction in order to ensure the homogeneity of the U.S. population: see Higham, *Strangers in the Land*; Kraut, *Silent Travelers*; and Jacobson, *Whiteness of a Different Color*.

58. See, for example, Sternberg, *Report of the Surgeon-General of the Army, 1900*, 95. See also Utley, *Frontier Regulars*; Olch, "Medicine in the Indian-fighting Army"; and Gillett, *The Army Medical Department*, chapter 3. It is important to understand that while the army was rarely responsible for the care of reservation Indians, it quickly took up early Philippine public health provision. (Health care on the reservations was the responsibility of the Bureau of Indian Affairs, which despite identical initials had no connection with the Bureau of Insular Affairs, responsible for the Philippines.) In *Facing West*, Drinnan, however, emphasizes similarities more generally in the acquisition and government of Indian territories and the Philippines.

59. In 1900, there were eighty-three agency physicians and two hospitals for some two hundred thousand American Indians. In general, those physicians who were not utterly feckless concentrated on treating advanced tuberculosis. Jones contrasts the neglect of Native American health, especially the prevention of disease, with the more efficient, and separate, medical care of troops on the frontier, conducted by officers who soon would work in the Philippines (*Rationalizing Epidemics*, esp. chapter 6). Indian health care remained neglected until President Taft, returned from the Philippines, in 1912 set out to improve conditions on the reservations. He had learned that "the tide can be turned, that the danger of infection among the Indians themselves and to the several millions of white persons now living as neighbors to them can be greatly reduced" ("Special Message to Congress, Sept. 12, 1912," quoted in Jones, *Rationalizing Epidemics*, chapter 6). See also Kunitz, "The History and Politics of U.S. Health Care Policy for American Indians"; and Trennert, *White Man's Medicine*.

60. But see Williams, "United States Indian Policy and the Debate Over Philippine Annexation."

61. Munson, *The Principles of Sanitary Tactics*, 35, 37.

62. Lippincott to Sternberg, March 31, 1899, p.7, RG 112-E26-57592-A, NARA.

63. Maus, "Military Sanitary Problems in the Philippine Islands," September 1, 1908, p.7, RG 112-E26-18668-27, NARA.

64. Guthrie, "Observations on the Philippines," 148.

65. D. T. E. Casteel to wife, 14–20 October, 1900, Casteel papers, U.S. Army Military History Institute, Carlisle Barracks, Penn., quoted in Linn, *United States Army and Counter-Insurgency*, 17. Casteel also observed that "The defense of the enemy was natural undergrowth as far as seen, they firing from within the edge of the woods" (Report of Action at Tanay, January 26, 1900, RG 350-764-284, NARA).

66. Young, *General's General*, 253.

67. Crane, "The Fighting Tactics of Filipinos," 497, 502, 506, 503.

68. Report, November 16, 1901, p. 4, RG 395-2423, NARA. The anonymous officer continued: "By reason of the rough and wooded character of its terrain, [the surrounding country] gives protection to bands of insurgents and ladrones."

69. Guthrie, "Observations on the Philippines," 144.

70. Ibid., 141.

71. Lippincott, "Reminiscences of the Expedition," 172.

72. J. J. Curry to Commanding Officer, First Reserve Hospital, January 2, 1900, RG 112-E26-57592-69, NARA; Greenleaf to Sternberg, January 3, 1900, RG 112-E26-57592-69, NARA. For a report on the laboratory activities, see Strong to Chief Surgeon, Division of the Philippines, October 15, 1900, RG 112-E26-68075-E, NARA. Strong later became director of the biological laboratory of the Philippine Bureau of Science and the first professor of tropical medicine at Harvard. See Chernin, "Richard Pearson Strong and Manchurian Epidemic of Bubonic Plague"; Cueto, "Tropical Medicine and Bacteriology in Boston and Peru"; and Anderson, "Richard Pearson Strong."

73. Curry, "The Diseases of the Philippine Islands: Report to the Surgeon General," c. 1900, p. 9, RG 112-E26-68075-G, NARA.

74. Strong to Sternberg, January 3, 1901, RG 112-E26-68075-J, NARA. In late 1899 and early 1900, after disengaging from Hoyt at the front, Simon Flexner and Llewelys Barker had conducted research on cadavers at the First Reserve Hospital laboratory, trying to isolate microorganisms. See Flexner and Barker, "Report of a Special Commission Sent to the Philippines" and "The Prevalent Diseases in the Philippines"; and Barker, "Medical Commission to the Philippines." Barker was "deeply impressed by the excellent organization of the medical and surgical work of the Army" (*Time and the Physician*, 66). For the correspondence between W. H. Welch and Flexner, see Welch papers, box 16, folder 12, Alan Mason Chesney Archives, Johns Hopkins Medical School.

75. Maus, "Monthly Report of the Board of Health for the Philippine Islands," February 1902, RG 350-3465-4, NARA. For the international context, see Edger, *The Present Pandemic of Plague*.

76. Manson, *Tropical Diseases* (1898), 152.

77. Herzog, *The Plague*, 19. W. G. Liston of the Indian Medical Service had documented rat-flea transmission of plague in 1902–3. On presumed modes of transmission, see also *Infectious Diseases: Period of Incubation, Quarantine and Infection; Sources of Infection*. Health Bulletin No. 1 (Manila: Bureau of Printing, 1903).

78. Headquarters' Provost Marshall General, Office of the Board of Health, Circular Letter No. 11, June 30, 1901, RG 350-3234-2, NARA.

79. Maus, "Monthly Report of the Board of Health for the Philippine Islands," February 1902, p. 2, RG 350-3465-4, NARA.

80. Office of the Board of Health, Circular Letter No. 5, "Ambulatory Plague," April 8, 1901, RG 350-2394-2, NARA. The notion of ambulatory plague was later challenged in Herzog and Hare, *Does Latent or Dormant Plague Exist?*

81. Office of the Board of Health, Circular Letter No. 3, "A Brief Synopsis of Bubonic Plague for Early Diagnosis," March 7, 1901, RG 350-2394-2, NARA.

82. Office of the Board of Health, Circular Letter No. 5, "Ambulatory Plague," April 8, 1901, RG 350-2394-2, NARA. By 1908, the consensus was that fleas were the vectors of the plague bacillus and rats its usual host.

83. *Report of the Secretary of the Interior to the Philippine Commission, for the Year Ending August 31, 1902* (Manila: Bureau of Public Printing, 1902), 13–14, 27. Cholera was reported in India in 1900; within a year it had spread to the Straits Settlements; in March 1901 it was found in Hong Kong. The disease later attacked Batavia in June and entered Yokohama a few months afterward. See Major Charles Lynch, "Asiatic Cholera," Circular No. 24, Headquarters Division of the Philippines, April 11, 1902, RG 350-4981-5, NARA; and Marshall, *Asiatic Cholera in the Philippines Islands.*

84. Worcester, *The Philippines Past and Present*, 334. See also his *History of Asiatic Cholera in the Philippine Islands.* His comments were meant as a reflection on Maus's competence: for Maus's response, see Maus to Adjutant General, December 21, 1908, RG 94-1488119-B, NARA.

85. On the Spanish response to cholera in 1882 (and later in 1888–89), see Capelo y Juan, *Manila, la Higiene y el Cólera*; del Rosario and Lopez Rizal, *Some Epidemiological Features of Cholera in the Philippines*, esp. 3–6; Bantug, *A Short History of Medicine in the Philippines under the Spanish Regime*, 64–77; Marcelo C. Angeles, "History of the Public Health System in the Philippines," c. 1967, Department of Health Archives, Republic of the Philippines, 1–4; and Enrico Azicate, "Medicine in the Philippines: An Historical Perspective," M.A. thesis, University of the Philippines, 1989, 72–83. The files in "Memorias Médicas," Philippine National Archives, Manila, contain much valuable information. De Bevoise estimates that 10 percent of the population of Manila died in the 1882 epidemic (*Agents of Apocalypse*, chapter 7). *Agents of Apocalypse* covers the Spanish response in more detail.

86. In April, the cholera section of San Lazaro was abandoned because of "ground infection" and the patients all moved out to Santa Mesa, which was closed in May. Afterward a cholera hospital was established in Ermita, closer to the city. Captain E. A. Southall took charge of the hospital even though he was "suffering from chronic dysentery the whole time." See Maus, *Report of the Board of Health for the Philippines Islands and the City of Manila*, April 1902, 2. See also Ileto, "Cholera and the Origins of the American Sanitary Order"; and Sullivan, "Cholera and Colonialism in the Philippines."

87. Headquarters Division of the Philippines, General Orders No. 66, March 25, 1902, RG 350-4981-4, NARA; Ken de Bevoise, "The Compromised Host: The Epidemiological Context of the Philippine-American War" (PH.D. dissertation, University of Oregon, 1986), 166–69. The burning of dwellings continued a well-established mili-

tary practice designed to deter collaboration with *insurrectos*. When Captain D. C. Cabell came to Albay in June 1901, he detected support from local villagers for the *insurrectos*, so he recommended that "orders be given to burn all these houses and bring in their occupants" (Cabell to Adjutant, Subdistrict of Albay, June 23, 1901, RG 350-2423, NARA).

88. Maus, *Report of the Board of Health for the Philippines*, March 1902, 1–3. See also the health regulations issued by Maus on April 10, 1901 (RG 350-3465-7, NARA).

89. Maus, *Report of the Board of Health for the Philippines*, March 1902, 1, 3. The high case mortality suggests either low host resistance (perhaps a result of malnutrition or concomitant infection) or a failure to diagnose or report mild cases. For sensitive American accounts of the epidemic, see Fee, *A Woman's Impressions of the Philippines*, 220 f.; Moses, *Unofficial Letters of an Official's Wife*, 221–42; and Mrs. W. H. Taft, *Recollections of Full Years*, 253–60.

90. Johnson, who fancied himself a "squaw man," did however develop "a fascination for [the Philippines'] pleasant clime as a whole, and some feeling of attachment toward these people who were generally hospitable and easy to become friendly with" ("My Life in the Army, 1899 to 1920" [Typescript 1952, rev. 1960], 63, 102, U.S. Army Military History Institute, Carlisle Barracks, Penn.).

91. Winfred T. Denison, secretary of interior, to Major-General Thomas H. Barry, August 31, 1915, RG 94-2115ACP93, NARA.

92. Maus, *Report of the Board of Health for the Philippines*, March 1902, 2.

93. Ibid. If not carefully diluted, benzozone burned the mucosa of the gastrointestinal tract.

94. Edger, "Special Report," pp. 1–3, RG 112-E26-90497-19, NARA, quoted in De Bevoise, "Compromised Host," 249. The medical officer was following the orders issued as Headquarters Division of the Philippines, General Orders No. 66, March 25, 1902, RG 350-4981-4, NARA.

95. George De Shon papers, U.S. Army Military History Institute, Carlisle Barracks, Penn. See also the 1902 diary of Perry L. Boyer, M.D., at the U.S. Army Military History Institute, Carlisle Barracks, Penn.

96. C. F. de Mey, "Cholera Report, May 30, 1902," in Dean C. Worcester, "Annual Report of the Secretary of the Interior to August 31, 1902," in *Reports of the Philippine Commission, 1902* (Washington D.C.: Government Printing Office, 1903), 412–13.

97. Maus, *Report of the Board of Health for the Philippines*, March 1902, 2. Worcester described opponents of the measures as "a few evil-intentioned persons, both foreign and native, who welcomed every opportunity to make trouble" (*Philippines, Past and Present*, 335).

98. Anna Page Russell Maus, "Old Army Days" (Typescript, c. 1920s), Halstead-Maus family papers, U.S. Army Military History Institute, Carlisle Barracks, Penn., n.p. Mrs. Maus claimed her husband had to "fight tropical diseases among a people utterly ignorant of the first principles of sanitation and infection."

99. Wright to Elihu Root, secretary of war, July 20, 1902, p. 8, Elihu Root papers, C 164, Library of Congress, quoted in De Bevoise, "Compromised Host," 240–41.

100. Maus, *Report of the Board of Health for the Philippines*, March 1902.

101. Pardo de Tavera to W. H. Taft, May 5, 1902, RG 350-3465-5, NARA. Pardo de Tavera was an honorary, and uninfluential, member of the Board of Health. He had studied medicine at Santó Tomás and the Sorbonne and became involved in the Philippine nationalist movement. Anticlerical and liberal, he quickly moved to collaborate with the American colonial state. In 1899 he founded *La Democracia* and became the first president of the Colegio médico-farmacéutico de Filipinas; the following year he set up the generally agreeable Federal Party. See Guerra, *El Médico Político*, 150–52.

102. Winfred T. Denison to Major-General Thomas H. Barry, August 31, 1915, RG 94-2115ACP93, NARA.

103. Maus, *Report of the Board of Health for the Philippines*, April 1902, 2.

104. Ibid., May 1902, 1; and ibid., January 1903, 3.

105. Worcester, *History of Asiatic Cholera*. The end of the epidemic was not officially declared until April 1904.

106. Louis D. Baun to mother, May 13, 1902, Baun letters, ms 80–75 z, Bancroft Library, University of California-Berkeley.

107. Heiser, *An American Doctor's Odyssey*, 34.

108. Ibid., 37. The threat to the "Occidental" was never far from the minds of the senior American administrators. According to Taft, "If the United States is to continue its governmental relations with the Philippines for more than a generation, and its business and social relations indefinitely, the fact that Americans can lead healthful lives in the Philippines is important of itself" (*Special Report of W. H. Taft*, 281).

109. Heiser, "Unsolved Health Problems," 177.

110. Ibid., 172.

111. Heiser, *An American Doctor's Odyssey*, 151.

112. Williams, *The United States Public Health Service*; Mullan, *Plagues and Politics*; and Fairchild, *Science at the Borders*. The origins of the PHS were actually in the Coast Guard, a paramilitary organization, and its institutional power within the United States remained marginal during most of this period.

113. Heiser, *An American Doctor's Odyssey*, 77. See Anderson, "Victor George Heiser." As director of quarantine in the islands (1903–05), Heiser had acquired a reputation as a zealous, tightfisted bureaucrat. Luke Wright, the governor, was "anxious to have Heiser chief of Bureau of Health speedily with a view to cutting expenses for the next fiscal year. Do not wish to hurt Carter's feelings by suggesting return. Could you not order him [Carter] home for duty?" (Wright to Secretary of War, March 29, 1905, RG 350-3267-18, NARA). Heiser's first impressions of Filipinos had been bad: he wrote to his cousin Sue, "The little brown brothers as they are called, are a lazy shiftless lot. The only thing the men seem to take an interest in is chicken fights and about all the women do is smoke big black cigars. It is mighty seldom that you can catch any of them at work" (June 5, 1903, Heiser papers, American Philosophical Society, B:H357.p).

114. Heiser, *An American Doctor's Odyssey*, 76.

115. I discuss this development in more detail in *The Cultivation of Whiteness*, chapter 2.

116. Haber, *Efficiency and Uplift*; and Wiebe, *The Search for Order*. Wiebe argues that

"the heart of progressivism was the ambition of the new middle class to fulfill its destiny through bureaucratic means" (166).

117. The emblematic text is Taylor, *Principles of Scientific Management*. See Galambos, "The Emerging Organizational Synthesis in American History," and "Technology, Political Economy and Professionalization." On the general move to efficiency and business models in medicine during this period, see Rosen, "The Efficiency Criterion in Medical Care"; Kunitz, "Efficiency and Reform in the Financing and Organization of American Medicine"; Vogel, "Managing Medicine"; Madison, "Preserving Individualism in the Organizational Society"; and Sturdy and Cooter, "Science, Scientific Management, and the Transformation of Medicine in Britain."

118. Worcester, *Philippines, Past and Present*, 354.

119. Heiser, "Sanitation in the Philippines," 133.

3. "ONLY MAN IS VILE"

1. Balfour, "Tropical Problems in the New World," 83. Balfour had recently returned from the Sudan, where he was director of the Wellcome Tropical Research Laboratories; he became director of the London School of Hygiene and Tropical Medicine. Balfour was referring to Chamberlain, "Observations of the Influence of the Philippine Climate on White Men," 429; and "Some Features of the Physiological Activity of White Races."

2. May has described the contribution of American educators to colonial governance in *Social Engineering in the Philippines*.

3. Ronald Ross, "Discussion," in Balfour, "Tropical Problems," 110.

4. Balfour, "Tropical Problems," 86. This is a minor misquotation of Bishop Heber's hymn, extolling Ceylon. Balfour, however, remained skeptical; see his "The Problem of Acclimatization."

5. Livingstone, "Climate's Moral Economy."

6. Codorniu y Nieto, *Topografía Médica*, 10, 32. On the related concern about the degeneration of European horses in the archipelago, see Bankoff, "A Question of Breeding."

7. Codorniu y Nieto, *Topografía Médica*, 37, 109, 46.

8. Ibid., 121.

9. Jagor, *Travels in the Philippines*, 25, 29, 263. Thus were southern Europeans implicated in the myth of the lazy native: see Alatas, *The Myth of the Lazy Native*.

10. Suarez Caopalleja, *La salud del Europeo*, 33, 74. Interestingly, Suarez is also concerned with the acclimatization of *criollos* to Spain, an indication of the mobility of population between the parts of the empire. For a more pessimistic contemporary view of Spanish prospects in the tropics, see Gonzalez, *Filipinas y sus inhabitantes*. Yet even as Gonzalez asserts that the European "can be considered as a truly exotic plant in that burning soil," he boasts of his eight years of good health in the archipelago (25).

11. Suarez Caopalleja, *La salud del Europeo*, 78, quotations on 88. Still, Suarez thought that acclimatization would always effect at least a slight modification in Spanish bodies and mentality. He regarded the inaptitude of *criollos* and *mestizos* for science as an especially telling sign of intellectual deterioration (88).

12. *Affairs in the Philippine Islands: Hearings before the Committee on the Philippines of the United States Senate.* Senate Document 331. 57th Congress, 1st Session, 1902 (Washington, D.C.: Government Printing Office, 1902), 3 vols., 1:343, 395.

13. *Affairs in the Philippine Islands,* 1:391, 395.

14. Taft, "Special Report of the Secretary of War on the Philippines," 281.

15. Bancroft, *The New Pacific,* 251, 403, 430.

16. Morris, *Our Island Empire,* 355. Morris was a prolific Aryanist and a biographer of Theodore Roosevelt.

17. Griffis, *America in the East,* 47, 46–47.

18. *Report of the Philippine Commission to the President,* 4 vols., in *Senate Journal,* 56th Congress, 1st session, January 31, 1900, 2:231.

19. L. F. Barker in *Report of the Philippine Commission,* 2:237, 238, 239. Later in San Francisco, on their way back to the East Coast, Flexner and Barker reported on the response to the epidemic of bubonic plague in that city.

20. Herbert Ingram Priestley to mother, October 6, 1901, Herbert Ingram Priestley letters 1901–04, 94/13 cz, Bancroft Library, University of California-Berkeley. Priestley became a historian of the Spanish empire in North America and the director of the Bancroft Library at Berkeley. (I discuss Priestley's nervousness in more detail in chapter 5.)

21. Conger, *An Ohio Woman in the Philippines,* 50, 133–34. Conger later trained as an osteopath.

22. Atkinson, *The Philippine Islands,* 151, 146. Large-scale white colonization was not, it seems, seriously contemplated in Washington, D.C. But see R. Macarthy Williamson to Roosevelt, November 29, 1906 — on the use of Italian migrants — in RG 350-873-2, NARA. In response to A. J. Garrissen's plans to colonize Mindanao (January 9, 1912), Colonel Frank Macintyre, the chief of the Bureau of Insular Affairs, wrote, "The Philippine government encourages the taking up of its public lands, by homestead, lease, or purchase, and will use every facility at its command to protect anyone engaged in any legitimate enterprise in the Islands" (RG 350-873-3, NARA).

23. Woodruff, "The Neurasthenic States Caused by Excessive Light," 1006. I discuss Woodruff's theories of "tropical neurasthenia" in more detail in chapter 5. For Woodruff's career and many contretemps, see RG 94-1946APC87, NARA. Taft in a letter to Worcester (February 26, 1914) refers to "that fellow Woodruff, of the Medical Corps, who went crazy on the subject of colors in the tropics" in D. C. Worcester papers, Aa/2/Ac, box 1, Bentley Historical Library, University of Michigan.

24. Woodruff, *The Effects of Tropical Sunlight Upon the White Man,* 278.

25. Woodruff, *Expansion of Races,* 257, 274. Jordan in *Imperial Democracy* had made similar claims, though they lacked Woodruff's medical rationale. The natural historian (and president of Stanford University) wrote that "civilization is. . . . suffocated in the tropics," (45) and the torrid zone was "Nature's asylum for degenerates" (93). "The Anglo-Saxon in the tropics deteriorates through the survival of the indolent and the loss of fecundity" (95).

26. Harrison to Woodruff, November 7, 1913, letters, box 36, Francis Burton Harrison papers, Library of Congress. See also Woodruff to Harrison, August 26, 1913.

27. Twain, "To the Person Sitting in Darkness."

28. De Witt, "A Few Remarks Concerning the Health Conditions of Americans in the Philippines," 56. De Witt ended his career as brigadier general and an assistant to the surgeon general.

29. Washburn, "The Relation between Climate and Health," 499, 505. Washburn relied in particular on the optimistic views of Felkin, *On the Geographical Distribution of Tropical Diseases.*

30. Washburn, "The Relation between Climate and Health," 506, 507, 513.

31. Wood, quoted in ibid., 515.

32. McDill, "Presidential Address," quoted in Taft, "Special Report of the Secretary of War on the Philippines," 281. On the history of the Philippine Islands Medical Association, see Stauffer, *The Development of an Interest Group*, chapter 1; and de la Cruz, *History of Philippine Medicine.*

33. Surgeon General, U.S. Army, to Chief Surgeon, Division of the Philippines, June 13, 1906, RG 112-68075-25, NARA. I have described the first Army Board (1899–1902) in chapter 2; a later board (1922–30) was housed in the Bureau of Science. Among the more important figures on the army boards were Lt. Richard P. Strong, Capt. Percy F. Ashburn, Lt. Charles Craig, Capt. James M. Phalen, Capt. Edwin D. Kilbourne, Maj. Weston P. Chamberlain, and Capt. Edward D. Vedder. On the board, see Ashburn and Craig, "The Work of the Army Board for the Study of Tropical Diseases"; [Ashburn], "A Synopsis of the Work of the Army Medical Research Boards"; and Gillett, *The Army Medical Department, 1865–1917*, chapter 11. The board confirmed the mosquito theory of dengue transmission and did important work on the nutritional basis of beriberi.

34. Aron, "Investigations of the Action of the Tropical Sun," 102.

35. Gibbs, "A Study of the Effect of Tropical Sunlight upon Men," 92.

36. Shaklee, "Experimental Acclimatization to the Tropical Sun."

37. James M. Phalen and H. J. Nichols, "Outline of an Experiment for US Soldiers Serving in the Philippines," 1909, RG 112-68075-68, NARA.

38. Phalen, "An Experiment with Orange-red Underwear."

39. Davy, *Researches, Physiological and Anatomical*, 1:812.

40. Rattray, "On Some of the More Important Physiological Changes Induced in the Human Economy by Change of Climate."

41. Chamberlain, "Observations of the Influence of the Philippine Climate." See also his "Some Features of the Physiological Activity of White Races."

42. Phalen and Nichols, "Outline of an Experiment."

43. Musgrave and Sison, "Blood Pressure in the Tropics." Musgrave, the director of the Philippine General Hospital, later became professor of pediatrics at the University of California in San Francisco. The Filipinos in this study were students and local police.

44. Chamberlain, "A Study of the Systolic Blood Pressure and the Pulse Rate," 481.

45. See Davidson, ed., *Hygiene and Diseases of Warm Climates*, and Daniels and Wilkinson, *Tropical Medicine and Hygiene.*

46. Chamberlain, "The Red Blood Corpuscles and the Hemoglobin of Healthy Adult

American Males," 484. Chamberlain was challenging the pathological findings of a colleague, Lt. W. A. Wickline. See Wickline to Chief Surgeon, Department of Luzon, June 24, 1907, RG 112-E26, 48453, NARA.

47. Chamberlain and Vedder, "A Study of Arneth's Nuclear Classification of Neutrophils in Healthy Adult Males." During this period Vedder and Chamberlain were also investigating the dietary causes of beriberi and the use of rice polishings in its treatment. See Vedder, *Beriberi*.

48. Weston P. Chamberlain, "Quarterly Report of the US Army Board of Study," June 30, 1910, RG 112-68075-81, NARA.

49. We now know that the eosinophilia was a result of hookworm infection: see chapter 7.

50. See chapter 5.

51. See the summary in Havard, *Manual of Military Hygiene*, chapter 57. This optimism in part reflected and confirmed a more general medical confidence in European self-projection in the tropics, which emerged with the new tropical medicine in Britain at the end of the nineteenth century. See, for example, Sambon, "Remarks on Acclimatization in Tropical Regions." It also perhaps indicates the earlier medical success, a generation or more before, in the United States in dissolving southern distinctiveness and creating a more homogeneous national disease habitat: see Warner, "The Idea of Southern Medical Distinctiveness."

52. Latour, "Give Me a Laboratory and I Will Raise the World," 154.

53. Heiser, "The Progress of Medicine in the Philippines."

54. For other examples of the recuperation of racial categories through the study of acquired immunity, see Sternberg, *Infection and Immunity*, 24; and Clemow, *The Geography of Disease*, 5. For an account that mutes the racialism of "acquired immunity," see Mendelsohn, "Medicine and the Making of Bodily Inequality."

55. Washburn, "Health Conditions in the Philippines," 273.

56. Freer, *The Philippine Experiences of an American Teacher*, 188.

57. Freer, "A Consideration of Some of the Modern Theories of Immunity," 74.

58. Louis Mervin Maus, "Military Sanitary Problems in the Philippine Islands," September 5, 1908, p. 4, RG 112-E26-18668-27, NARA. (This is the typescript of a lecture presented at the annual meeting of the American Association of Military Surgeons.)

59. Bean, *The Racial Anatomy of the Philippine Islanders*, 513. Bean became professor of anatomy at Tulane.

60. Buckland, *In the Land of the Filipino*, 231.

61. Fee, *A Woman's Impressions of the Philippines*, 236.

62. W. Cameron Forbes, Journals, October 19, 1907, 2:324–25, Forbes papers, fMS Am 1365, Houghton Library, Harvard University, Cambridge, Mass.

63. Freer, *Philippine Experiences*, 144.

64. Conger, *Ohio Woman*, 159, 51, 148.

65. W. P. Chamberlain to Surgeon General, June 24, 1905, RG 112-E26-72605-31, NARA. As Robert Joy points out, the first person to document carrier status (ironically, his own) was Brigadier General George M. Sternberg, M.D., in "A Fatal Form of Septacemia in the Rabbit Produced by Subcutaneous Injection of Human Saliva." Frie-

drich Loeffler identified diphtheria carriers in 1884. On the development of the idea of carrier status in the 1890s by Robert Koch and William H. Park, see Winslow, *The Conquest of Epidemic Disease*, chapter 16.

66. P. E. Garrison et al., "Medical Survey of Taytay." On the "latent malaria" of Philippine scouts, see James M. Phalen to C. E. Woodruff, March 4, 1903, RG 112-E26-77872-33, NARA.

67. Chamberlain et al., "Examination of Stools and Blood among the gorots."

68. P. E. Garrison, "The Prevalence and Distribution of the Animal Parasites of Man in the Philippine Islands," 205.

69. Headquarters, Third Brigade, Department of Luzon, Circular No. 7, March 2, 1903, RG 112-E26-77872-33, NARA.

70. Manson, *Tropical Diseases* (1914), 368.

71. Vaughan, *Infection and Immunity*, 179. Zinsser discusses the limitations of the immunities of race in *Infection and Resistance*, chapter 3.

72. Castellani and Chalmers, *Manual of Tropical Medicine*, 115.

73. LeRoy, *Philippine Life in Town and Country*, 54.

74. Moses, *Unofficial Letters of an Official's Wife*, 222.

75. Chief Surgeon, Philippines Division, to Surgeon General, December 31, 1909, GR 112-E26-24508–120, NARA. See also the "Report on Typhoid Fever," September 30, 1909, RG 112-E26-68075-73, NARA.

76. Chief Surgeon, Philippines Division, to Surgeon General, December 31, 1909, p. 13, GR 112-E26-24508-120, NARA.

77. Quoted in Chief Surgeon, Philippines Division, to Surgeon General, December 31, 1909, p. 21, RG 112-E26-24508-120, NARA. On the use of the Widal test to diagnose typhoid, see Heiser, "Typhoid Fever in the Philippine Islands."

78. Quoted in Chief Surgeon, Philippines Division, to Surgeon General, December 31, 1909, p. 17, RG 112-E26-24508-120, NARA.

79. Quoted in Chief Surgeon, Philippines Division, to Surgeon General, December 31, 1909, p. 23, RG 112-E26-24508-120, NARA.

80. Craig, "Observations upon Malaria," 525. Craig is better known for his work on the parasitic amoebae of man.

81. Ibid.

82. Charles F. Craig, Report, quoted in Chief Surgeon, Philippines Division, to Surgeon General, March 7, 1908, p. 10, RG 112-E26-24508-38, NARA.

83. Craig, "Observations upon Malaria," 525.

84. Colonial scientists also conducted extensive vaccine and therapeutic experimentation on Filipino prison inmates during this period. Perhaps the most notorious of these studies was Richard P. Strong's inoculation of twenty-four inmates at Bilibid with a new live cholera vaccine that had somehow become contaminated with plague organisms. A virulent plague culture had been accidentally mixed with the cholera cultures. All the men sickened, and thirteen died. After an investigation, Strong was exonerated. Strong had, though, conducted the inoculations "in the convalescent ward [where] he ordered all the prisoners there to form a line . . . without telling them what he was going to do, nor consulting their wishes in the matter" ("Report of the

General Committee," 1 March 1907, p. 11, RG 350-4341-21, NARA). Neither cholera nor plague was prevalent in the prison at the time. The investigating committee suggested that Strong had forgotten "the respect due every human being in not having asked the consent of persons inoculated." It enjoined the governor-general to order that no one would be subjected to "experiment without prior determination of the character of that experiment by authorities . . . nor without having first gained the expressed consent of the person subject to it" ("Report of the General Committee," March 1, 1907, p. 18, RG 350-4341-21, NARA). See Chernin, "Richard Pearson Strong and the Iatrogenic Plague Disaster." Chernin (1001) points out that Strong's earlier study of plague immunization (1905), also conducted without consent, has been presented as a case study in human experimentation in Katz, *Experimentation with Human Beings*.

85. Antityphoid immunization was available from 1911 for troops stationed in the Philippines, but not for Filipinos (and not for American civilians either): see Frederick Russell, *The Results of Anti-Typhoid Vaccination in the Army*.

86. Heiser, "Unsolved Health Problems," 174–75.

87. Ibid., 175.

88. *Annual Report of the Bureau of Health for the Philippine Islands, July 1, 1912–June 30, 1913* (Manila: Bureau of Printing, 1913), 61.

89. Chapin, "Dirt, Disease and the Health Officer," 21, 24. A report on Chapin's visit to Havana can be found in the *Providence Medical J.* 2 (1902): 103–05. Chapin, a friend of William Crawford Gorgas, paid close attention to colonial public health work. See also Cassedy, *Charles V. Chapin and the Public Health Movement*.

90. Chapin, "The Fetich of Disinfection," 75. See also Chapin, *Sources and Modes of Infection*.

91. Winslow, "Man and the Microbe," 9. Winslow was professor of public health at Yale.

92. Leavitt, *Typhoid Mary*. On the new public health, see Hill, *The New Public Health*; Rosen, *A History of Public Health*; Rosenkrantz, *Public Health and the State*; Leavitt, *Healthiest City*; Rogers, "Germs with Legs"; Duffy, *The Sanitarians*; and Porter, *Health, Civilization and the State*. Nancy Tomes also describes a shift in interest from dust and fomite infection to a concern with healthy carriers and contact infection during the first two decades of the twentieth century. See Tomes, *The Gospel of Germs*. Tomes tends to emphasize the ways in which germs overcame social divisions, rather than sharpened them.

93. Taft, "Address of President Taft," 505.

94. Ibid.

95. Shah, *Contagious Divides*. See also Trauner, "The Chinese as Medical Scapegoats in San Francisco"; McClain, "Of Medicine, Race and American Law"; and Craddock, *City of Plagues*.

96. Howard, "The Negro as a Distinct Ethnic Factor in Civilization," 424, quoted in Fredrickson, *The Black Image in the White Mind*. A few other southern physicians began to urge "the development and upbuilding of the minds, morals and bodies of a 'child race,'" in order to protect whites from Negro tuberculosis (Harris, "Tuber-

culosis in the Negro," 837). See also Galishoff, "Germs Know No Color Line"; Brown, "Purity and Danger in Color"; and Abel, "From Exclusion to Expulsion."

97. Kraut, *Silent Travelers*; Markel, *Quarantine!*; and Fairchild, *Science at the Borders*. See also Higham, *Strangers in the Land*.

98. Monnais-Rousselot, *Médecine et Colonisation*, 170, 165.

99. Manderson, *Sickness and the State*; and Gouda, *Dutch Culture Overseas*.

100. Davisakd Puaksom, "Modern Medicine in Thailand: Germ, Body, and the Medicalized State" (Unpublished ms., c. 2004).

101. Liu, "Building a Strong and Healthy Empire"; and Lo, *Doctors Within Borders*.

102. Arnold, *Colonizing the Body*. Operating through the Rockefeller Foundation, Heiser and other ex-Philippines health officers had a profound influence on these regional developments in the 1920s and 1930s: see Conclusion.

103. See, for example, Anon., "Stand Off Heiser's Men at the Point of a Gun: Filipino Family in Santa Cruz Would Die Rather than Be Disinfected," *Manila Times* (July 1, 1907), 1.

104. Musgrave, "Progress of Medicine in the Philippines," 143.

105. Herzog, "The Brain Weight of Filipinos," 42, 47.

106. McLaughlan, "The Suppression of a Cholera Epidemic in Manila," 55.

107. Heiser, "Unsolved Health Problems," 176.

108. Thomas W. Jackson, "Sanitary Conditions and Needs in Provincial Towns," *PJS* 3B (1908): 431–38, at 432, 435–36.

109. *Cablenews-American* (May 30, 1909).

110. Shaler, "The Future of the Negro in the Southern States," 151. On Shaler, the "forefather of American geography," see Livingstone, "Science and Society."

111. Shaler, "The Transplantation of a Race," 521. Shaler was surprised at how well Africans—those "tropical exotics"—had acclimatized to North America. They had withstood their "trials of deportation in a marvelous way," with no particular liability to disease or impairment of fecundity (514). He supposed this was because slave-owners had sensitively managed their health and breeding (518).

112. Bullard, "Some Characteristics of the Negro Volunteer," 29. When Arthur A. Snyder, M.D., volunteered as a surgeon with one of the "immune regiments," the surgeon general asked him if he was "an immune." As he was white, his application initially was rejected—he had to be "an immune or nothing." Later he received a posting in a nonimmune regiment. See Arthur Augustine Snyder, "Experiences of a Contract Surgeon," ms., n.d., p. 1, Spanish-American War Survey, U.S. Army Military History Institute, Carlisle Barracks, Penn.

113. Bullard, "Some Characteristics of the Negro Volunteer," 30–31. Bullard had ensured that "men with a larger proportion of white blood [were] rejected" (30). See also Gatewood, *Black Americans and the White Man's Burden*, esp. 297–309.

114. Rhodes, "The Utilization of Foreign Troops in Our Foreign Possessions," 6, 7. The exception refers to what we now know as dengue.

115. Ibid., 7. See also Seaman, "Native Troops for Our Colonial Possessions."

116. Fortune, "The Filipino," 202–3. Roosevelt had appointed Fortune in 1902 to investigate labor and race relations in the insular possessions. Also in favor of Negro

colonization was Scarborough, "The Negro and Our New Possessions." Opposed
was Lemus, "The Negro and the Philippines." By 1903, there was little official
interest in the idea. See Moore, "Senator John Tyler Morgan and Negro Colonization in the Philippines"; and Gatewood, *Black Americans*.

117. *Congressional Record*, 57th Congress, 1st Session, May 7, 1902, 5103. But studies
continued. See, for example, the report of the comparative fitness of white and
colored troops in Assistant Surgeon General to Chief of Staff, U.S. Army, April 27,
1907, RG 112-E26-48453-D, NARA.

4. EXCREMENTAL COLONIALISM

1. Bureau of Health, *The Disposal of Human Wastes in the Provinces*, 4–5

2. De Witt, "A Few Remarks Concerning the Health Conditions of Americans in the
Philippines," 56.

3. Marshall, *Asiatic Cholera in the Philippine Islands*, 9.

4. See especially Corbin, *The Foul and the Fragrant*. Laporte has suggested that "apprenticeship in smelling [was] directed entirely toward excrement" (*Histoire de la
Merde*, 60) and that the rise of a strong state led to the privatizing and constrained
circulation of smell-producing excrement.

5. Vigarello argues that the microbe "materialized" the risk previously associated with
odor, in *Concepts of Cleanliness*, 203. On "excremental vision," see Brown, "The
Excremental Vision."

6. Chapin, "Dirt, Disease and the Health Officer," 21.

7. Munson, *The Theory and Practice of Military Hygiene*. See chapter 1.

8. Douglas, *Purity and Danger*, 35. William James, in his lecture "The Sick Soul," also
refers to the challenge that "matter out of place" presents to any system — "evil" can
thus be represented as "an alien unreality, a waste element, to be sloughed off and
negated," and the "ideal" is "marked by its deliverance from all contact with this
diseased, inferior, and excrementitious stuff" (113). Of course James warns us
against "medical materialism," that is, reducing symbolic systems to a medical
explanation. (James was a friend and correspondent of some of the senior colonial
administrators in the Philippines, in particular W. Cameron Forbes.)

9. See Stallybrass and White, "The City: The Sewer, the Gaze and the Contaminating
Touch," in *The Politics and Poetics of Transgression*.

10. The emphasis of this chapter differs slightly from a previous version: see Anderson,
"Excremental Colonialism." See also Mbembe, "The Banality of Power"; Lee, "Toilet Training the Settler Subject"; and Esty, "Excremental Postcolonialism."

11. On abjection, "which modernity has learned to repress, dodge or fake" (26), see Kristeva, *Powers of Horror*. She describes the abject as "something rejected from which
one does not part, from which one does not protect oneself as from an object" (4).

12. See, for example, Heiser, "Sanitation in the Philippines." On the necessary preliminary performance of rottenness, see De Certeau, "The Institution of Rot," in
Heterologies, 42.

13. Elias, *The Civilizing Process*. Bourdieu has argued more generally that the reformation of manners "extorts the essential while seeming to demand the insignificant,"

ensuring that "the concessions of *politeness* always contain *political* concessions" (*Outline of a Theory of Practice*, 90).

14. On the body as a medium of social expression, see Mauss, "Techniques of the Body." The relation I am sketching here between the "technologies of domination of others" and the "technologies of the self," Foucault, in his later work, has called "governmentality." See "Governmentality"; "The Political Technology of Individuals" in *Technologies of the Self*; "Body/Power," in *Power/Knowledge*; and *Discipline and Punish*.

15. Phelan, "Sanitary Service in Surigao," 3, 7, 6, 18, 17, 10, 17.

16. Munson, "Cholera Carriers in Relation to Cholera Control," 5, 9. See also Shöbl, "Observations Concerning Cholera Carriers."

17. Paul C. Freer, *Eighth Annual Report of the Director of the Bureau of Science, For the Year Ending August 1, 1909* (Manila: Bureau of Printing, 1910), 16. Alvin J. Cox, *Thirteenth Annual Report of the Director of the Bureau of Science, For the Year Ending December 31, 1914* (Manila: Bureau of Printing, 1915), 11, 12.

18. Sanitary engineering — the construction of sewers and a clean water supply — offered to limit contact with native excreta, but these major projects did not much alter conditions in Manila until 1910, and then only in the more prosperous districts. In the rest of the archipelago, behavior change remained the only alternative — and a cheaper one too.

19. P. E. Garrison, "The Prevalence and Distribution of the Animal Parasites of Man," p. 208.

20. Benjamin J. Edger, "Some Medical and Sanitary Experiences" [c. 1904], p. 7, RG 112-E26-72605-27, NARA. See also "Report of Major Franklin A. Meacham, chief surgeon 3rd military district of the Department of Northern Luzon, to Chief Surgeon Department of Northern Luzon, May 31, 1900," in Sternberg, *Report of the Surgeon-General of the Army*, 1900, 140.

21. Chamberlin, *The Philippine Problem*, 113–14.

22. Strong et al., "Medical Survey of the Town of Taytay."

23. Edger, "Some Medical and Sanitary Experiences," 5, 15.

24. Moses, *Unofficial Letters of an Official's Wife*, 14, 16, 221, 226. More generally, see Rafael, "Colonial Domesticity."

25. Conger, *An Ohio Woman in the Philippines*, 51, 70.

26. Mearns, *A Philippine Romance*, 77. Naturally, Patricia felt out of place among these "barbarous people just emerging from centuries of superstition, fear and medievalism" (36).

27. Dauncey, *An Englishwoman in the Philippines*, 242. Mrs. Dauncey, a terrible English snob, lamented that the manners of bourgeois white Americans were those of "ordinary European peasants" (12), and she disparaged the "half-finished, skin-deep, hustling modernity of Americanized Manila" (133). It seemed to her "a pity that such rough diamonds should represent to these natives the manners and intellect of a great and ruling white nation" (13).

28. On the grotesque, defecating body and its opposite, see Bakhtin, *Rabelais and His World*. Bakhtin, however, argues for the authenticity of the grotesque folkloric, and the communal bodies he describes are isolated by the fracture lines of class, not race.

29. Haraway describes a similar masculine American relation to the natural world in "Teddy Bear Patriarchy: Taxidermy in the Garden of Eden, New York City, 1908–1936," in *Primate Visions*.

30. The "American sublime" is a rhetorical sublime, not the metaphysics of the unpresentable. It is a colonial displacement of the "sublimated spectacle of national empowerment" that Wilson has described in *American Sublime* and in "Technoeuphoria and the Discourse of the American Sublime," 208.

31. Lefebvre, *The Production of Space*, esp. 285–91. Lefebvre describes the production of abstract space from the sixteenth century, as it in part supplanted the "space of accumulation," typically the marketplace.

32. See RG 350-3466-0, NARA. Act No. 607 (June 30, 1903) transferred the serum laboratory of the Board of Health to the Bureau of Government Laboratories. Act No. 1407 (October 26, 1905) reorganized the laboratories into the Bureau of Science. See Velasco and Baens-Arcega, *The National Institute of Science and Technology, 1901–1982*; Quisumbing, "Development of Science in the Philippines"; and Anderson, "Science in the Philippines."

33. Act No. 156, section 2, RG 350-3466-0, NARA.

34. Act No. 156, section 2, p. 10, RG 350-3466-0, NARA.

35. Freer, *Description of the New Buildings of the Bureau of Government Laboratories*, 8.

36. Ibid., 13. This is the original building, still standing on the campus of the Philippines Medical School. In 1912, a new wing was opened to contain a division of mines, the section of fisheries and fish products, the entomological collections and laboratories, and a new herbarium and library. See Paul C. Freer, *Tenth Annual Report of the Director of the Bureau of Science, for the year ending August 1, 1911* (Manila: Bureau of Printing, 1912), 3–5.

37. Freer, *Description of the New Buildings*, 21.

38. Freer, *Third Annual Report of the Director of the Bureau of Science, 1903–04* (Manila: Bureau of Printing, 1904), 16–18.

39. Freer, *Description of the New Buildings*, 29. Freer described the herbarium as "a card catalogue of the economic and scientific aspects of Philippine botany" (*Fourth Annual Report of the Director of the Bureau of Science, 1904–05* [Manila: Bureau of Printing, 1905], 4).

40. Freer, *Third Annual Report, 1903–04*, 11.

41. Ibid., 26.

42. LeRoy, *Philippine Life in Town and Country*, 290.

43. Hayden, *The Philippines: A Study in National Development*, 644.

44. Latour, "Give Me a Laboratory and I Will Raise the World."

45. Freer, *Third Annual Report, 1903–04*, 24.

46. Bakhtin, *Rabelais*, 23.

47. Although such places do not seem to have retained the "utopian folk element"—the reveling, games, clowning, and so on—that Bakhtin found in an earlier European carnivalesque, entering the market undoubtedly continued to produce a discomforting sense of a suspension of hierarchy, a sense of freedom and familiarity (Bakhtin, *Rabelais*, 217–76). See Stallybrass and White, *Transgression*, on the carnivalesque as

a mode of understanding (6–19). They suggest that "repugnance and fascination are the twin poles of the process in which a *political* imperative to reject and eliminate the debasing 'low' conflicts powerfully and unpredictably with a desire for this Other" (4–5). This vulnerable assumption of superiority actually depends on the construction of the low Other.

48. LeRoy, *Philippine Life in Town and Country*, 54; Roosevelt, *The Philippines: A Treasure and a Problem*, 233; Williams, *The United States and the Philippines*, 125; and Freer, *The Philippine Experiences of an American Teacher*, 7–8. For a similar account of the "filth" and the "swarming masses of people" in primitive markets, see Lévi-Strauss, *Tristes tropiques*, 143–45.

49. Mayo, *The Isles of Fear*, 174. According to the *Proposed Sanitary Code*, 1920, Sect. 49, "Every person engaging in the dispatching, transportation, handling or manipulation of food products . . . shall be provided with a certificate from the district health officer . . . [to] show that he is in good health and he is not a carrier of pathogenic germs" (22).

50. J. F. Smith to Secretary of War, November 22, 1908, RG 350-3465-91, NARA. In the early 1900s, when Buckland visited the Visayas, he found "not a knife, fork, nor spoon, nor a tumbler in the whole barrio. I had to eat with a piece of bamboo cut in the form of a paddle" (*In the Land of the Filipino*, 184).

51. Heiser, *Annual Report of the Bureau of Health of the Philippine Islands, July 1, 1912–June 30, 1913* (Manila: Bureau of Printing, 1914), 29.

52. Fox, *Handbook for Sanitary Inspectors*.

53. Heiser, *Annual Report of the Bureau of Health of the Philippine Islands, July 1, 1912–June 30, 1913* (Manila: Bureau of Printing, 1914), 29–30. Heiser argued that the "habit of eating with the fingers" was the "largest factor in the transmission of cholera and intestinal diseases" ("Unsolved Health Problems," 176).

54. Heiser, *Annual Report, 1912–13*, 28. The *tienda* proprietors generally were a cause of considerable concern: "The tienda owner . . . shall wear clean clothes with or without an apron. The hands must be kept clean and the finger nails short and well trimmed." So too were street peddlers: "The peddler must be neatly dressed. His hands should be clean and the nails short" (Bantug, Gabriel, and Aguelles, *A Simple Manual for Sanitary Inspectors*, 12, 14).

55. Heiser, *Annual Report, 1912–13*, 67–68.

56. [Miller], *Interesting Manila*, 191. In more ways than the metaphysical, then, "the Anglo-Saxon lives in the concrete, the Oriental in the shadows" (17).

57. Carpenter, *Through the Philippines and Hawaii*, 24.

58. John D. Long, director of health, to W. H. Greenleaf, Jan. 7, 1918, RG 350-3465-97, NARA, provides a detailed account of these activities. See also Vicente de Jesús, "Circular W-82," Philippine Health Service, Manila, Nov 20, 1924, RG 350-3465-132, NARA; and Heiser to commissioner of education, Dept. of the Interior, Washington, D.C., Sept. 27, 1913, RG 350-3465-55, NARA.

59. John D. Long to W. H. Greenleaf, Jan. 7, 1918, RG 350-3465-97, NARA.

60. Bureau of Education and Philippine Health Service, *Health: A Manual for Teachers*, consolidates instructions to teachers from the previous decade.

61. Ibid., 33.

62. Ibid., 49.

63. Ibid., 5. On the development of the water closet in the late nineteenth century, see Wright, *Clean and Decent*; and Goubert, *The Conquest of Water*, 91–97. The water closet is an invention of the last decades of the nineteenth century: Wright goes so far as to call 1870 the "annus mirabilis of the water closet" (201). On the enclosure of the bathroom as a private space, from 1880 onward, see Vigarello, *Concepts of Cleanliness*, 215–25.

64. Heiser, "Unsolved Health Problems," 173.

65. Bureau of Health, *Cholera Measures*, 4.

66. Heiser, "Unsolved Health Problems."

67. *Disposal of Human Wastes*, 5–7.

68. Ibid., 7–9.

69. Large parts of Manila were sewered between 1905 and 1910. See *Annual Report of the Municipal Board of the City of Manila* (Manila: Bureau of Printing, 1910), 81.

70. Willets, "Conditions Affecting Batanes Islands," 51. Still, one was less likely to be as embarrassed on the boat to Capiz as Buckland was in 1903: "A walk around the deck failed to disclose any of the conveniences that Americans have come to regard as absolute necessities. There was not a sign of a bathroom nor even of a lavatory any place on the main deck" (*Land of the Filipino*, 62).

71. McLaughlin, "The Suppression of a Cholera Epidemic in Manila," 49, 50.

72. Bureau of Health. *Proposed Sanitary Code*, 15–17. The director of health in his report for the fiscal year 1919 had urged "preferential attention [be] given to the disposal of human wastes" (p. 15, RG 350-3465-108, NARA). A further description of the "Antipolo system of toilet" is provided in Tianco (under the direction of Long), *Philippine Health Service Sanitary Almanac for 1919 and Calendars for 1920 and 1921*, 13, 16–19.

73. Rizal, *Noli Me Tangere*, 166–92.

74. Dauncey, *An Englishwoman in the Philippines*, 52.

75. Moses, *Unofficial Letters*, 45, 17, 67. On public gatherings as sites of resistance, see Ileto, *Pasyon and Revolution*.

76. Bureau of Health, "Sanitary Measures in Connection with Local Fiestas," Provincial Circular No. 124, Oct. 6, 1915, RG 350-3465-86, NARA. On the dangers of fiestas, see also Marshall, "Asiatic Cholera," 8.

77. Bureau of Health, "Sanitary Measures in Connection with Local Fiestas."

78. Ibid. See also *Annual Report Bureau of Health for the Philippine Islands, 1912–1913*, 33.

79. *The Philippines Carnival, Manila, February 3–8, 1908*, RG 350-5453-2, NARA. Gomez was the son of the Filipino statistician at the Bureau of Health.

80. O'Reilly, "Manila's Grand Annual Carnival," 55. O'Reilly, ironically, concluded: "Come, ye globe trotters, and enjoy our contagious enthusiasm!" (59).

81. Harry Debnam, "The Philippine Carnival: Being an Official Report of its Organization, Purpose and Success," pp. 14, 26, RG 350-5453-9, NARA.

82. J. F. Smith to Chief, Bureau of Insular Affairs, March 5, 1908, RG 350-5434-5, NARA.

83. "Manila Carnival" 1909, n.p., RG 350-5453-13, NARA.

84. W. Cameron Forbes to Edwards, Bureau of Insular Affairs, June 17, 1909, RG 350-5453-14, NARA.

85. W. Cameron Forbes to Major Frank MacIntyre, Bureau of Insular Affairs, December 6, 1910, RG 350-5453-24, NARA.

86. W. Cameron Forbes to Jacob M. Dickinson, February 19, 1910, RG 350-5453-30, NARA. Still, these institutional carnivals played on a few extraordinary symbolic inversions. In *The Carnival Spirit*, a gossip sheet published daily during the 1911 carnival, "Hemlock Jones," the carnival detective, reported that he found Dr. Victor Heiser "on the Main Street carrying a hypodermic syringe and injecting cholera germs into the arms of luckless persons who came within his grasp" (RG 350-5453-38, NARA). Perhaps memories of R. P. Strong's use of contaminated vaccine at Bilibid were still fresh.

87. H. S. Howland to Secretary, Philippine Carnival Association, April 30, 1908, p. 4, RG 350-5453-12, NARA.

88. Editorial, *La Vanguardia* (January 19, 1911).

89. Editorial, *La Democracia* (February 8, 1911).

90. See Vaughan, "Ogling Igorots."

91. Editorial, *El Ideal* (January 23, 1912).

92. Editorial, *La Vanguardia* (January 27, 1912).

93. See, for example, *La Vanguardia* (January 30, 1912), *El Ideal* (February 1, 1912), and *La Vanguardia* (February 1, 1912).

94. Anon., "Highly Artistic Red Cross Carnival," 95.

95. Anon., "The 1918 Philippine Red Cross Carnival," 196, 197.

96. Anon. "The 1918 Philippine Red Cross Carnival," 198.

97. Anon., "Commercial Exhibits," 3.

98. Anon., "The Carnival and the Student," 6. For a report emphasizing sanitation in the 1922 Carnival (and describing the first "Health Parade"), see Anon., "Manila Carnival and Commercial-Industrial Fair."

99. "Clean-Up Week." Provincial Circular (Unnumbered), Oct. 21, 1914 RG 350-3465- 80, NARA. Clean-Up Week was also observed in many U.S. towns. Frank Crone instructed teachers in the Philippines to explain to their students the meaning of Clean-Up Week. "If 'Clean-Up Week' is carried out successfully the Philippines will be cleaner than ever before in their history," he declared. "Public health will be improved accordingly" ("Clean-Up Week." Board of Education Circular No. 142, Nov. 3, 1914, RG 350-3465-80, NARA).

100. "Clean-Up Week." Provincial Circular (Unnumbered), Nov. 2, 1915, RG 350-3465-80, NARA.

101. *Clean-Up Week: A Patriotic Message to all Patriotic Citizens* (Manila: Bureau of Printing, 1922), RG 350-3465-80, NARA. This pamphlet also suggests that "unsanitary condition is not compatible with our national pride and aspiration."

102. "Clean-Up Week." Public Welfare Board Circular, Oct. 30, 1920, RG 350-3465-80, NARA.

103. Ibid.

104. *Clean-Up Week: A Patriotic Message*, 8. Clean-up Week was still popular in the

1930s: see Davis, "Significance of Clean-Up Week." Davis, the governor-general of the islands, pointed out that "the formation of health habits is an important factor in the prevention of diseases. Health habits include sanitation, personal cleanliness, plenty of fresh air, good nourishing food, sleep, sunshine, and exercise" (7). See also the delightfully specific *Organization and Activities of Clean-Up Week for 1924* (Manila: Bureau of Printing, 1924), RG 350-3465-80, NARA. This is prefaced with a "proclamation" from Leonard Wood, then governor-general: he insists that "unattractive unsanitary surroundings are inconsistent with the best traditions and ideals of a progressive people" (5).

105. These are not, however, commonly regarded as sites where the nation may be imagined. See Benedict Anderson, *Imagined Communities*; and Chatterjee, *The Nation and Its Fragments*. Of course both Benedict Anderson and Chatterjee are arguing about the sources of nationalism, which should be distinguished from what I describe here: the creation of a certain sort of civic mentality, that is, the colonial project of making proper, though never quite authentic, national subjects.

106. Joaquin, "Sa loob ng Manila," 455.

107. Walker and Sellards, "Experimental Entamoebic Dysentery." William H. Welch had recommended Sellards, a Hopkins graduate, as a man with "a good training in laboratory work in bacteriology and pathology . . . a gentleman of high character" (RG 350-19335-7, NARA). Sellards was later a physician at Hopkins and Harvard. See Sellards, "Bonds of Union between Tropical Medicine and General Medicine."

108. Douglas, *Purity and Danger*, 165. "Epistemological clarity" is from Stallybrass and White, *Transgression*, 108.

5. THE WHITE MAN'S PSYCHIC BURDEN

1. "Journal," n.d [c. March 1912], vol. 5, p. 121, fMS Am 1365, W. C. Forbes papers, Houghton Library, Harvard University. On Forbes, see Stanley, "William Cameron Forbes."

2. Forbes to A. L. Lowell, Oct. 24, 1912, Dean's File (T. M.) 1908–23, Code 11: 597, Rare Book Room, Countway Medical Library, Harvard Medical School.

3. Adjutant general, Philippines Division, to P. M. Ashburn, March 15, 1912, RG 112-E26-68075-123, NARA. P. M. Ashburn to adjutant general, March 18, 1912, RG 112-E26-68075-123, NARA.

4. Roosevelt, *The Philippines*, 245.

5. Beard, *A Practical Treatise on Nervous Exhaustion (Neurasthenia)*. Rosenberg has suggested that Beard's work illustrates "the utility of scientific metaphor and authority in helping rationalize a rapidly changing and stress-filled world" ("George M. Beard and American Nervousness," 98). On the rise of the diagnosis of neurasthenia in America, see also Sicherman, "The Uses of a Diagnosis"; Gosling, *Before Freud*; and Lutz, *American Nervousness 1903*. See also Showalter, *The Female Malady*, esp. chapter 5; Oppenheim, *"Shattered Nerves"*; and Gijswijt-Hofstra and Porter, eds., *Cultures of Neurasthenia from Beard to the First World War*. On the related "discovery of fatigue" by European scientists after 1890, see Rabinbach, *The Human Motor*.

6. On tropical neurasthenia in other imperial contexts, see Kennedy, "The Perils of the Midday Sun."

7. See Vaughan, *Curing Their Ills*; Ernst, *Mad Tales from the Raj*, and "European Madness and Gender in Nineteenth-century British India"; McCulloch, *Colonial Psychiatry and "the African Mind"*; Sadowsky, *Imperial Bedlam*; and Mills, *Madness, Cannabis, and Colonialism*. For a perceptive review essay, see Keller, "Madness and Colonization."

8. Hartnack, "Vishnu on Freud's Desk"; Nandy, "The Savage Freud"; and Sudhir Kakar, "Encounters of the Psychological Kind."

9. In American studies they are rarely recognized as such: both Bederman and Rotundo emphasize the importance of the *idea* of empire in reshaping masculinity but do not study the *experience* of empire. See Bederman, *Manliness and Civilization*; and Rotundo, *American Manhood*. Yet Rafael has remarked on the Philippines as a "terrain for the testing and validation of white masculinity" ("Colonial Domesticity"). See also Mrozek, "The Habit of Victory"; and Kaplan, "Romancing the Empire."

10. See Bederman's helpful remarks on the redefining of manhood in terms of racial dominance in the United States, in *Manliness and Civilization*.

11. Nandy, *The Intimate Enemy*; Hyam, *Empire and Sexuality*, 72; and Sinha, *Colonial Masculinities*. On the mutually reinforcing categories of gender and empire, see also Callaway, *Gender, Culture and Empire*; Sangari and Vaid, *Recasting Women*; Hansen, ed., *African Encounters with Domesticity*; Chaudhuri and Strobel, eds, *Western Women and Imperialism*; and Nussbaum, *Torrid Zones*. All of these studies refer to the British Empire.

12. Stoler, *Race and the Education of Desire*, 62, 99, 32. See especially Stoler, "Rethinking Colonial Categories," "Carnal Knowledge and Imperial Power," and "Sexual Affronts and Racial Frontiers."

13. Rosenberg, "Sexuality, Class and Role in Nineteenth-century America"; Lears, "The Destructive Element"; Kimmel, "The Contemporary 'Crisis' in Masculinity in Historical Perspective"; and Griffen, "Reconstructing Masculinity from the Evangelical Revival to the Waning of Progressivism."

14. Bederman, *Manliness and Civilization*; and Rotundo, *American Manhood*. On the flexibility of gender categories, see Scott, "Gender: A Useful Category of Historical Analysis."

15. James, "The Moral Equivalent of War," 323. On James's own breakdown, see Feinstein, "The Use and Abuse of Illness in the James Family Circle." For similar prescriptions, see Roosevelt, *The Strenuous Life*.

16. The phrase is of course from Kipling's poem "The White Man's Burden."

17. Rafael, "White Love," 200. See also Rafael, *White Love, and Other Events in Filipino History*.

18. Much recent postcolonial criticism has valorized heterogeneity and hybridity: see, for example, Bhabha, *The Location of Culture*; McClintock, *Imperial Leather*; and Young, *Colonial Desire*.

19. The quotation is from Williams, *Empire as a Way of Life*. See also Kaplan, "'Left Alone with America,'" 14.

20. See Kagan, *Life and Letters of Fielding H. Garrison*; the Fielding H. Garrison Memorial Number of the *Bulletin of the History of Medicine* 5 (1937): 299–403; and Brieger, "Fielding H. Garrison: The Man and His Book." Garrison was a leading figure in the study of medical history in the United States; the Fielding H. Garrison lecture is delivered each year at the annual meeting of the American Association of the History of Medicine. The Army Medical Library was the forerunner of the National Library of Medicine.

21. Garrison-Mencken correspondence, box 5, F. H. Garrison papers, Ms c 166, History of Medicine Division, National Library of Medicine, Bethesda, Md. I am grateful to Elizabeth Toon for suggesting I look at the Garrison-Mencken correspondence.

22. Garrison frequently boasts about his alcohol consumption. He liked "above all the local beer, which is well-brewed and of which I usually absorb two bottles a day in the 'wet' (typhoon) season. There are also Burgundies, Spanish (Rioja) clarets, and even some Rhine wines, also chartreuses, benedictines, and other cordials galore." The Scotch "flows in rivers" (July 29, 1923).

23. "Review of the Year 1906," 51; "Review of the Year 1907," 241; "Review of the Year 1908," 105; in cartons 2 and 3, David Prescott Barrows papers, mss c-B 1005, Bancroft Library, University of California at Berkeley. Barrows had studied anthropology at the University of Chicago. During his stay in the Philippines, Barrows was losing a political battle over the direction of the school system. He returned to the United States as a professor of education at Berkeley; and in 1919–23 he was president of the University of California.

24. Herbert I. Priestley to mother, October 5, 1902; October 19, 1902; December 21, 1902; January 2, 1903; March 9, 1903, Priestley papers, mss 94/13 cz, Bancroft Library, University of California at Berkeley.

25. Havard, "Is Mortality Necessarily Higher in Tropical than in Temperate Climates?" 17, 20. Havard was an assistant surgeon general of the army. This is probably the earliest article on tropical neurasthenia in the Philippines. But see Tucker, "Neurasthenia in Anglo-Indians." Tucker suggested that in India too there is "a continual strain upon the machinery of [British] bodies from the influence of a tropical climate" (44). Beard had doubted that neurasthenia was present in the tropics because of the absence of any civilization in the region (*Nervous Exhaustion*, 189).

26. Temkin, "The Scientific Approach to Disease: Specific Entity and Individual Sickness."

27. Woodruff, "The Neurasthenic States Caused by Excessive Light," and *The Effects of Tropical Sunlight Upon the White Man*. I discuss Woodruff's theories in more detail in chapter 3. For a similar explanation of the "lack of self-control," "profound nervous depression," and "irritability of temper" that prevailed in sunny parts of the United States, see Watkins, "Neurasthenia among Blondes in the Southwest," 1374. (Watkins was stationed with Woodruff at Plattsburgh Barracks, New York.) Woodruff was probably responding to the theories of Sterne, "Neurasthenia and Its Treatment by Actinic Rays."

28. See Pick, *Faces of Degeneration*.

29. Woodruff, *Expansion of Races*, 257, 274.

30. "Charles E. Woodruff," RG 94-1946APC87, NARA. This file contains Woodruff's medical records, including the "Report" of March 31, 1910.

31. Fales, "Tropical Neurasthenia,"586, 583. Fales also thought that attacks of dengue fever and alcoholism frequently "predisposed to nerve exhaustion" (585). Fales had spent three years as a medical inspector in the islands and become dissatisfied both with the opportunities for private practice there and with "favoritism" in the Bureau of Health. See his "The American Physician in the Philippine Civil Service." Castellani and Chalmers in their *Manual of Tropical Medicine* rely heavily on Fales for their description of tropical neurasthenia (1065). For another evocative account of the "mental and physical stagnation and retrogression" of whites in the tropics, see Edwin P. Wolfe, "Report on Research Work on the Effects of Tropical Climate on the White Race" [c. 1906], RG 112-E26-72605-75, NARA.

32. Fales, "Tropical Neurasthenia," 591. Warnings of the damage to the mental apparatus of white children are commonplace and persistent: "In the case of European children living in the tropics the whole nervous system seems to be in a condition of unstable equilibrium so that, apart from illness, fretfulness and peevishness are common, and a condition often approaching hysteria may even be encountered" (Balfour, "Personal Hygiene," 5).

33. Huntington, *Civilization and Climate*, 8, 42, 44. The lack of will power was often the reason for fits of anger: "their power of self-control is enfeebled" (44).

34. Collini, "The Idea of 'Character' in Victorian Political Thought." Oppenheim explains the importance of "will or "managerial force" as an organizing principle for the nervous system in "*Shattered Nerves*" (42–43).

35. Fales, "American Physician," 514. See also Fales "Tropical Neurasthenia," 584. Fales estimated that 50 percent of women and 30 percent of men in the American community in Manila became neurasthenic.

36. Francis B. Harrison to secretary of war, September 30, 1914, letters, box 43, Francis Burton Harrison papers, Library of Congress.

37. King, "Tropical Neurasthenia," 1519. King was an assistant surgeon with the U.S. Public Health and Marine Hospital Service. For an analysis of similar explanations of female neurasthenia in the United States and Britain, see Showalter, *Female Malady*, esp. chapter 5; and Oppenheim, "*Shattered Nerves*." On tropical menstrual irregularities, see Mackinnon, "Diseases of Women in the Tropics."

38. For example, Moses, *Unofficial Letters of an Official's Wife*; Dauncey, *An Englishwoman in the Philippines*; and Mrs. W. H. Taft, *Recollections of Full Years*.

39. See Rafael, *White Love*.

40. Bernard Moses thought it was because the men of the army showed a "lack of wide intellectual range" — though "formally polite . . . to the best of knowledge and memory they never say anything" (February 8, 1901, Diary, vol. 2. Moses papers, mss 308x M911 di, Bancroft Library, University of California-Berkeley).

41. Eli L. Huggins to sisters, January 18, 1901, Huggins papers, mss 81/51 p, Bancroft Library, University of California-Berkeley. Huggins retired in 1903 as brigadier general. See Huggins, "Custer and Rain-in-the-Face"; and Foreman, "General Eli Lundy Huggins." Dean C. Worcester, in his struggle with Col. L. M. Maus, claimed that the

director of health had suffered in the effort to control a cholera epidemic, and "he had become excessively nervous and had at times been very depressed. On two occasions he had shed tears in my office when discussing difficulties of minor importance" (D. C. Worcester to adjutant-general, March 2, 1909, p. 8, RG 94-67091-a220, NARA). Not surprisingly, Colonel Maus denied this accusation.

42. William P. Banta, "Medical History of ALS, Oct. 2, 1901," and Richard McDonald, "Personal Report, Feb. 5, 1902," AGO file, RG 94-403201, NARA.

43. William P. Banta, "Medical History of WB, Oct. 2, 1901" AGO file, RG 94-403202, NARA.

44. Gimlette, "Notes on a Case of 'Amok.'" For other local "culture-bound" syndromes, all regarded as evidence of "mental degeneracy," see Musgrave and Sison, "Mali-mali, a Mimic Psychosis in the Philippine Islands." See also Winzeler, "Amok: Historical, Psychological, and Cultural Perspectives"; Ee, "Amok in Nineteenth-century British Malaya History"; and Ugarte, " 'Like a Mad Dog': The Perceived Savageness of 'the Malay.' "

45. Foreman, *The Philippine Islands*, 140. See also Ugarte, "Muslims and Madness in the Southern Philippines." Ugarte distinguishes premeditated *juramentado* or *jihad* from *amok*.

46. Osler, "The Nation and the Tropics," 1401, 1405. Osler, one of the leading physicians of the late nineteenth century, had recently left the United States to take up the Regius Chair of Medicine at Oxford.

47. "Report of the Secretary of War on the Philippines," in *Report of the Philippine Commission to the President*, 1907 (Washington, D.C.: Government Printing Office, 1908), 3:287. See also Worcester, *The Philippines, Past and Present*, 358–87; and Reed, *City of Pines*. The Spanish had built a small sanitarium nearby at La Trinidad, but a commission led by Worcester and Luke E. Wright, with Frank Bourns and L. M. Maus as medical advisors, in 1900 decided to develop Baguio. Although a civil sanitarium operated there from 1902, the road was opened only in 1905. On other hill stations, see Kennedy, *The Magic Mountains*.

48. "Report of the Secretary of War," 288.

49. W. Cameron Forbes, quoted in V. G. Heiser, *Annual Report of the Bureau of Health for the Philippine Islands, July 1912–June 1913* (Manila: Bureau of Printing, 1913), 63. Interestingly, this report extols the advantages of Baguio while condemning Filipino recourse to Sibul Springs. Heiser refers to the "unsanitary conditions and undesirable features which prevail at the Sibul baths" (31). He conceded that the sulfurous water may have a specific effect on "chronic gastritis of a catarrhal nature" (32), but Filipinos, in their ignorance, took it also for "moist skin diseases, low-grade ulcers, herpes, dyspepsia, . . . chronic dysentery, liver diseases, and menstrual disorders" (64).

50. Atkinson, *The Philippine Islands*, 153.

51. John F. Minier to Harriet C. Huggins, August 15, 1912, mss 76/157p, Bancroft Library, University of California-Berkeley.

52. Carpenter, *Through the Philippines and Hawaii*, 86.

53. Worcester to Miss C. E. Worcester, February 5, 1908, box 1, Worcester papers, Bentley Historical Library, University of Michigan.

54. Worcester, *Philippines*, 379, 387n.
55. H. R. Hoff to Surgeon General, Washington, D.C., Mar. 7, 1908, p. 31, RG 112-E26-24508-100, NARA.
56. Ibid., 32.
57. Ibid., 33.
58. Victor G. Heiser to Walter Wyman, Surgeon General U.S. Public Health Service, Jan. 14, 1908, Letterbook, 1901–13, vol. 15, Heiser papers, B:H357.p, American Philosophical Society.
59. Heiser, *An American Doctor's Odyssey*, 74.
60. But see Brooke, "Baguio as a Health Resort."
61. Charles Burke Elliott, Diary, June 10, 1912, Library of Congress. Elliott was secretary of commerce and police between 1910 and 1912. When he left the Philippines later in 1912 he took "the cure" at Carlsbad, where his physician detected evidence of tropical residence. Forbes made perfunctory efforts to welcome elite Filipinos to Baguio, but in general they found it too cold.
62. Editorial, *El Ideal* (April 22, 1911).
63. Editorial, *El Ideal* (June 6, 1911) . McDonnell was editor of the *Cablenews*; Hathaway was Forbes's secretary. See also the criticism in the June 21 issue; and the concern about the cost of American self-indulgence in *La Vanguardia* (October 6, 1911). Randy David has recently defended the investment in Baguio, arguing that "the American governors knew that leisure was a complement to the work ethic" (*Philippine Daily Inquirer* [December 30, 2001]).
64. Memorandum Book No. 1 (Army and Navy Club, Philippines), Garrison papers, Ms C 166, History of Medicine Division, National Library of Medicine. Garrison's later memoranda books consist mostly of literary quotations and clinical descriptions, without passages of self-analysis.
65. Garrison returned to Baltimore, his nervousness apparently under control once he was back in the United States.
66. On the selective appropriation of Freud in America, see Hale, *Freud and the Americans*. Interestingly, Garrison (who had read Freud in German) seems far more receptive than most early American psychoanalysts to Freud's theories of infantile sexuality.
67. Stone, "Shellshock and the Psychologists." See also Hale, *The Rise and Crisis of Psychoanalysis in the United States*, esp. chapter 1.
68. Thompson, " 'Tropical Neurasthenia': A Deprivation Psychoneurosis," 319.
69. Ibid., 325. See also Beard's later emphasis on "sexual neurasthenia."
70. V. B. Green-Armytage, "Discussion," in Acton, "Neurasthenia in the Tropics," 7. Acton was professor of bacteriology at the Calcutta School of Tropical Medicine and Hygiene; Green-Armytage was a gynecologist.
71. Hill, "Neurasthenia in the Tropics," 234. Berkeley Hill was superintendent of the European Mental Hospital at Ranchi, Bihar, between 1919 and 1934. In 1922, he was one of fifteen psychiatrists brought together by Girindrasekhar Bose to form the Indian Psychoanalytic Society. See Hartnack, "British Psychoanalysts in Colonial India," and "Vishnu on Freud's Desk." Nandy refers to Berkeley Hill as the "first Westerner to attempt a psychoanalytic study of the Hindu modal personality and the first Westerner to use psychoanalysis as a form of cultural critique in India" ("Savage

Freud," 96). But if critique at all, it was a strangely complicit one: see Hill, "The 'Colour-question' from a Psychoanalytic Standpoint."

72. C. J. Singapore "Mental Irritability and Breakdown in the Tropics," *BMJ* i (March 13, 1926): 503–04. The bishop observed, "Countries such as British Malaya are now distinctly healthy, but 'nerves' are as frequent a cause of breakdown as ever," 503. See later contributions, under the same title, by A. F. MacCallan, *BMJ* i (March 20, 1926): 545–46; Andrew S. McNeil and R. van Someren, *BMJ* i (March 27, 1926): 595–96; R. Murray Barrow and J. W. Thomson, *BMJ* i (April 3, 1926): 634–35; H. M. Hanschell, M. Iles, and E. Rivaz Hunt, *BMJ* i (April 10, 1926): 676–77; George Mahomed and K. Vaughan, *BMJ* i (April 24, 1926): 760–61; Andrew S. McNeil, *BMJ* i (May 8 and 15, 1926): 846–47; Q. B. de Freitas, M. Jackson, and L. D. Parsons, *BMJ* i (May 22, 1926): 884; and J. W. Lindsay, *BMJ* i (May 29, 1926): 920. An editorial ("The White Man in the Tropics," *BMJ* i [May 29, 1926]: 909–10) was optimistic about the prospects for settling a working white race in the tropics but pointed out that "shibboleths die hard" (910).

73. Hill, "Mental Hygiene of Europeans in the Tropics," 392. Hill had married an Indian in order to escape his neuroses.

74. Joseph R. Darnell, "Sojourn in Zamboanga" [typescript, c. 1949], U.S. Army Military History Institute, Carlisle Barracks, Penn, 190, 195. Fugate had arrived in the Philippines in 1903 and remained there until 1938, when he was murdered.

75. Historians are prone to structure such breakdowns of male identity as feminization, but I would argue that male neurasthenia connoted disorder and fragmentation so profound as to subvert the sort of coherence that *feminization* implies. To be called unmanned is not always to be named woman. On the coding of aporias in grand narratives as feminine, see Jardine, *Gynesis: Configurations of Women and Modernity*.

76. For an ethnographic project to retrieve embodied memory, see Kleinman and Kleinman, "How Bodies Remember."

77. For example, there is still the folk diagnosis of "going troppo" in northern Australia and perhaps similar popular residuals in other tropical settler societies (see Anderson, *The Cultivation of Whiteness*, chapter 6). Recently there has been renewed critical attention to white male ambivalence in colonial settings: Nandy has described Kipling's "pathetic self-hatred and ego construction which went with colonialism" ("The Psychology of Colonialism," 209); and Bhabha observes that "the colonizer is himself caught in the ambivalence of paranoic identification" (*Location of Culture*, 61). Bhabha argues that by avoiding the earlier emphases on personal responsibility and on the recovery of masterful identity, it may be possible "to redeem the pathos of cultural confusion into a strategy of political subversion" (61).

78. Musgrave, "Tropical Neurasthenia, Tropical Hysteria and Some Special Tropical Hysteria-like Neuropsychoses," 399, 400, 401.

79. Musgrave clung to a mechanistic theory of Filipino neurasthenia which emphasized simple racial incompetence, but a later generation of colonial psychiatrists would render the male native conflicted, or hybrid, and therefore psychoanalyzable. Just as Freud had discovered the tropics within the European mind, colonial psychoanalysts like Berkeley Hill began to argue that the elite native might yet develop a superego. For later developments in "socioanalysis," see Fanon, *Black Skin, White Masks*; and

Memmi, *The Colonizer and the Colonized*. For more on critical colonial psycho-analysis, see Gates, "Critical Fanonism." Gates notes that in Fanon's work, "the Freudian mechanisms of psychic repression are set in relation to those of colonial repression" (466). Similarly, Bhabha has referred to "Fanon's sociodiagnostic psychiatry" ("Remembering Fanon," xx). For an interesting account of Fanon's "socio-therapy," see Vergès, "Chains of Madness, Chains of Colonialism."

6. DISEASE AND CITIZENSHIP

1. On the history of the Culion leper colony, see Thomas, *A Study of Leprosy Colony Policies*, chapter 7; [Wade, ed.], *Culion: A Record of Fifty Years Work with the Victims of Leprosy at the Culion Sanitarium*; Chapman, *Leonard Wood and Leprosy in the Philippines*; and Anderson, "Leprosy and Citizenship."

2. Mr. V. to Rev. Frederick Jansen, May 8, 1927, Culion Museum. On the transfer of Estela, see Casimiro B. Lara, M.D., to Director of Health, Manila, February 25, 1927, Culion Museum.

3. See Elias, *The Civilizing Process*. See also Bauman, *Modernity and Ambivalence*; and Burkitt, "Civilization and Ambivalence." On similar reformism at the Iwahig Prison Colony, see Michael Salman, "The United States and the End of Slavery in the Philippines, 1898–1914: A Study of Imperialism, Ideology, and Nationalism" (PH.D. dissertation, Stanford University, 1993), esp. chapter 23. Zinoman has criticized the efforts of Salman and others to "locate in colonial environments a system of power relations marked by the pervasive circulation of disciplinary practices throughout the social body" (*The Colonial Bastille*, 7). Yet he later concedes that Vietnamese "incarceration promoted certain characteristically modern attitudes toward society and human nature" (131).

4. On nationalism's tendency to forget, see Renan, *Qu'est-ce qu'une nation?*

5. Chakrabarty, "Of Garbage, Modernity and the Citizen's Gaze."

6. Victor G. Heiser, "The Culion Leper Colony: One of the Outgrowths of Our Occupation of the Philippine Islands," December 14, 1914, p. 6, Heiser collection, B:H357.p, American Philosophical Society.

7. Heiser Diaries, July 13, 1914, Heiser collection, B:H357.p, American Philosophical Society.

8. Stoler, "Tense and Tender Ties," 832.

9. Ibid.

10. Foucault, *Discipline and Punish*, 144.

11. Foucault, *Abnormal*, 46.

12. Foucault, *Discipline and Punish*, 199. For a complication of this argument, see Pegg, "Le corps et l'authorité: la lèpre de Badouin IV."

13. Vaughan, "Without the Camp: Institutions and Identities in the Colonial History of Leprosy," in *Curing Their Ills*, 79.

14. Kipp, "The Evangelical Uses of Leprosy," 176. For another account of leper evangelizing, see Kakar, "Leprosy in British India, 1860–1940." See also Harriet Jane Deacon, "A History of the Medical Institutions on Robben Island, Cape Colony, 1846–1910" (PH.D., University of Cambridge, 1994), esp. chapter 6; Buckingham,

Leprosy in Colonial South India; and Obregón, *Batallas contra la lepra*, and "The Anti-leprosy Campaign in Colombia."

15. Heiser later claimed that the attitude of Filipinos "fluctuated between a great horror of [leprosy] amounting almost to a panic, and the greatest callousness" (*An American Doctor's Odyssey*, 220). On the developing bacteriological understanding of leprosy in the Philippines at the end of the Spanish period, see M. Rogel, "Lepra en Visayas," *El Boletín de Cebú* (Dec. 15, 1895), (Dec. 22, 1895), and (Dec. 29, 1895).

16. MacNamara, "Leprosy," 426, 448, 448–49.

17. Gatewood, "Report on the International Conference on Leprosy," 155, 158. He had attended the First International Leprosy Conference in Berlin, which recommended the segregation of lepers. See also Pandya, "The First International Leprosy Conference, Berlin, 1897"; and Robertson, "Leprosy and the Elusive M. leprae."

18. Manson, *Tropical Diseases* (1898), 412, 417. Difficulties in transmitting the disease through inoculation led to disputes over the degree of contagiousness, but few authorities doubted that infection would eventually take place. Heiser concurred that "prolonged intimate contact" was necessary for infection, but he was understandably far more optimistic about the feasibility of segregation ("Tropical Diseases," 195, 204).

19. Manson, *Tropical Diseases* (1914), 627. On the supposed susceptibility of "dressed natives" to tuberculosis (caused by another mycobacterium), see Packard, *White Plague, Black Labor*.

20. Dean C. Worcester, "Report of the Committee Appointed to Select a Site for a Leper Colony," Jan. 1, 1902, pp. 447, 449, RG 350-1972-2, NARA. Worcester, the secretary of the interior, was chairman of the search committee.

21. D. C. Worcester to J. E. Reighard, April 23, 1903, box 4, Reighard papers, Bentley Library, University of Michigan Historical Collections, Ann Arbor.

22. Heiser, "The Culion Leper Colony," 1–2. See also, Victor G. Heiser to Secretary of the Interior, Memorandum, 1911, RG 350-1972-31, NARA.

23. H. B. Wilkinson to Commissioner of Public Health, September 1, 1903, Wilkinson folder, U.S. Medical Corps box, Spanish-American War survey, U.S. Army Military History Institute, Carlisle Barracks, Penn.

24. Case report, RG 350-1972-16, NARA. Heiser, *An American Doctor's Odyssey*, 235.

25. Heiser, "Culion Leper Colony," 5.

26. Heiser, *An American Doctor's Odyssey*, 220.

27. Victor G. Heiser, Diary, Sept 1, 1908, Heiser collection, B:H357.p, American Philosophical Society. On accusations of insidious harm as a technique of exclusion and control, see Douglas, "Witchcraft and Leprosy: Two Strategies of Exclusion."

28. C. E. MacDonald to Isadore Dyer, M.D., August 15, 1908, Charles Everett MacDonald papers, U.S. Army Military History Institute, Carlisle Barracks, Penn.

29. Richard Johnson, "My Life in the Army, 1899–1922" (typescript, 1952), 107, 108, Johnson papers, U.S. Army Military History Institute, Carlisle Barracks, Penn.

30. See Victor G. Heiser, "Memorandum of Leper Collecting Trip," June–July 1913, Heiser collection, B:H357.p, American Philosophical Society. See also, Teofilo Corpus, "Experiences in Collecting Lepers," *Philippine Health Service Monthly Bulletin* 4 (October 1924): 450. The accusation of leprosy became a potent weapon in local

disputes. Thus when Teodulfo Ylaya wrote a scathing play about Vicente Sotto, a Cebuano politician, he was denounced as a leper. Sotto ensured that Ylaya was consigned to Culion in 1907, where he remained for the rest of his life. (I am grateful to Mike Cullinane for this information.)

31. Heiser, "Culion Leper Colony," 7. Between 1912 and 1924, a few dozen Chamorro lepers from Guam were transferred to Culion: see Hattori, *Colonial Dis-Ease*, chapter 3. Heiser estimated that there were over fifty thousand lepers in Japan, few of whom had been isolated; in China, the problem was still the responsibility of missionaries; in Java, too, the government had done little. In India the number of lepers was so great that the financial burden would far surpass the resources of the Indian treasury. Only in the Federated Malay States had the government tried systematically to isolate lepers: a colony was planned at Pulau Jerajak. See Victor G. Heiser, "Leprosy in the East: Its Treatment and Prevention," Nov. 3, 1915, pp. 10–11, Heiser collection, B:H357.p, American Philosophical Society.

32. *Saturday Evening Post* (Feb. 2, 1918).

33. Mayo, *The Isles of Fear*, 154.

34. Victor G. Heiser, "Hospital No. 66" [c. 1938], p. 14, Heiser collection, B:H357.p, American Philosophical Society.

35. Goffman, *Asylums*.

36. Wade and Avellana Basa, "The Culion Leper Colony," 402. Avellana Basa was the director of the colony in 1919–25; Wade, a pathologist from Tulane, was the resident physician in 1922–31 — he stayed on and died there in 1968.

37. Ibid., 399. See also Ernest R. Gentry, "Report of a Leper-Collecting Trip in the Philippine Islands," 1912, RG 112-E26-68075-123, NARA.

38. Long, "Health in the Philippine Islands," 50.

39. MacNamara, "Leprosy," 451.

40. Manson, *Tropical Diseases* (1898), 419.

41. Ibid., 420–21, 419. The reference to specific therapy for syphilis was dropped in later editions. On the search for a "specific therapeutics," see Warner, *The Therapeutic Perspective*.

42. Heiser, "Fighting Leprosy in the Philippines," 311, 312. Eliodoro Mercado, of San Lazaro Hospital, had prepared the first injectable form of chaulmoogra in 1910, but Heiser took most of the credit for his invention. Snodgrass describes unsuccessful early attempts made in the Philippines to treat the disease with x-rays (*Leprosy in the Philippine Islands*, 27). For an overly optimistic discussion of x-ray treatment, see Heiser, "The Progress of Medicine in the Philippine Islands." See also Lara, *Leprosy Research in the Philippines*. Lara was a physician at Culion in 1922–62 and director in 1947–55.

43. Snodgrass, *Leprosy*, 27. Unusually, Snodgrass had trained in homeopathy and bacteriology.

44. Ibid., 28.

45. Manson, *Tropical Diseases* (1914), 634.

46. Ibid., 637. For more on the results of nastin treatment and of immunological therapies, see Strong, "Leprosy."

47. Heiser, "Tropical Diseases," 203.

48. Ibid.

49. Victor G. Heiser, "Leprosy in the East: Its Treatment and Prevention," Nov. 3, 1915, pp. 10–11, 16, Heiser collection, B:H357.p, American Philosophical Society. The first female suffrage in the rest of the macrocolony occurred in 1916.

50. Heiser, "Hospital No. 66," p. 5, Heiser collection, B:H357.p, American Philosophical Society.

51. Heiser, "Fighting Leprosy," 316–17.

52. Heiser, *An American Doctor's Odyssey*, 236. See Snodgrass, *Leprosy in the Philippine Islands*.

53. Heiser, *An American Doctor's Odyssey*, 236.

54. Wade and Avellana Basa, "Culion Leper Colony," 406.

55. A. J. McLaughlin to Mrs. G. H. Burwell, April 5, 1909, RG 350-1972-10, NARA.

56. Snodgrass, *Leprosy in the Philippine Islands*, 25.

57. Goffman describes the institutional theatrical in *Asylums*, 99; Stewart describes the theatricality of the miniature in *On Longing*; and Bhabha refers to the performativity of "people" in the narrative address of the nation in "DissemiNation: Time, Narrative and the Margins of the Modern Nation," in *The Location of Culture*, esp. 145–46. On the "exhibitionary order," see Mitchell, *Colonising Egypt*.

58. Heiser, "Fighting Leprosy," 318.

59. Heiser, "Leprosy in the East," 17–18. See also Wilson, "Industrial Therapy in Leprosy."

60. Heiser, "Leprosy in the East," 17–18.

61. Heiser, "Hospital No. 66," p. 4, Heiser collection, B:H357.p, American Philosophical Society. When Dr. T. C. Wu visited from China in 1930 he found a "happy colony of people whose principal idea in life is to get cured. . . . The bright light of hope has permeated the horizon of consciousness and changed the whole aspect of the people" ("Fighting Leprosy in the Philippines," 7). I am grateful to Angela Leung for this reference.

62. Heiser, "Fighting Leprosy," 318, 320.

63. Heiser, "Memorandum of Leper Collecting Trip," 1. Yet when the evangelist Rev. James B. Rodgers visited Culion, he admired the same gardens ("Culion, the Leper Colony of the Philippines," *Silliman Truth* [Negros Oriental], [May 1, 1911], pp. 2, 4, RG 350-1972-19, NARA).

64. "Culion and Its Inhabitants," *La Vanguardia* (August 27, 1912).

65. "What Is Happening in Culion?" *El Ideal* (September 16, 1912).

66. "The Culion Lepers," *La Vanguardia* (October 2, 1912).

67. Burgess, *Who Walk Alone*, 92, 94, 101. Burgess won the National Book Award for this work.

68. Ibid., 142, 180.

69. Ibid., 220, 221, 245.

70. Ibid., 266.

71. Frederick Hoffman to Forrest F. Dryden, March 10, 11, 1915, Special Reports on Leper Colonies, Hoffman papers, MS/B/247, National Library of Medicine, Bethesda, Md. Hoffman, well known as a race theorist in North America, was selecting

a site for the federal leprosarium. Edmond claims "Molokai was less a model colony than a monstrous reflection of the real thing" ("Abject Bodies/Abject Sites," 139).

72. Gussow, *Leprosy, Racism, and Public Health: Social Policy in Chronic Disease*, 147. Carville began with ninety inmates, and the most it ever contained was four hundred. For an account of Carville in the 1930s, see Stein, with Blochman, *Alone No Longer*. See also Gussow and Tracy, "Stigma and the Leprosy Phenomenon: The Social History of a Disease in the Nineteenth and Twentieth Centuries." Culion also served as a model for the leper colony at Trujillo Alto, Puerto Rico, which opened in 1926, replacing the deplorable old colony at Isla de Cabras. The scale of the new Puerto Rico colony limited its activities: there were only forty-three inmates in 1926. See Levinson, "Beyond Quarantine: A History of Leprosy in Puerto Rico, 1898–1930s."

73. A protestant missionary, Rev. Paul F. Jansen, was stationed at Culion permanently through the 1920s, successfully evangelizing the Catholic lepers, with the tacit approval of the medical authorities. Previously, Dr. George "Skypilot" Wright had visited the colony regularly from the Presbyterian Mission in Manila.

74. Sergio Osmeña, a leading nationalist politician, was a Cebuano like so many of the lepers. He became vice president of the Philippine Commonwealth in 1935–44 and then president in 1944–46. Manuel Roxas defeated him in 1946 in the first elections for the presidency of the independent Philippines.

75. Chapman, *Leonard Wood and Leprosy in the Philippines*, esp. 83–84. See Wood, "Progress Fighting Leprosy at Culion." In 1921, Wood inaugurated a more intensive treatment program at Culion. Over 4,000 lepers were injected weekly with the ethyl esters of chaulmoogra oil. It was claimed that by 1925 a total of 196 cases were sent away as cured and 499 were bacteriologically negative and undergoing the required two years' observation period for release. See Callender, "The Leprosy Problem in the Philippine Islands"; and *Annual Report of the Philippine Health Service, Fiscal Year 1922* (Manila: Bureau of Printing, 1923), 15. By the early 1920s, Bayer had developed "antileprol," a derivative of chaulmoogra oil, which was better tolerated orally, and it soon displaced the parenteral oil. See Stitt, *Diagnostics and Treatment of Tropical Diseases*, 266. After Wood's death, American supporters established in 1927 the Leonard Wood Memorial for the Eradication of Leprosy. In 1931, H. W. Wade organized a conference in Manila that led to the establishment of the International Leprosy Association and the *International Journal of Leprosy*, which he edited. See Anon., "Leprologists form International Leprosy Association," *Manila Daily Bulletin* (January 22, 1931), 1.

76. Anon., "Quezon Tells Medicos Culion Costs Too Much," *Manila Times* (December 17, 1923), 1. Dr. José Albert, a liberal pediatrician and former revolutionary, also condemned Culion as "anachronistic, unjustified, and ultrascientific" (*The Experiment of Leper Segregation in the Philippines*, 2).

77. Anon., "Quezon Pays His Respects to Major Hitchens," *Manila Times* (December 19, 1926), 1. The voluntary efforts were organized through the Philippine Islands Anti-Tuberculosis Society; I discuss tuberculosis further in chapter 8. The annual appropriation for Culion did not fall below one million pesos until 1931, and it was sharply reduced in later years.

78. See Quezon, *The Good Fight*. Quezon was president of the new Philippine Commonwealth from 1935 until his death in exile.

79. Diary of Dr. Heiser's Trip Around the World, October 1930-May 1931, January 18–
20, 1931, pp. 111–12, 5.27, unit 63, room 104, RG 12.1, RFA, RAC.

80. Diary of Dr. Heiser's Trip Around the World, 1932–33, Dec. 21, 1932, p. 62, 5.27,
unit 63, room 104, RG 12.1, RFA, RAC.

81. "Will Continue Segregation in Leprosy Work," *Manila Bulletin* (October 7, 1936).
The activists pointed out that after thirty years of strict segregation, there had been
no decrease in the admission of new cases to Culion.

82. "Police Force Helpless as Mob Rushes," *Manila Bulletin* (April 1, 1932). Marriage
had been restricted in 1929, when the number of births increased; the sanctions were
lifted in 1934.

83. "Hearing in the Colony Hall," July 26, 1935, pp. 1–4, Joseph R. Hayden papers,
Bentley Library, University of Michigan Historical Collections. For another account
linking medicalization with unrest, see Kakar, "Medical Developments and Patient
Unrest in the Leprosy Asylum, 1860–1940."

84. Chakrabarty, *Provincializing Europe: Postcolonial Thought and Historical Difference*.

85. Brownell, "American Ideas of Citizenship," 975. Brownell claimed U.S. policy was
"the subject of scoff by every other colonizing nation" because it "considers each of
the subject people to be a human being, entitled to certain unalienable rights, which
we not only freely grant, but *teach to him*" (975, emphasis added). See also Brownell,
"Turning Savages into Citizens."

86. Jenks, "Assimilation in the Philippines, as Interpreted in Terms of Assimilation in
America," 789. Jenks, formerly the chief of the Bureau of Ethnology, thought that in
the archipelago more generally, "to accomplish all this against their natural inertia of
race, and the inertia of social and physical environment is not a task that can be
completed by the year 1921" (789). Culion was designed to disturb this "inertia."

87. Brownell, "American Ideas of Citizenship," 975.

88. During the war, the Japanese effectively quarantined Culion, and more than a quarter of the inhabitants starved to death. In 1947, sulfone drugs were introduced; and
in 1948, Culion was declared a municipality. There were, however, still over two
hundred lepers in Culion in 2001.

89. Foucault, *Discipline and Punish*, 298.

7. LATE-COLONIAL PUBLIC HEALTH AND FILIPINO "MIMICRY"

1. V. G. Heiser, "Notes of 1916 Trip," July 19, 1916, vol. 2, p. 537, 58.5, room 102,
Hei 2, RFA, RAC.

2. Heiser lamented that Harrison had "the same peculiar and intangible view of things
as of yore" ("Notes of 1916 Trip," August 10, 1916, vol. 2, pp. 573–74). Harrison
later described Heiser as "a shrewd intriguer" (Journal, 27 February 1936, in Ono-
rato, ed., *Origins of the Philippine Republic: Extracts from the Diaries of Francis
Burton Harrison*, 58).

3. Heiser, "Notes of 1916 Trip," July 28, 1916, vol. 2, p. 553.

4. Heiser, "Notes of 1916 Trip," August 7, 1916, vol. 2, p. 570.

5. V. G. Heiser, Diary of Dr. Heiser's World Trip, October 1927-May 1928, March 27, 1928, p. 166, 5.27, unit 63, room 104, RG 12.1, RFA, RAC.

6. Heiser, "Notes of 1916 Trip," August 31, 1916, vol. 2, p. 621.

7. V. G. Heiser, Diary of Dr. Heiser's World Trip 1925–26, November 22, 1925, p. 130, 5.27, unit 63, room 104, RG 12.1, RFA, RAC.

8. V. G. Heiser, Diary of Dr. Heiser's Trip Around the World, October 1930-May 1931, Jan. 6, 1931, p. 91, 5.27, unit 63, room 104, RG 12.1, RFA, RAC.

9. V. G. Heiser, Diary of Dr. Heiser's Trip Around the World, October 1930-May 1931, Jan. 8, 1931, p. 96.

10. C. H. Yaeger to V. G. Heiser, June 10, 1933, folder 94, box 7, series 242, RG 1.1, RFA, RAC.

11. Douglas, *Purity and Danger*. See also James, "Lectures Six and Seven: The Sick Soul," 113.

12. Wilson, *Constitutional Government in the United States*, 52–53. Rafael has summarized this American colonial principle: "The self that rules itself can only emerge by way of an intimate relationship with a colonial master who sets the standards and practices of discipline to mold the conduct of the colonial subject" (*White Love and Other Events in Filipino History*, 22). See also Miller, *"Benevolent Assimilation": The American Conquest of the Philippines 1899–1903*.

13. Bhabha makes the more general point in "Of Mimicry and Man."

14. Elias, *The Civilizing Process*.

15. Benjamin, "On the Mimetic Faculty"; Taussig, *Mimesis and Alterity*; and Rafael, "Mimetic Subjects." On Rockefeller activities in the tropics, see Farley, *Bilharzia*, chapter 5; Cueto, ed., *Missionaries of Science*; Palmer, "Central American Encounters with Rockefeller Public Health, 1914–21"; Birn, "A Revolution in Rural health?" and "Revolution, the Scatological Way"; and Birn and Solorzano, "Public Health Policy Paradoxes."

16. For examples of the historical and anthropological study of development practitioners after World War II, see Ferguson, *The Anti-Politics Machine*; Escobar, *Encountering Development*; Cooper and Packard, eds., *International Development and the Social Sciences*; and Gupta, *Postcolonial Developments*. All of these studies treat development as though it emerged only in the 1940s and pay little attention to colonial antecedents. As Escobar notes, "The period between 1920 and 1950 is still ill understood from the vantage point of the overlap of colonial and developmentalist regimes of representation" (27). The lack of attention to U.S. colonial policy is especially surprising given the prominence of American development institutions and agencies after World War II.

17. Harrison to Gen. Frank McIntyre, chief, Bureau of Insular Affairs, November 15, 1915, RG 350-4981-123A, NARA.

18. Leslie A. I. Chapman to Guy N. Rohrer, October 4, 1915, RG 350-4981-123A, NARA.

19. Hards to G. N. Rohrer, 10 August 1915, RG 350-4981-123A, NARA.

20. Harrison to Gen. Frank McIntyre, November 15, 1915, RG 350-4981-123A, NARA.

21. Victor G. Heiser, *Annual Report of the Bureau of Health for the Philippine Islands, July 1, 1912, to June 30, 1913* (Manila: Bureau of Printing, 1913), 3–6.

22. Sullivan, *Exemplar of Americanism*; and Worcester, *The Philippines, Past and Present*.

23. Heiser, "Sanitation in the Philippines," 124.

24. Heiser, *An American Doctor's Odyssey*, 192, 194.

25. Heiser, *An American Doctor's Odyssey*, 195, 198.

26. Kafka, "A Report to an Academy," in *The Metamorphosis, In the Penal Colony and Other Stories*.

27. Pardo de Tavera, "Filipino Views of American rule," 74. Pardo de Tavera, who came from a wealthy *mestizo* family, had trained in medicine in Paris. See Paredes, "The Ilustrado Legacy: The Pardo de Taveras of Manila"; Santiago, "The First Filipino Doctors of Medicine and Surgery (1878–97)"; and Gaerlan, "The Pursuit of Modernity: Trinidad H. Pardo de Tavera and the Educational Legacy of the Philippine Revolution."

28. Pardo de Tavera, *El Legado del ignorantismo*, 33, 36, 4, 5, 41. This is the text of an address to the annual teachers' assembly at Baguio.

29. T. H. Pardo de Tavera, "The Conservation of the National Type," 11th Annual Commencement Address, University of the Philippines, April 4, 1921, pp. 19–20, 13, 22, Pardo de Tavera Collection, B2 E16, Rizal Library, Ateneo de Manila. On the various understandings of self-government among Filipino elites, see Go, "Colonial Reception and Cultural Reproduction."

30. Forbes to James, January 30, 1905, Forbes papers, bMS Am 1092 (262–68), Houghton Library, Harvard University.

31. Forbes to James, June 15, 1905, Forbes papers, bMS Am 1092 (262–68), Houghton Library, Harvard University.

32. Stanley refers to a "collaborative compromise" emerging in the first decade of American colonial government and institutionalized in the second, in his edited collection, *Reappraising an Empire*, 2. See also Robinson, "Non-European Foundations of European Imperialism." Etherington also suggests the importance of peripheral political negotiations when he calls for "an historical sociology of colonial bureaucracies" (*Theories of Imperialism*, 270). On the role of local elites in "modernization," see Johnson, "Imperialism and the Professions."

33. Wilson, *Constitutional Government*, 52.

34. Harrison, *Inaugural Address*, 4–5.

35. Harrison, *The Corner-Stone of Philippine Independence*, 81, 44.

36. Zaide, *Philippine Political and Cultural History*, 2:248. The total population was approximately eight million plus. Agoncillo and Alfonso point out that in 1913 Filipinos were already occupying 71 percent of civil service positions, but usually at the lower levels (*Short History of the Philippine People*).

37. Heiser, *An American Doctor's Odyssey*, 56.

38. Worcester, *Philippines*, 685, 693, 695. Worcester complained that "seldom, if ever, have health officials been more viciously and persistently attacked than have Dr. Heiser and myself. The assaults on us have been the direct result of a firm stand for a new sanitary order of things" (444).

39. H. L. Kneedler to Woodrow Wilson, March 25, 1913, RG 350-2394-35, NARA. See also Alatas, *The Myth of the Lazy Native*.

40. Charles H. Yeater to Daniel R. Williams, August 28, 1917, David P. Barrows papers, mss c-b 1005, Bancroft Library, University of California at Berkeley. Williams later wrote to Barrows, "You know, and I know, that the masses of Filipinos have neither the numbers, capacity nor industry to compete against or protect themselves from their more virile neighbors to the North" (October 4, 1924). Williams was referring to the Japanese occupying Taiwan.

41. *New York Herald* (September 17, 1916).

42. Vicente de Jesús to Gen. Frank McIntyre, March 3, 1920, RG 350-3465-105, NARA. See also Eschscholtzia and Haymond, *An Analysis of Certain Causes of Mortality in the Philippine Islands*.

43. Vicente de Jesús to Gen. Frank McIntyre, March 3, 1920, RG 350-3465-105, NARA.

44. Ibid. The death rate in 1921 did go down to 21.14 per 1,000 of population.

45. On Heiser's involvement in the hospital disputes of 1912, see D. C. Worcester to Governor-General, January 31, 1912, RG 350-21274-15, NARA; and Dean C. Worcester's Private Annotated Copy of the Attempt to Transfer Jurisdiction over the Philippine General Hospital from the Bureau of Health . . . , box 1, Worcester papers, Bentley Historical Library, University of Michigan Historical Collections.

46. F. McIntyre, Memorandum, November 1915, RG 350-59-81, NARA.

47. Winfred T. Denison to David P. Barrows, November 28, 1914, Barrows papers, mss c-b 1005, Bancroft Library, University of California at Berkeley.

48. Winfred T. Denison to T. Roosevelt, November 27, 1914, Barrows papers, mss c-b 1005, Bancroft Library, University of California at Berkeley.

49. Winfred T. Denison to David P. Barrows, March 27, 1915, Barrows papers, mss c-b 1005, Bancroft Library, University of California at Berkeley.

50. United States Special Mission of Investigation to the Philippine Islands, *Report on the Special Mission on Investigation to the Philippine Islands to the Secretary of War* (Washington, D.C.: Government Printing Office, 1922), 21.

51. Heiser, *An American Doctor's Odyssey*, 417, 419.

52. Wood, *Report of the Governor-General of the Philippines, 1925*, 5. In 1919 Americans comprised 6 percent of all government personnel, including teachers; in 1925, 3.1 percent. Wood did, however, make some efforts to "stem the slowly-moving landslip which our friend Harrison left for us" (Wood to Forbes, 9 March 1924, Forbes papers, bMS Am 1364, Houghton Library, Harvard University). See also Hagedorn, *Leonard Wood: A Biography*.

53. For science and Philippine nationalism, see Ileto, "Outlines of a Non-linear Emplotment of Philippines History." Lo observes a similar generational disposition in colonial Taiwan in *Doctors Within Borders*.

54. Vicente de Jesús to F. McIntyre, March 5, 1920, RG 350-3465-105, NARA.

55. Hernando, "The Environment in Relation to Infectious Diseases," in his *Management of Communicable Diseases*, 5–7.

56. V. de Jesús, "Narrative Summary of the Cholera Situation in the Provinces and Manila," Sept. 19, 1914, RG 350-4981-114, NARA.

57. Calderón, "Faulty Maternity Practices and Their Influence upon Infant Mortality."

58. De Jesús, *Proposed Sanitary Code*, 7.

59. De Jesús, "Narrative Summary of the Cholera Situation."

60. Philippine Health Service, Memorandum, July 1929, RG 350-3465-165, NARA.

61. Paul C. Freer, *Eighth Annual Report of the Director of the Bureau of Science for the Year ending August 1, 1909* (Manila: Bureau of Printing, 1910), 16.

62. Cole, "*Necator americanus* in the Natives of the Philippine Islands"; P. E. Garrison, "The Prevalence and Distribution of the Animal Parasites of Man in the Philippine Islands"; Phalen and Nichols, "Notes on the Distribution of *Filaria nocturna* in the Philippine Islands"; R. E. Hoyt, "Results of Three Hundred Examinations of Feces with Reference to the Presence of Amoebae"; P. E. Garrison and Llamas, "The Intestinal Worms of 385 Filipino Women and Children in Manila"; Stitt, "A Study of the Intestinal Parasites Found in Cavite Province." Stitt later wrote the major American text in tropical medicine, *The Diagnostics and Treatment of Tropical Diseases*.

63. Willets, "A Statistical Study of Intestinal Parasites in Tobacco Haciendas of the Cagayan Valley."

64. Ettling, *The Germ of Laziness*. See also Cassedy, "The 'Germ of Laziness' in the South, 1901–1915." Ashford disclaimed Stiles's influence: see his letter to Major Lynch, November 16, 1909, RG 112-E26-106177-21, NARA.

65. Bailey K. Ashford, "Porto Rico Sanitary Commission," July 24, 1905, p. 3, RG 112-E26-106177-S, NARA.

66. Ettling, *The Germ of Laziness*.

67. Ibid. See also Ashford, *A Soldier in Science*; and Trigo, "Anemia and Vampires: Figures to Govern the Colony, Puerto Rico, 1880–1904."

68. Charles T. Nesbitt, "The Health Menace of Alien Races," *The World's Work* 28 (November 1913): 74–75, quoted in Ettling, *The Germ of Laziness*, 173.

69. C. W. Stiles, *Hookworm Disease and the Negroes* (Hampton, Va.: Hampton Normal and Agricultural Institute, 1909), 4, quoted in Ettling, *The Germ of Laziness*, 172. The term "ecological détente" is Ettling's (172).

70. Anon. [Wickliffe Rose], "Visit to Manila" (June 1–7, 1914), p. 2, folder 121, series 242, RG 5, RFA, RAC.

71. J. D. Long, *Report of the Philippine Health Service for the Fiscal Year from January 1 to December 31, 1915* (Manila: Bureau of Printing, 1916), 56. Long was director of health in the Philippines from 1915 until 1918 and was succeeded by Vicente de Jesús.

72. Long, *Report of the Philippine Health Service*, 57. For more on toilet design, see chapter 4.

73. Heiser, Diary of Dr. Heiser's World Trip 1925–26, November 25, 1925, p. 132.

74. Heiser to Jerome D. Greene, secretary Rockefeller Foundation, February 20, 1915, folder 61, subseries 2, series 1, RG 5, RFA, RAC.

75. See chapter 8.

76. Heiser to Leonard Wood, May 26, 1922, folder 122, series 242, RG 5, RFA, RAC.

77. Charles N. Leach to V. de Jesús, May 10, 1923, folder 122, series 242, RG 5, RFA, RAC. Leach at the time was director of Rockefeller Foundation activities in the Philippines.

78. [C. N. Leach], "Methods Suggested for Carrying Out a Hookworm Campaign in the Philippine Islands" [1922], folder 122, series 242, RG 5, RFA, RAC.

79. E. L. Munson to Leonard Wood, October 7, 1922, folder 126, series 242, RG 5, RFA, RAC.

80. Heiser to Leonard Wood, October 22, 1921, folder 127, series 242, RG 5, RFA, RAC.

81. W. S. Carter to G. E. Vincent, pres. Rockefeller Foundation, January 28, 1923, folder 34, box 4, series 242, RG 1.1, RFA, RAC.

82. W. S. Carter to Alan Gregg, January 29, 1923, folder 34, box 4, series 242, RG 1.1, RFA, RAC

83. E. B. McKinlay, "Report concerning the Bureau of Science," Manila, 1927, folder 1, box 1, series 242, RG 1.1, RFA, RAC.

84. C. F. Moriarty to Heiser, April 11, 1928, p. 31, folder 94, box 7, series 242, RG 1.1, RFA, RAC. The Rockefeller Foundation set up similar rural health centers in India after 1934.

85. Heiser to C. H. Yaeger, July 11, 1929, folder 95, box 7, series 242, RG 1.1, RFA, RAC.

86. Heiser, Diary of Dr. Heiser's Trip Around the World, October 1930-May 1931, January 11, 1931, p. 103.

87. C. H. Yaeger to Heiser, December 31, 1929, folder 95, box 7, series 242, RG 1.1, RFA, RAC.

88. C. H. Yaeger to Heiser, July 2, 1929, folder 4, box 1, series 242, RG 1.1, RFA, RAC. The unit in Laguna was closed in 1932, when funds became scarce as a result of the depression.

89. C. H. Yaeger to Heiser, March 4, 1932, folder 96, box 7, series 242, RG 1.1, RFA, RAC.

90. V. G. Heiser, Diary of Dr. Heiser's Trip Around the World, 1932–33, December 11, 1932, p. 52, 5.27, unit 63, room 104, RG 12.1, RFA, RAC.

91. Paul F. Russell to Heiser, September 5, 1933, folder 96, box 7, series 242, RG 1.1, RFA, RAC.

92. Limjuco, "Hygiene in the Community," 23, 21.

93. Yaeger to Heiser, May 26, 1933, folder 96, box 7, series 242, RG 1.1, RFA, RAC.

94. Yaeger to Heiser, May 28, 1932, folder 96, box 7, series 242, RG 1.1, RFA, RAC.

95. Yaeger to Heiser, February 11, 1930, folder 100, box 7, series 242, RG 1.1, RFA, RAC.

96. Yaeger to Heiser, June 17, 1932, folder 101, box 8, series 242, RG 1.1, RFA, RAC.

97. Yaeger to Heiser, April 12, 1934, folder 96, box 7, series 242, RG 1.1, RFA, RAC.

98. Heiser, Memorandum on Conference with Dr. Jacobo Fajardo, January 9, 1930, folder 8, box 1, series 242, RG 1.1, RFA, RAC. As far as I know, this is the only time Heiser refers to "the masses," rather than the Filipino: it may be an aberration or it may indicate a shift in his attitudes — an embrace of social medicine — during the 1930s.

99. Sison, "Educating Our Educators," 123, 124.

100. Fajardo, "Commencement Address," 174, 175. For an account of earlier hygiene education in the schools, see chapter 4. Fajardo was a great favorite of Heiser's, who was disappointed when the director of health was forced to resign in 1936 after allegedly taking a bribe from a leper.

101. Yaeger to Heiser, May 23, 1933, folder 9, box 1, series 242, RG 1.1, RFA, RAC. Pigg quotes an aid advisor in Nepal during the 1990s: "Our own staff don't even boil their drinking water. How are we going to educate villagers?" (" 'Found in Most

Traditional Societies': Traditional Medical Practitioners between Culture and Development," 259).

102. Yaeger to F. F. Russell, May 2, 1933, folder 9, box 1, series 242, RG 1.1, RFA, RAC.

103. Yaeger to F. F. Russell, February 8, 1935, folder 11, box 1, series 242, RG 1.1, RFA, RAC.

104. Heiser, Diary of Dr. Heiser's Trip Around the World, 1932–33, January 4, 1933, p. 74.

105. Heiser to F. F. Russell, January 31, 1931, folder 100, box 7, series 242, RG 1.1, RFA, RAC. Russell, the director of the International Health Division from 1923 to 1935, preferred laboratory research to demonstration units: see Farley, *To Cast Out Disease*.

106. Heiser, Diary of Dr. Heiser's Trip Around the World, October 1930-May 1931, February 4, 1931, p. 143.

107. Heiser, Diary of Dr. Heiser's Trip Around the World, October 1930-May 1931, January 11, 1931, p. 103.

108. Paul F. Russell to Heiser, April 4, 1932, folder 67, box 6, subseries 1, series 242, RG 1.1, RFA, RAC.

109. Heiser to Paul F. Russell, August 10, 1933, folder 67, box 6, subseries 1, series 242, RG 1.1, RFA, RAC.

110. Heiser, Diary of Dr. Heiser's World Trip, October 1927-May 1928, March 27, 1928, p. 164.

111. Heiser, Diary of Dr. Heiser's World Trip, October 1927-May 1928, March 28, 1918, p. 167.

112. Administration, Programs and Policy — IHB, box 3, series 908, RG 3, RFA, RAC.

113. Tomes, *Gospel of Germs*, 19.

114. As Bhabha reminds us, "Colonial mimicry is the desire for a reformed, recognizable Other, as a subject of a difference that is almost the same but not quite" ("Of Mimicry and Man," 126). For a complication of this argument, see McClintock, *Imperial Leather*, 61–71. According to Glenn, women comics dominated American stage mimicry during this period. It is therefore tempting to relate the figure of the mimic to the notion of the feminine, but there is far more evidence that Filipinos were cast as children, not as women. See Glenn, " 'Give Me an Imitation of Me': Vaudeville Mimics and the Play of the Self."

115. Recto, "Most Ignominious Surrender," 18–19.

116. Recto, "Our Mendicant Foreign Policy," 82.

117. Recto, "Our Lingering Colonial Complex," 90, 91.

118. Freud, "The Uncanny."

8. MALARIA BETWEEN RACE AND ECOLOGY

1. Victor G. Heiser, Memorandum re. Conference with Dr. Jacobo Fajardo, January 9, 1930, folder 8, box 1, series 242, RG 1.1, RFA, RAC. In 1928, after talks with the governor's health advisors, Heiser writes in his diary, "If these amateurs could only understand something of the lack of economic resources, and that at this stage building them up would do more to improve health than direct hygienic measures"

(Diary of Dr. Heiser's Trip Around the World, October 1927–May 1928, March 18, 1928, p. 154, 5.27, Unit 63, Room 104, RG 12.1, RFA, RAC).

2. Victor G. Heiser, Memorandum, February 2, 1932, p. 1, folder 9, box 1, series 242, RG 1.1, RFA, RAC.

3. Diary of Dr. Heiser's Trip Around the World, October 1930–May 1931, January 7, 1931, p. 94, 5.27, Unit 63, Room 104, RG 12.1, RFA, RAC. Edward L. Munson, however, remained convinced that while "tuberculosis is rife . . . improvement depends chiefly on changes in the basic habits of life of the people" (Memorandum to Leonard Wood, governor-general, October 7, 1922, folder 126, series 242, RG 5, RFA, RAC). He was referring principally to expectoration.

4. Headquarters, Third Brigade, Department of Luzon, Circular No. 7, March 2, 1903, RG 112-E26-77872-33, NARA. See chapter 3.

5. Craig, "Observations upon Malaria," 525.

6. Ross, *Memoirs, with a Full Account of the Great Malaria Problem and its Solution*; Harrison, *Mosquitoes, Malaria and Man*; and Haynes, *Imperial Medicine: Patrick Manson and the Conquest of Tropical Disease*. Ross believed in the drinking-water theory of transmission as late as 1897: see his letter to Manson, May 3, 1897, in Bynum and Overy, eds., *The Beast in the Mosquito: The Correspondence of Ronald Ross and Patrick Manson*, 163–66. Ross had wondered if "the disease is communicated by the *bite* of the mosquito" (May 27, 1896, 116); but Manson advised him that "it may be that the mosquito conveys the parasite in biting but I do not think so" (October 12, 1896, 124).

7. Ross, *Memoirs*; and Worboys, "Manson, Ross and Colonial Medical Policy." For a debate on the medical uses of segregation during this period, see Curtin, "Medical Knowledge and Urban Planning in Tropical Africa," and Cell, "Anglo-Indian Medical Theory and the Origins of Segregation in West Africa."

8. De Bevoise provides an excellent account of the epidemiology and underlying causes of malaria in the colonial Philippines in *Agents of Apocalypse*.

9. Page, "Malaria and Mosquitoes at Lucena Barracks, Philippine Islands."

10. Chamberlain, "Analysis of One Hundred and Twenty Cases of Malaria Occurring at Camp Gregg, Philippine Islands."

11. W. D. Crosby, "Record of the Medical History of Camp Stotsenberg" (1904), 104, quoted in Russell, *Malaria and Culicidae in the Philippine Islands*, 15. Stotsenberg, later Clark Air Base, was in Pampanga, Luzon. It included the foothills of the Zambales mountains.

12. Chief Surgeon, Philippines Division, to Surgeon General, Washington, D.C., March 14, 1907, pp. 9–10, RG 112-E26-24508-38, NARA.

13. Chief Surgeon, Philippines Division, to Surgeon General, Washington, D.C., March 14, 1907, pp. 10, 13, RG 112-E26-24508-38, NARA.

14. Craig, "Observations on Latent and Masked Malarial Infections," "Observations upon Malaria," and "A Study of Latent Malarial Infection." See chapter 3. We now know that some clinical immunity to malaria is achieved after one or two infections; antiparasitic immunity is rarer and requires many infections. The high rate of thalassemia and frequency of HbE in the Philippines would also have provided some

Filipinos with protection from the disease. See Carter and Mendis, "Evolutionary and Historical Aspects of the Burden of Malaria."

15. Craig, "The Importance to the Army of Diseases Transmitted by Mosquitoes and Methods for their Prevention."

16. Bureau of Health, *Annual Report for the Year Ending August 31, 1905* (Manila: Bureau of Printing, 1906).

17. Dunbar, "Antimalarial Prophylactic Measures and Their Results."

18. Bureau of Health, *Annual Report for the Year Ending June 30, 1911* (Manila: Bureau of Printing, 1911), 48–49.

19. Joint Commission of Representatives, "Sanitary Survey of San José Estates and Adjacent Properties on Mindoro Island," 187, 188.

20. Bureau of Health, *Insects and Disease*, 12–14.

21. Seale, "The Mosquito Fish, *Gambusia affinus* in the Philippine Islands." Of course, this introduction proved completely useless.

22. Bureau of Health, *Annual Report for the Year Ending December 31, 1914* (Manila: Bureau of Printing, 1915), 170.

23. Walker and Barber, "Malaria in the Philippine Islands I."

24. Barber, Raquel, Guzman, and Rosa, "Malaria in the Philippine Islands II," 243.

25. Russell, *Man's Mastery of Malaria*; and Harrison, *Mosquitoes, Malaria and Man*.

26. J. W. W. Stephens, in "Discussion of the Prophylaxis of Malaria," *British Medical J.* ii (1904): 629–31, at 629, 631. See also Christophers and Stephens, "The Native as the Prime Agent in the Malarial Infection of Europeans." For more on the racializing of malaria transmission in India, see Arnold, "'An Ancient Race Outworn': Malaria and Race in Colonial India, 1860–1930"; and Bynum, "Malaria in Inter-war British India." On malaria and segregation policies in Africa, see Dumett, "The Campaign against Malaria and the Expansion of Scientific Medical and Sanitary Services"; and MacKinnon, "Of Oxford Bags and Twirling Canes: The State, Popular Responses and Zulu Antimalaria Assistants."

27. Ronald Ross, in "Discussion of the Prophylaxis of Malaria," 635. See also Ross, *The Prevention of Malaria*.

28. Ross, *Studies on Malaria*, 137, 78. As late as 1936, Paul F. Russell noted that: "Mian Mir proved nothing, but it weighed heavily with officialdom" ("Malaria in India: Impressions from a Tour," 653).

29. Watson, *The Prevention of Malaria in the Federated Malay States*, 10, 360. This technique of mosquito reduction would have been ineffective in decreasing malaria in the Philippines.

30. Ronald Ross, "Preface," to Watson, *Prevention of Malaria*, lx.

31. But see the report to the Army Board for the Study of Tropical Diseases from the 1909 Bombay Medical Congress, at which Christophers and Stephens had complained that the "human factor" in malaria had been neglected in favor of larval destruction, and Ross "replied with vigor" (Anon., "The Bombay Medical Congress," p. 2, RG 112-E26-68075-68, NARA). The delegate from the Philippines recommended an emphasis on mosquito control, "done with American thoroughness and attention to detail" (3).

32. Delaporte, *The History of Yellow Fever*.

33. Ross, *Studies on Malaria*, 127. See Gorgas, *Sanitation in Panama*; and Gorgas and Hendrick, *William Crawford Gorgas, His Life and Work*. Gorgas became surgeon general of the army and later advised the Rockefeller Foundation on yellow fever control programs in South America.

34. Russell, *Man's Mastery of Malaria*, 145. The term *ecological* was not part of the vocabulary of tropical medicine before the 1920s, but it is hard to describe this understanding of malaria in any other way.

35. Hackett, *Malaria in Europe: An Ecological Study*.

36. Farley, *To Cast Out Disease: A History of the International Health Division of the Rockefeller Foundation, 1913–1951*; and Schneider, ed., *Rockefeller Philanthropy and Modern Biomedicine: International Initiatives from World War I to the Cold War*.

37. Rose, "Field Experiments in Malaria Control," 1414. Rose directed the International Health Board from 1913 to 1923. In 1914, Rose had sought advice from Ross and Watson: see Russell, "The United States and Malaria: Debits and Credits."

38. Rose, "Field Experiments in Malaria Control," 1416, 1417.

39. Ibid., 1417–18. The scope of southern vector control programs widened in the 1920s, as local communities took them over. By 1922, the Rockefeller Foundation was aiding malaria control in 163 counties in 10 states. See Humphreys, *Malaria: Poverty, Race and Public Health in the United States*.

40. Bass, "A Discussion of Malaria Carriers and the Important Role They Play in the Persistence and Spread of Malaria"; and Graves, "The Negro as a Menace to the Health of the White Race."

41. Rose, "Field Experiments in Malaria Control," 1418–20.

42. Stapleton, "Internationalism and Nationalism: The Rockefeller Foundation, Public Health, and Malaria in India, 1923–51," 134. See also Stapleton, "Dawn of DDT"; Farley, *To Cast Out Disease*; and Pauline A. Mead, "The Rockefeller Foundation: Operations and Research in the Control and Eradication of Malaria" (New York: Rockefeller Foundation, 1955 [typescript at RAC]). Stapleton points out that the Sardinian experiment was the culmination of the foundation's antimalaria program. The International Health Division closed in 1951.

43. Farley makes another, related distinction, arguing that hookworm was a means to an end and malaria an end in itself ("The International Health Division of the Rockefeller Foundation: The Russell Years, 1920–1934").

44. Barber and Hayne, "Arsenic as a Larvicide for Anopheline Larvae." On the development of Paris Green—copper aceto-arsenite—in the 1920s, see Whorton, "Insecticide Spray Residues and Public Health, 1865–1938." The first large-scale use of Paris Green was in the Philippines in 1924.

45. Tiedemann, "Malaria in the Philippines." See also Paul F. Russell, "Final Report on the Malaria Investigations of the International Health Division of the Rockefeller Foundation in the Philippine Islands, 1921–1934," p. 7, box 72, 3, series 242I, RG 5, RFA, RAC. A few years later it was established that *A. minimus* was probably the sole effective vector.

46. "Annual Report 1930," box 71, 3, series 242I, RG 5, RFA, RAC; and Russell, "Final Report on the Malaria Investigations."

47. J. J. Mieldazis to W. A. Sawyer, May 26, 1928, box 70, 3, series 242, RG 5, RFA, RAC. It was in this period that Vedder claimed that Philippine experience showed that quinine prophylaxis was a "complete washout," and selective mosquito control was the only answer to malaria ("Report on the Seventh Congress of the Far Eastern Association of Tropical Medicine," 280).

48. Diary of Dr. Heiser's World Trip, 1925–26, November 30, 1925, p. 151, 5.27, unit 63, room 104, RG 12.1, RFA, RAC.

49. Diary of Dr. Heiser's World Trip, October 1927–May 1928, March 27, 1928, p. 162, 5.27, unit 63, room 104, RG 12.1, RFA, RAC.

50. C. H. Yaeger to V. G. Heiser, July 29, 1929, folder 63, box 6, series 242I, RG 1.1, RFA, RAC.

51. Persis Putnam to W. A. Sawyer, January 18, 1928, folder 63, box 6, series 242I, RG 1.1, RFA, RAC.

52. Heiser to F. F. Russell, May 8, 1928, folder 63, box 6, series 242I, RG 1.1, RFA, RAC.

53. C. H. Yaeger to V. G. Heiser, July 29, 1929, folder 63, box 6, series 242I, RG 1.1, RFA, RAC.

54. C. H. Yaeger, "Annual Report of the Rockefeller Foundation for the Philippine Islands, 1929," pp. 17, 11, box 70, 3, series 242, RG 5, RFA, RAC.

55. Diary of Dr. Heiser's World Trip, October 1927–May 1928, March 27, 1928, p. 162, 5.27, unit 63, room 104, RG 12.1, RFA, RAC.

56. Diary of Dr. Heiser's Trip Around the World, October 1930–May 1931, January 2, 1930, p. 80, 5.27, unit 63, room 104, RG 12.1, RFA, RAC.

57. Heiser to Jacobo Fajardo, September 6, 1927, folder 63, box 6, series 242I, RG 1.1, RFA, RAC.

58. C. Manalang, "Brief Report on the Results of Paris Green Control in the Philippines," 1928, folder 80, box 7, series 242I, RG 1.1, RFA, RAC.

59. Diary of Dr. Heiser's Trip Around the World, 1932–33, December 29, 1932, p. 67, 5.27, unit 63, room 104, RG 12.1, RFA, RAC. See Lovewell, "Malaria at Camp Stotsenberg, P.I."; Parsons, "Malaria Control at Camp Stotsenberg, P.I."; and Simmons, St John, and Reynolds, "Malaria Survey at Camp Stotsenberg, P.I."

60. Paul F. Russell to V. G. Heiser, October 11, 1933, folder 2, box 1, series 242, RG 1.1, RFA, RAC.

61. Selskar M. Gunn, "Report on Visit to the Philippines," August 26, 1933, folder 4, box 1, series 242, RG 1.1, RFA, RAC.

62. Heiser to F. F. Russell, January 31, 1931, folder 66, box 6, series 242I, RG 1.1, RFA, RAC. W. V. King was also active at the bureau during this period as an entomologist, working on mosquitoes.

63. Paul F. Russell to V. G. Heiser, January 21, 1930, folder 65, box 6, series 242I, RG 1.1, RFA, RAC.

64. Paul F. Russell to V. G. Heiser, March 23, 1932, folder 67, box 6, series 242I, RG 1.1, RFA, RAC. Ironically, Russell complained that the malaria control section of the Philippine Health Service was "more concerned with research than with practical control measures" (Russell, "Final Report on the Malaria Investigations," 18).

65. Paul F. Russell to V. G. Heiser, April 4, 1932, folder 67, box 6, series 242I, RG 1.1, RFA, RAC.

66. Michael Salman, "The United States and the End of Slavery in the Philippines, 1898–1914: A Study of Imperialism, Ideology and Nationalism" (PH.D. dissertation, Stanford University, 1993).

67. Heiser to Paul F. Russell, August 22, 1934, folder 69, box 6, series 242I, RG 1.1, RFA, RAC.

68. Paul F. Russell to V. G. Heiser, February 15, 1934, and C. H. Yaeger to F. F. Russell, February 7, 1935, folder 71, box 6, series 242I, RG 1.1, RFA, RAC. See also C. H. Yaeger, "Final Report—Malaria Control at Iwahig, Palawan, Philippine Islands, 1933–34," folder 72, , box 6, series 242I, RG 1.1, RFA, RAC. The hospital admission rate for malaria in August 1933 was 246; in August 1934 it was 62. On Atebrin use among U.S. troops from 1933, see Simmons et al., *Malaria in Panama*.

69. Russell, *Malaria and Culicidae in the Philippine Islands*, 55.

70. Paul F. Russell, "Malaria in the Philippine Islands," 174. Frederick F. Russell, the director of the International Health Division, had previously complained about working with "backward peoples" ("War on Disease, Particularly Yellow Fever and Malaria," 11). He stressed that for quinine treatment to succeed, the population must be "small, very intelligent and under perfect control" (31).

71. Manalang, "Malaria Transmission in the Philippines II." Manalang was concerned that the mosquitoes could fly farther than 1.5 km., which was the usual coverage of Paris Green spraying.

72. Russell, *Malaria and Culicidae in the Philippine Islands*, 55, 56, 60.

73. Russell, "Malaria in the Philippine Islands," 176.

74. Russell, "Malaria in India: Impressions from a Tour," 662, 658, 664.

75. Russell and Knipe, "Malaria Control by Spray-killing Adult Mosquitoes." See also Paul F. Russell, "Malaria Investigations—Madras: A Résumé of Activities, 1936–1940," folder 88, box 11, series 464, RG 1.1, RFA, RAC. Pyrethrum sprays were introduced in the 1930s and used from 1938 in Rockefeller projects in India.

76. Russell, "Malaria in the Philippine Islands," 176.

77. On the "central role of technical expertise in malaria control from 1930 to 1960," see Stapleton, "Technology and Malaria Control, 1930–1960: The Career of Rockefeller Foundation Engineer Frederick W. Knipe," 59. Similarly, Najera, a former director of the Malaria Action Program of the World Health Organization, has noted that "the overwhelming emphasis was on the creation of an efficient operational mechanism for the spraying of insecticides and the collection of blood slides" ("Malaria Control: Present Situation and Need for Historical Research," 220). On the development of international health services between the wars, see Allen, "World Health and World Politics"; Howard-Jones, *International Health Between the Two Worlds*; and Weindling, ed. *International Health Organizations*.

78. Najera observes that the antimalaria campaign "reveals in its own terminology its origin from the military, in concepts such as campaign, attack, logistics, armamentarium, brigades, squads, strategy and tactics" ("Malaria Control," 225).

79. On military metaphor, see Edmund Russell, *War and Nature: Fighting Humans and Insects with Chemicals from World War I to Silent Spring*. These different "military"

strategies map roughly onto the debate between advocates of vertical (or specific) and horizontal (or primary health care) approaches to disease control in the developing world: see, for example, Bradley, "The Particular and the General: Issues of Specificity and Verticality in the History of Malaria Control." Predictably, some British and European malariologists displayed a lingering commitment to working with the human factor in malaria. They felt that specific vector control projects might deprive native peoples of their acquired immunity to malaria, thus making fresh outbreaks of the disease more devastating. See Corbellini, "Acquired Immunity against Malaria as a Tool for the Control of the Disease"; and Dobson, Malowany, and Snow, "Malaria Control in East Africa: The Kampala Conference and the Pare-Taveta Scheme." Most historians, though, date the interest in primary health care to the 1970s: Cueto, "The Origins of Primary Health Care and Selective Primary Health Care"; and Litsios, "The Christian Medical Commission and the Development of the World Health Organization's Primary Health Care Approach."

80. Hackett, "Malaria Control through Anti-mosquito Measures in Italy," 478, 482, 493. Hackett had worked with the International Health Board since 1914, mostly on hookworm in Guatemala and health policy in Brazil. On the continuing conflict in Europe between malariologists favoring antimosquito measures and those wanting quininization and social improvement, see Evans, "European Malaria Policy in the 1920s and 1930s: The Epidemiology of Minutiae."

81. Hackett, "Biological Factors in Malaria Control," 343, 350. Hackett and Russell later wrote together on the principle of "species sanitation" and the use of "naturalistic methods" (Hackett, Russell, Scharf, and White, "The Present Use of Naturalistic Measures in the Control of Malaria").

82. Farley, *To Cast Out Disease*. See also Soper and Wilson, *Anopheles gambiae in Brazil, 1930–1940*; and Packard and Gadelha, "A Land Filled with Mosquitoes: Fred L. Soper, the Rockefeller Foundation, and the *Anopheles gambiae* Invasion of Brazil." Interestingly, Packard and Gadelha criticize the "inattention to the human dimension of malaria" and point out that the "landscape portrayed in these documents [on mosquito eradication] is almost devoid of humans" (205).

83. Litsios, "René Dubos and Fred L. Soper: Their Contrasting Views on Vector and Disease Eradication"; and Packard, "'No Other Logical Choice': Global Malaria Eradication and the Politics of International Health in the Post-war Era."

84. Russell, *Man's Mastery of Malaria*, 257.

85. Russell, West, Manwell, *Practical Malariology*.

86. Hackett, *Malaria in Europe*, 266.

87. Strong, "The Importance of Ecology in Relation to Disease," 308.

88. Burnet, *Biological Aspects of Infectious Disease*, 159, 284. On Burnet, one of the leaders of the new disease ecology, see Anderson, "Natural Histories of Infectious Disease: Ecological Vision in Twentieth-century Biomedical Science."

CONCLUSION

1. On social medicine in the twentieth century, see Rosen, *From Medical Police to Social Medicine*; Porter, *Health, Civilization and the State*.

2. Anderson, *The Cultivation of Whiteness*. For a comparison of Australian and Philippines racial and national hygiene projects, see Anderson, "States of Hygiene: Race 'Improvement' and Biomedical Citizenship in Australia and the Colonial Philippines."

3. Deutschman, "Public Health and Medical Services in the Philippines"; de la Cruz, *History of Philippine Medicine and the* PMA; and Dayrit, Santos Ocampo, and de la Cruz, *History of Philippine Medicine, 1899–1999*.

4. Cohen, "Public Health in the Philippines"; and Dayrit, Santos Ocampo, and de la Cruz, *History of Philippine Medicine*.

5. As Michel Foucault argues, "A whole series of colonial models was brought back to the West, and the result was that the West could produce something resembling colonization . . . on itself" (*"Society Must be Defended,"* 103).

6. *First Annual Report of the Department of Public Health [Illinois], July 1, 1917, to June 30, 1918* (Springfield, Ill.: State Printers, 1919), 19. The phrase "public health is purchasable" was a commonplace of the New York City and State Health Departments when Hermann M. Biggs directed them in the early twentieth century. See Winslow, *The Life of Hermann M. Biggs*. Stern traces the direct medical influences of Panama and the Panama-Pacific Exhibition in *Eugenic Nation*.

7. Heiser, *An American Doctor's Odyssey*; and Duffy, *A History of Public Health in New York City*, 271. Reform and reorganization of the New York City Health Department had begun earlier under Dr. Sigismund S. Goldwater, but Emerson greatly increased the momentum.

8. William Everett Musgrave papers, UCSF, mss 27–5.

9. Gonzalez Flores, *Historia de la influencia extranjera en el desenvolvimiento educacional y científico de Costa Rica*, 160; Palmer, *From Popular Medicine to Medical Populism*, 155–81. I am grateful to Steve Palmer for drawing this to my attention. On Milwaukee public health, see Leavitt, *The Healthiest City*.

10. The San Francisco Department of Public Health even established a Bureau of Tropical Medicine in 1911 because "numbers of Asians immigrating to this country are afflicted with or carry with them germs of diseases which are endemic to Oriental countries" (*Annual Report of the Department of Public Health, San Francisco, California, July 1, 1910–June 30, 1911* [San Francisco: Neal Publishing, n.d.], 7). To get an idea of the range of public health activities in the United States during this period, see Chapin, *A Report on State Health Work*. Even in 1913, American sanitary science was "still largely in the experimental stage" (3), with great variation in public health activities, from the extensive work of authorities in New York, Massachusetts, and Pennsylvania to almost nothing in states like New Mexico, Wyoming, Arkansas, and Florida.

11. Rosenkrantz, *Public Health and the State*, 142.

12. *Forty-Sixth Annual Report of the State Board of Health of Massachusetts* (1914) (Boston: Wright and Potter, 1915), 2. There had been part-time district officers since 1907.

13. *First Annual Report of the State Department of Health of Massachusetts* (1915) (Boston: Wright and Potter, 1916), 8, 22–23. The phrase "public health is purchasable" (10) again betrays another great influence on the reform of U.S. public health departments during this period: the New York City Health Department.

14. McLaughlin, assisted by Tobey, *Personal Hygiene: The Rules of Right Living*, 63.

15. Many of the American scientists at the Manila Bureau of Science did, however, go on to distinguished careers in pathology and microbiology: W. B. Wherry became professor of bacteriology at the University of Ohio; Paul G. Woolley, professor of pathology at the same institution; Maximilian Herzog, professor of pathology at Northwestern University; and H. T. Marshall, professor of pathology at the University of Virginia.

16. Some of Heiser's former colleagues expressed disappointment with these curiously depopulated reminiscences. S. M. "Sam" Lambert wondered why it was not entitled "Alone in the Orient" (*A Yankee Doctor in Paradise*, 4).

17. Victor G. Heiser, "Conquering Industrial Diseases" (c. 1940), p. 11, Heiser papers, American Philosophical Society B: H357.p. Heiser argued that an "industrial health program . . . bids fair to take such issues [of labor conditions] out of the grievance picture and place management in an improved bargaining position" ("Industrial Health Programs are Good Business," 1947, p. 6, Heiser papers, American Philosophical Society B: H357.p).

18. "It is high time," he wrote, "for Americans to get some of the brawn of their pioneer forbears and quit being dainty, steam-heated, rubber-tired, beauty-rested, effeminized, pampered sissies" (*Toughen Up America*, 21).

19. See, for example, his comments on the habitual carelessness of "Negro workers" in a radio talk: "Conquering Industrial Diseases" (c. 1940), p. 1, Heiser papers, American Philosophical Society B: H357.p.

20. James D. Sobredo, "From American 'Nationals' to the 'Third Asiatic Invasion': Racial Transformation and Filipino Exclusion (1898–1934)" (PH.D. dissertation, University of California-Berkeley, 1998); Deverell, "Plague in Los Angeles, 1924: Ethnicity and Typicality"; and Abel, "'Only the Best Class of Immigration': Public Health Policy toward Mexicans and Filipinos in Los Angeles, 1910–1940."

21. Choy, *Empire of Care: Nursing and Migration in Filipino-American History*.

22. See Hewa, *Colonialism, Tropical Disease and Imperial Medicine: Rockefeller Philanthropy in Sri Lanka*; and Farley, *To Cast Out Disease*.

23. Long was on epidemic duty in San Francisco in 1914 and 1921. See Williams, *The United States Public Health Service, 1798–1950*. Richard Strong was another major figure in international health development. In 1920, he established the medical department of the League of Red Cross Societies and later became a leading promoter of the League of Nations Health Organization.

Bibliography

MANUSCRIPT AND PHOTOGRAPH COLLECTIONS

Philippines

Archives Section, Department of Health, Republic of the Philippines, Manila
Angeles, Marcelo C. "History of the Public Health System in the Philippines."
Unpublished ms., c. 1967

Culion Museum, Palawan
Patient Records

Philippine National Archives, Manila
Memorias Medicas
Sanidad

Rizal Library, Ateneo de Manila
American Historical Collection
T. H. Pardo de Tavera Papers

California

Bancroft Library, University of California, Berkeley
David Prescott Barrows Papers
Louis D. Baun Papers
Eli L. Huggins Papers
John F. Minier Papers
Bernard Moses Papers
Herbert I. Priestley Papers

Special Collections, University of California, San Francisco
Alice Burrell Papers
William E. Musgrave Papers

Delaware

Hagley Museum and Library, Wilmington
National Association of Manufacturers Papers

Maryland

Alan Mason Chesney Archives, The Johns Hopkins Medical School, Baltimore
The Johns Hopkins University Commission for the Study of the Prevalent Diseases
of the Philippine Archipelago
William C. Welch Papers

History of Medicine Division, National Library of Medicine, Bethesda
   Fielding H. Garrison Papers
   Charles R. Greenleaf Papers
   Frederick Hoffman Papers

United States National Archives and Records Administration, College Park
   RG 94: Records of the Adjutant General's Office, 1780s–1917
   RG 111-FG: Photographs of Scenes in the Philippines, c. 1899–c. 1903
   RG 112-E25: Records of the Office of the Surgeon General, Army
   RG 165-PW: Prints of the Philippine Insurrection, 1899–1903
   SWS: Spanish-American War Photographs, 1898–99
   RG 200-PI: Allan N. Webster Photographic Collection Relating to the Philippine
      Islands, 1898–99
   RG 350: War Department, Bureau of Insular Affairs
   RG 350-BS: Photographs of the Philippines Islands, c. 1907–c. 1918
   RG 350-P: Photographs of the Philippines Islands, 1898–1935
   RG 350-PC: Photographs of the Philippine Islands, c. 1902–1928

Massachusetts

Countway Medical Library, Harvard Medical School, Boston
   Richard P. Strong Papers

Houghton Library, Harvard University, Cambridge
   William Cameron Forbes Papers

Massachusetts Archives, Boston
   Health and Human Services Records

Michigan

Michigan Historical Collections, Bentley Library, University of Michigan, Ann Arbor
   Joseph R. Hayden Papers.
   J. E. Reighard Papers
   Dean C. Worcester Papers

New York

Rockefeller Foundation Archives, Rockefeller Archive Center, Sleepy Hollow
   RG 1: Projects, 1912–89
   RG 2: General Correspondence, 1927–89
   RG 5: International Health Board/Division
   RG 12: Officers' Diaries

Pennsylvania

American Philosophical Society, Philadelphia
   Victor G. Heiser Papers

United States Army Military History Institute, Carlisle Barracks
   Darnell, Joseph R. "Sojourn in Zamboanga." Unpublished ms., c. 1947
   George De Shon Papers

Johnson, Richard. "My Life in the Army, 1899–1922." Unpublished ms., c. 1952

Halstead-Maus Family Papers

Charles Everett MacDonald Papers

Snyder, Arthur Augustine. "Experiences of a Contract Surgeon." Unpublished ms.

Spanish-American War Survey: U.S. Medical Corps Box

Washington, D.C.

United States Library of Congress

Charles Burke Elliott Papers

Francis Burton Harrison Papers

PUBLISHED PRIMARY SOURCES

Acton, Hugh W. "Neurasthenia in the Tropics." *Indian Medical Gazette* 62 (1927): 1–7.

Albert, José. *The Experiment of Leper Segregation in the Philippines.* Manila: n.p., n.d. [1920].

Alden, Charles H. "The Special Training of the Medical Officer, with Brief Notes on Army Medical Schools Abroad and at Home." *TAMS* 4 (1894): 675–89.

Anon. "Highly Artistic Red Cross Carnival." *Philippine Review* (January 1918): 95.

———. "Commercial Exhibits." *Philippines National Weekly* (February 9, 1918): 3.

———. "The Carnival and the Student." *Philippines National Weekly* (February 9, 1918): 6.

———. "The 1918 Philippine Red Cross Carnival." *Philippine Review* (March 1918): 196–200.

———. "Manila Carnival and Commercial-Industrial Fair." *American Chamber of Commerce J.* 2 (1922): 9–12.

———. "Quezon Tells Medicos Culion Costs Too Much." *Manila Times* (December 17, 1923).

———. "Quezon Pays His Respects to Major Hitchens." *Manila Times* (December 19, 1926).

———. "Leprologists Form International Leprosy Association." *Manila Daily Bulletin* (January 22, 1931).

Aron, Hans. "Investigations of the Action of the Tropical Sun on Men and Animals." *PJS* 6 (1911): 101–23.

Ashburn, Percy M. *The Elements of Military Hygiene, Especially Arranged for Officers and Men of the Line.* Boston: Houghton Mifflin, 1909.

Ashburn, Percy M., and Charles F. Craig. "The Work of the Army Board for the Study of Tropical Diseases in the Philippine Islands." *Military Surgeon* 21 (1907): 38–49.

Ashford, Bailey K. *A Soldier in Science.* New York: William Morrow, 1934.

Atkinson, Fred W. *The Philippine Islands.* Boston: Ginn, 1905.

Bache, Dallas. "The Location of Sites for, and the Construction of, Military Posts in Relation to Proper Sanitation." *JAMS* 5 (1895): 413–30.

Balfour, Andrew. "Tropical Problems in the New World." *Trans. Society of Tropical Medicine and Hygiene* 8 (1915): 75–108.

———. "The Problem of Acclimatisation." *Lancet* 205 (1923): 84–87.

Balfour, Andrew. "Personal Hygiene." In *The Practice of Medicine in the Tropics*, edited by W. Byam and R. G. Archibald, 3 vols., 1:1–26. London: Henry Frowde and Hodder and Stoughton, 1923.

Bancroft, Hubert Howe. *The New Pacific*. New York: Bancroft, 1899.

Bantug, J. P., P. Gabriel, and M. Arguelles. *A Simple Manual for Sanitary Inspectors*. Manila: Bureau of Printing, 1923.

Barber, M. A., A. Raquel, A. Guzman, and A. P. Rosa. "Malaria in the Philippine Islands II." *PJS* 10 (1915): 177–245.

Barber, M. A., and T. B. Hayne. "Arsenic as a Larvicide for Anopheline Larvae." *U.S. Public Health Reports* 36 (1921): 3027.

Barker, Lewellys F. *Time and the Physician: The Autobiography of Lewellys F. Barker*. New York: G. P. Putnam's Sons, 1942.

———. "Medical Commission to the Philippines." *Bulletin of the Johns Hopkins Hospital* 11 (1900): 26–30.

Bass, C. C. "A Discussion of Malaria Carriers and the Important Role They Play in the Persistence and Spread of Malaria." *Southern Medical J.* 8 (1915): 182–84.

Bean, Robert Bennett. *The Racial Anatomy of the Philippine Islanders*. Philadelphia: J. B. Lippincott, 1910.

Beard, George M. *A Practical Treatise on Nervous Exhaustion (Neurasthenia) and its Symptoms, Nature, Sequences, Treatment*. 2nd ed. New York: William Wood, 1880.

Berkeley Hill, Owen. "The 'Colour-question' from a Psychoanalytic Standpoint." In *Collected Papers*, 139–48. Calcutta: Book Co., 1933 [1923].

———. "Neurasthenia in the Tropics." *Indian Medical Gazette* 62 (1927): 228–37.

———. "Mental Hygiene of Europeans in the Tropics." In *Trans. of the 7th Congress of the Far Eastern Association of Tropical Medicine, December 1927*, edited by J. Cunningham, 1:389–99. Calcutta: Thacker's Press and Directories, 1928.

Beveridge, Albert J. "March of the Flag." In *The Meaning of the Times and Other Speeches*, 47–57. N.p.: Bobbs-Merrill, 1908 [1900].

———. "Our Philippine Policy." In *The Meaning of the Times and Other Speeches*, 58–88. N.p.: Bobbs-Merrill, 1908 [1900].

Billings, John Shaw. "The Military Medical Officer at the Opening of the Twentieth Century." *JAMS* 12 (1903): 349–57.

Birch, E. A. "Influences of Warm Climates on the Constitution." In *Hygiene and Diseases of Warm Climates*, edited by Andrew Davidson. Edinburgh: Pentland, 1893.

Birmingham, Henry P. "Some Practical Suggestions of Tropical Hygiene." *JAMS* 12 (1903): 45–54.

Board of Health. *Manual of the Board of Health for the Philippine Islands*. Manila: Bureau of Printing, 1911.

Boekmann, Edouard. "Some Remarks about Asepsis in Military Service." *TAMS* 5 (1895): 143–62.

Brooke, A. Y. "Baguio as a Health Resort." *Mid-Pacific Magazine* 23 (1922): 457–58.

Brown, Orlando J. "The Effects and Treatment of Heat and Sunstroke at Camps of Instruction." *JAMS* 5 (1895): 431–35.

Brownell, Atherton. "What American Ideas of Citizenship May Do for Oriental Peoples." *The Outlook* (Dec. 23, 1904): 975–85.

——. "Turning Savages into Citizens." *The Outlook* (Dec. 24, 1910): 921–31.

Bryan, William Jennings. *Bryan on Imperialism*. New York: Arno Press and New York Times, 1970 [1900].

Buckland, Ralph Kent. *In the Land of the Filipino*. New York: Every-Where, 1912.

Bullard, Robert L. "Some Characteristics of the Negro Volunteer." *JMSI* 29 (1901): 29–39.

——. "Small Maneuvers," *JMSI* 39 (1906): 57–67.

Bureau of Education and Philippine Health Service. *Health: A Manual for Teachers*. Manila: Bureau of Printing, 1928.

Bureau of Health. *Infectious Diseases: Period of Incubation, Quarantine and Infection; Sources of Infection*. Health Bulletin No. 1. Manila: Bureau of Printing, 1903.

——. *Cholera Measures*. Health Bulletin No. 7. Manila: Bureau of Printing, 1909.

——. *Insects and Disease*. Health Bulletin No. 11. Manila: Bureau of Printing, 1913.

——. *The Disposal of Human Wastes in the Provinces*. Health Bulletin No. 13. Manila: Bureau of Printing, n.d. [c. 1914].

——. *Sanitary Measures in Connection with Local Fiestas*. Provincial Circular No. 124 (Oct. 6, 1915).

——. *Proposed Sanitary Code*. Health Bulletin No. 22. Manila: Bureau of Printing, 1920.

Burgess, Perry. *Who Walk Alone*. New York: Henry Holt, 1940.

Burrill, Herbert L. "Is It Expedient to Have a Physical Examination of Men before Enlisting Them as State Troops?" *TAMS* 2 (1892): 133–37.

Calderón, Fernando. "Faulty Maternity Practices and Their Influence upon Infant Mortality." In *Proceedings of the First National Conference on Infant Mortality and Public Welfare, December 6–10, 1921*, 33–43. Manila: Bureau of Printing, 1922.

Callender, George R. "The Leprosy Problem in the Philippine Islands." *American J. Tropical Medicine* 5 (1925): 351–58.

Callwell, Charles C. E. *Small Wars: Their Principles and Practice*. 3rd ed. London: His Majesty's Stationery Office, 1906 [1896].

Capelo y Juan, Francisco. *Manila, la Higiene y el Cólera*. Manila: Colegio de Santo Tomás, 1883.

Carpenter, Frank G. *Through the Philippines and Hawaii*. Garden City, N.Y.: Doubleday, Page, 1925.

Carter, E. C. "Sanitary Conditions as Affecting Contracts for Works in the Philippine Islands." *Engineering News* 54 (1905): 544–47.

Castellani, Aldo, and Albert J. Chalmers. *Manual of Tropical Medicine*. London: Baillière, Tindall and Cox, 1910.

Chamberlain, Weston P. "Analysis of One Hundred and Twenty Cases of Malaria Occurring at Camp Gregg, Philippine Islands." *Boston Medical and Surgical J.* 154 (1906): 29–40.

——. "Observations of the Influence of the Philippine Climate on White Men of the Blond and Brunet Type." *PJS* 6 (1911): 427–63.

Chamberlain, Weston P. "A Study of the Systolic Blood Pressure and the Pulse Rate of Healthy Adult Males in the Philippines." *PJS* 6 (1911): 467–81.

——. "The Red Blood Corpuscles and the Hemoglobin of Healthy Adult American Males Residing in the Philippines." *PJS* 7 (1912): 483–88.

——. "Some Features of the Physiological Activity of White Races in the Philippine Islands." *American J. of Tropical Disease and Preventive Medicine* 1 (1913): 12–32.

Chamberlain, Weston P., et al. "Examination of Stools and Blood among the Igorots at Baguio, Philippine Islands." *PJS* 5B (1910): 505–14.

Chamberlain, Weston P., and Edward B. Vedder. "A Study of Arneth's Nuclear Classification of Neutrophils in Healthy Adult Males and the Influence thereon of Race, Complexion and Tropical Residence." *PJS* 6 (1911): 405–19.

Chamberlin, Frederick. *The Philippine Problem*. Boston: Little, Brown, 1913.

Chapin, Charles V. *Sources and Modes of Infection*. New York: John Wiley and Sons, 1910.

——. *A Report on State Public Health Work, Based on a Survey of State Boards of Health*. Chicago: AMA, n.d. [1915].

——. "Dirt, Disease and the Health Officer." In *The Papers of Charles V. Chapin*, M.D.: A Review of Public Health Realities, edited by Frederic P. Gorham and Clarence L. Scamman, 20–26. New York: Commonwealth Fund, 1934 [1902].

——. "The Fetich of Disinfection" In *The Papers of Charles V. Chapin*, M.D.: A Review of Public Health Realities, edited by Frederic P. Gorham and Clarence L. Scamman, 65–75. New York: Commonwealth Fund, 1934 [1905].

Christophers, S. R., and J. W. W. Stephens. "The Native as the Prime Agent in the Malarial Infection of Europeans." *Reports of the Malaria Committee of the Royal Society*, 3:3–19. London: Royal Society, 1900.

Clausewitz, Carl von. *On War*. Translated by Michael Howard and Peter Paret. Princeton: Princeton University Press, 1976 [1832].

Clemow, F. G. *The Geography of Disease*. Cambridge: Cambridge University Press, 1903.

Codorniu y Nieto, Antonio. *Topografía médica de las Islas Filipinas*. Madrid: Alejandro Gomez Fuentenebro, 1857.

Cole, C. L. "*Necator americanus* in the Natives of the Philippine Islands." *PJS* 2B (1907): 333–42.

Comisión Central de Manila. *Memoria complementaria de la sección 2 del programa: Pobladores aborígenes, razas existentes y sus variedad de religiones, usos y costumbres de los habitantes de Filipinas*. Manila: Imprenta del Colegio de Santo Tomás, 1887.

Conger, Emily Bronson. *An Ohio Woman in the Philippines*. Cleveland: Arthur H. Clark, 1904.

Corpus, Teofilo. "Experiences in Collecting Lepers." *Philippine Health Service Monthly Bulletin* 4 (October 1924): 450.

Craig, Charles F. "Observations on Latent and Masked Malarial Infections with an Analysis of 395 Cases." *American Medicine* 8 (1904): 757–61.

——. "Observations upon Malaria: Latent Infection in Natives of the Philippine Islands." *PJS* 1 (1906): 523–31.

——. "A Study of Latent Malarial Infection." *Yale Medical J.* 13 (1906–7): 349–63.

——. "The Importance to the Army of Diseases Transmitted by Mosquitoes and Methods for Their Prevention." *Military Surgeon* 26 (1910): 292–308.

Crane, C. J. "The Fighting Tactics of Filipinos." *JMSI* 31 (1902): 496–507.

Daniels, Charles W., and E. Wilkinson. *Tropical Medicine and Hygiene.* 2nd ed., 2 vols. New York: Wood, 1913–14.

Dauncey, Campbell. *An Englishwoman in the Philippines.* New York: E. P. Dutton, 1906.

Davidson, Andrew, ed. *Hygiene and Diseases of Warm Climates.* Edinburgh: Pentland, 1893.

Davis, Dwight D. "Significance of Clean-Up Week." *Monthly Bulletin Philippines Health Service, January 1930.* Manila: Bureau of Printing, 1930.

Davy, John. *Researches, Physiological and Anatomical.* 2 vols. London: Smith, Elder, 1839.

De Jesús, V. *Proposed Sanitary Code.* Health Bulletin No. 22. Manila: Bureau of Printing, 1920.

De Witt, Wallace. "A Few Remarks Concerning the Health Conditions of Americans in the Philippines." *Yale Medical J.* 11 (1904–05): 56–63.

Del Rosario, S. V., and L. Lopez Rizal. *Some Epidemiological Features of Cholera in the Philippines.* Philippine Health Service Bulletin No. 25. Manila: Bureau of Printing, 1922.

Dunbar, A. W. "Antimalarial Prophylactic Measures and Their Results at the Naval Station, Olongapo, P.I." *PJS* 5 (1910): 285–89.

Edger, J. M. *The Present Pandemic of Plague.* Washington, D.C.: Government Printing Office, 1908.

Fajardo, J. "Commencement Address." *Bulletin of the San Juan de Dios Hospital* 5 (1931): 173–75.

Fales, Louis H. "The American Physician in the Philippine Civil Service." *American Medicine* 9 (1905): 513–17.

——. "Tropical Neurasthenia and Its Relation to Tropical Acclimation." *American J. Medical Science* 133 (1907): 582–93.

Fee, Mary H. *A Woman's Impressions of the Philippines.* Chicago: A. C. McClurg, 1910.

Felkin, Robert W. *On the Geographical Distribution of Tropical Diseases in Africa.* Edinburgh: Clay, 1895.

Flexner, Simon, and Lewellys Barker. "Report of a Special Commission Sent to the Philippines by the Johns Hopkins University to Investigate the Prevalent Conditions of the Islands." *JMSI* 26 (1900): 421–33.

——. "The Prevalent Diseases in the Philippines." *Science* 11 ns (April 6, 1900): 521–28.

Forbes, William Cameron. *The Philippine Islands.* 2 vols. Boston: Houghton Mifflin, 1928.

Foreman, J. *The Philippine Islands.* Singapore: Kelly and Walsh, 1906.

Fortune, T. Thomas. "The Filipino." *Voice of the Negro* 1 (1904): 93–99, 199–203, 240–46.

Foster, Charles C. "Notes by a Medical Officer in the East." *TAMS* 6 (1896): 365–69.

Fox, Carroll. *Handbook for Sanitary Inspectors*. Manila: Bureau of Printing, 1914.

Freer, Paul C. *Description of the New Buildings of the Bureau of Government Laboratories*. Manila: Bureau of Printing, 1904.

——. "A Consideration of Some of the Modern Theories of Immunity." *PJS* 2B (1907): 71–82.

Freer, William B. *The Philippine Experiences of an American Teacher: A Narrative of Work and Travel in the Philippine Islands*. New York: Charles Scribner's Sons, 1906.

Galliéni, Joseph S. *La Pacification de Madagascar: opérations d'octobre 1896 à mars 1899*. Edited by F. Hellot. Paris: Chapelot, 1900.

Garrison, P. E. "The Prevalence and Distribution of the Animal Parasites of Man in the Philippine Islands, with a Consideration of Their Possible Influence upon the Public Health." *PJS* 3B (1908): 191–210.

Garrison, P. E., and R. Llamas. "The Intestinal Worms of 385 Filipino Women and Children in Manila." *PJS* 4B (1909): 185–87.

Garrison, P. E., et al. "Medical Survey of Taytay." *PJS* 4B (1909): 257–68.

Gatewood, James D. "Report on the International Conference on Leprosy." In *Report of the Surgeon-General, U.S. Navy, to the Secretary of the Navy, 1898*, 138–58. Washington, D.C.: Government Printing Office, 1898.

Gibbs, H. D. "A Study of the Effect of Tropical Sunlight upon Men, Monkeys, and Rabbits, and a Discussion of the Proper Clothing for the Tropics." *PJS* 7B (1912): 91–114.

Gimlette, John D. "Notes on a Case of 'Amok.'" *J. Tropical Medicine* 4 (1901): 195–96.

Gonzalez, R. *Filipinas y sus inhabitantes*. N.p.: n.pub., 1896.

Gorgas, William Crawford. *Sanitation in Panama*. London: Appleton, 1915.

Graves, Marvin L. "The Negro as a Menace to the Health of the White Race." *Southern Medical J.* 9 (1916): 407–13.

Greenleaf, Charles R. *An Epitome of Tripler's Manual and Other Publications on the Examination of Recruits*. 4th ed. Washington D.C.: Judd and Detweiler, 1898 [1884].

——. "The Practical Duties of an Army Surgeon in the Field, in Time of War." *TAMS* 2 (1892): 9–14.

——. "A Brief Statement of the Sanitary Work Accomplished So Far in the Philippine Islands, and of the Present Shape of the Sanitary Administration." *Public Health Papers and Reports: American Public Health Association* 27 (1901): 159.

Griffis, William Elliot. *America in the East: A Glance at Our History, Prospects, Problems and Duties in the Pacific Ocean*. New York: A. S. Barnes, 1899.

Griffith, Jefferson D. "Hospital Experience in the War with Spain." *JAMS* 8 (1899): 161–67.

Guthrie, Joseph A. "Some Observations While in the Philippines." *JAMS* 13 (1903): 141–49.

Hackett, L. W. *Malaria in Europe: An Ecological Study*. Oxford: Oxford University Press, 1937.

——. "Malaria Control through Anti-mosquito Measures in Italy." *Trans. of the Royal Society of Tropical Medicine and Hygiene* 22 (1929): 477–506.

———. "Biological Factors in Malaria Control." *American J. Tropical Medicine* 16 (1936): 341–52.

Hackett, L. W., P. F. Russell, J. W. Scharf, and R. Senior White. "The Present Use of Naturalistic Measures in the Control of Malaria." *Bulletin of the Health Organization of the League of Nations* 7 (1938): 1016–64.

Halley, George. "First-aid to the Wounded." *TAMS* 2 (1892): 129–32.

Hamilton, Louis M. "Jungle Tactics," *JMSI* 37 (1905): 23–28.

Hammond, William Alexander. *A Treatise on Hygiene, with Special Reference to the Military Service.* San Francisco: Norman, 1991 [1863].

Harris, Seale. "Tuberculosis in the Negro." *JAMA* 41 (1903): 834–38.

Harrison, Francis B. *Inaugural Address.* Manila: Bureau of Printing, 1913.

———. *The Corner-Stone of Philippine Independence: A Narrative of Seven Years.* New York: Century, 1922.

Havard, Valery. *Manual of Military Hygiene for the Military Services of the United States.* 3rd ed. New York: William Wood, 1917.

———. "Is Mortality Necessarily Higher in Tropical than in Temperate Climates?" *American Medicine* 9 (1905): 16–20.

Heiser, Victor G. *An American Doctor's Odyssey: Adventures in Forty-Five Countries.* New York: W. W. Norton, 1936.

———. *Toughen Up America.* New York: McGraw-Hill, 1941.

———. "The Progress of Medicine in the Philippine Islands." *JAMA* 47 (1906): 245–47.

———. "Unsolved Health Problems Peculiar to the Philippines." *PJS* 5 (1910): 171–78.

———. "Typhoid Fever in the Philippine Islands from the Sanitary Standpoint." *PJS* 7B (1912): 115–18.

———. "Sanitation in the Philippines." *J. Race Development* 3 (1912): 121–34.

———. "Fighting Leprosy in the Philippines." *World's Work* 31 (1916): 310–20.

———. "Tropical Diseases." In *Handbook of Medical Treatment*, edited by J. C. DaCosta, 1:189–399. Philadelphia: F. A. Davis, 1918.

Henderson, Thomas. *Hints on the Medical Examination of Recruits for the Army.* Philadelphia: Haswell, Barrington and Haswell, 1840.

Hernando, E. *Management of Communicable Diseases.* Health Bulletin No. 21. Manila: Bureau of Printing, 1919.

Herzog, Maximilian. *The Plague: Bacteriology, Morbid Anatomy, and Histopathology.* Manila: Bureau of Printing, 1904.

———. "The Brain-weight of Filipinos." *American Anthropologist* 10 (1908): 41–47.

Herzog, Maximilian, and Charles B. Hare. *Does Latent or Dormant Plague Exist Where the Disease Is Endemic?* Bureau of Government Laboratories Publication No. 20. Manila: Bureau of Printing, 1904.

Hill, Hibbert Winslow. *The New Public Health.* Minneapolis: Press of the Journal Lancet, 1913.

Hirsch, August. *Handbuch der Historisch-Geographischen Pathologie.* 2nd ed., 3 vols. London: New Sydenham Society, 1883.

Hoff, John van R. "Sanitary Organization in the United States Army." *TAMS* 6 (1896): 207–30.

———. "Scheme of Military Sanitary Organization." *JAMS* 7 (1897): 437–47.

Hoff, John van R. "Some Steps in the Organization and Instruction of the Medical Department of the Third Corps, U.S.V." *Proceedings 8th Annual Meeting of the Association of Military Surgeons of the U.S., Kansas City, 1899*, 106–38. Columbus, Ohio: Berlin Printing, 1900.

Howard, R. "Emotional Psychoses among Dark-skinned Races." *Trans. of the Society of Tropical Medicine and Hygiene* 3 (1910): 323–41.

Howard, William Lee. "The Negro as a Distinct Ethnic Factor in Civilization." *Medicine* 60 (1903): 418–28.

Hoyt, Henry F. *A Frontier Doctor*, edited by Doyce B. Nunis. Chicago: R. R. Donnelly and Sons, 1979 [1929].

——. "Observations upon and Reasons for a More Complete Physical Examination of Railway Employees." *Railway Surgeon* 4 (1895): 51–54.

——. "Appendix." In *Report of the Philippine Commission to the President*, 1:262–64. Washington D.C.: Government Printing Office, 1900.

Hoyt, R. E. "Results of Three Hundred Examinations of Feces with Reference to the Presence of Amoebae." *PJS* 3B (1908): 417–20.

Huggins, Eli L. "Custer and Rain-in-the-Face." *The American Mercury* 9 (1926): 338–43.

Huntington, Ellsworth. *Civilization and Climate*. New Haven: Yale University Press, 1915.

Jackson, Thomas W. "Sanitary Conditions and Needs in Provincial Towns." *PJS* 3B (1908): 431–38.

Jagor, Fedor. *Travels in the Philippines*. Manila: Filipiniana Books, 1965 [1873].

James, William. *The Varieties of Religious Experience*. Cambridge: Harvard University Press, 1985 [1901–02].

——. "Lectures Six and Seven: The Sick Soul." In *The Varieties of Religious Experience*, vol. 15 of *The Works of William James*, edited by Frederick H. Burkhardt, Fredson Bowers, and Ignas K. Skrupskelsis, 103–31. Cambridge: Harvard University Press, 1985 [1901–2].

——. "The Moral Equivalent of War." In *Essays on Faith and Morals*, 311–28. New York, 1943.

Jenks, Albert E. "Assimilation in the Philippines, as Interpreted in Terms of Assimilation in America." *American J. Sociology* 19 (1912): 773–91.

Joaquin, Nick. "Sa loob ng Manila." In *The Likhaan Anthology of Literature in English from 1900 to the Present*, edited by Gemino H. Abad, 445–60. Quezon City: University of the Philippines Press, 1998 [1988].

Joint Commission of Representatives from the College of Medicine and Surgery, University of the Philippines, the Bureau of Science, and the Bureau of Health. "Sanitary Survey of San José Estates and Adjacent Properties on Mindoro Island, P.I., with Special Reference to the Epidemiology of Malaria." *PJS* 9B (1914): 137–95.

Jordan, David Starr. *Imperial Democracy: A Study of the Relation of Government by the People, Equality Before the Law, and Other Tenets of Democracy, to the Demands of a Vigorous Foreign Policy and Other Demands of Imperial Dominion*. New York: D. Appleton, 1899.

Kafka, Franz. *The Metamorphosis, In the Penal Colony and Other Stories*. New York: Simon and Schuster, 1995.

Kemp, Franklin M. "Field Work in the Philippines." *JAMS* 9 (1900): 73–85.

Kidd, Benjamin. *The Control of the Tropics*. New York: Macmillan, 1898.

King, W. W. "Tropical Neurasthenia." *JAMA* 46 (1906): 1518–19.

Kipling, Rudyard. "The White Man's Burden." *McClure's Magazine* 12 (February 1899): 290–91.

Kulp, John S. "A Manila Military Hospital." *JAMS* 10 (1901–02): 225–38.

Lara, Casimiro B. *Leprosy Research in the Philippines: A Historical-Critical Review*. Manila: National Research Council, 1936.

Lemus, Rienzi B. "The Negro and the Philippines." *Colored American Magazine* 6 (1903): 314–18.

LeRoy, James A. *Philippine Life in Town and Country*. New York: G. P. Putnam's Sons, 1906.

———. *The Americans in the Philippines: A History of the Conquest and First Years of Occupation, with an Introductory Account of the Spanish Rule*. 2 vols. New York: AMS Press, 1970 [1914].

———. "The Philippines, 1860–1898 — Some Comment and Bibliographical Notes." In *The Philippines Islands 1493–1898*, edited by E. H. Blair and J. A. Robertson, 52:112–207. Cleveland: Arthur H. Clark, 1907.

Lévi-Strauss, Claude. *Tristes tropiques*. New York: Athenaeum, 1975 [1955].

Limjuco, Ignacia. "Hygiene in the Community." *Bulletin of the San Juan de Dios Hospital* 6 (1932): 21–25.

Lippincott, Henry. "Report of Lt.-Col. Henry Lippincott, Deputy Surgeon-general, U.S. Army, on the Condition of Medical Affairs in the Philippine Expeditionary Commands, Manila, August 31, 1898." In George M. Sternberg, *Report of the Surgeon-General of the Army to the Secretary of War*, 262–65. Washington, D.C.: Government Printing Office, 1898.

———. "Reminiscences of the Expedition to the Philippine Islands." *JAMS* 8 (1899): 168–74.

Long, J. D. "Health in the Philippine Islands." *Philippine Review* (January 1916): 49–51.

Lopes-Rizal, Leoncio. *Annual Report of the National Research Council of the Philippines*. Manila: Bureau of Printing, 1934–35.

Lovewell, C. H. "Malaria at Camp Stotsenberg, P.I." *Military Surgeon* 60 (1927): 688–700.

Lyautey, Hubert. "Du rôle social de l'officier." *Revue des deux mondes* 104 (March 11, 1891): 443–59.

———. "Du rôle coloniale de l'armée," *Revue des deux mondes* 157 (Feb. 15, 1900): 308–28.

Mackinnon, Grace. "Diseases of Women in the Tropics." In *The Practice of Medicine in the Tropics*, edited by W. Byam and R. G. Archibald, 3:2472–76. London: Henry Frowde and Hodder and Stoughton, 1923.

MacNamara, N. C. "Leprosy." In *Hygiene and Diseases of Warm Climates*, edited by Andrew Davidson, 426–52. Edinburgh: Pentland, 1893.

Manalang, C. "Malaria Transmission in the Philippines II." *PJS* 45 (1931): 367–81.

Manson, Patrick. *Tropical Diseases: A Manual of the Diseases of Warm Climates*. London: Cassell, 1898.

———. *Tropical Diseases: A Manual of the Diseases of Warm Climates*. 5th ed. London: Cassell, 1914.

Marshall, Thomas R. *Asiatic Cholera in the Philippines Islands*. Manila: Bureau of Public Printing, 1904.

Mason, Charles F. "Notes from the Experiences of a Medical Officer in the Tropics." *JAMS* 13 (1903): 306–14.

Maus, L. Mervin. "Report of Major L. M. Maus, Surgeon, U.S. Army, Chief Surgeon Second Division, Eighth Army Corps, to Chief Surgeon, Division of the Philippines, June 15, 1900." In George M. Sternberg, *Report of the Surgeon-General of the Army to the Secretary of War*, 116–29. Washington, D.C.: Government Printing Office, 1900.

———. "Venereal Diseases in the United States Army — Their Prevention and Treatment." *Military Surgeon* 27 (1910): 130–48.

———. "The Ethics, Scope, and Prerogative of the Army Medical Officer." *Military Surgeon* 28 (1911): 295–309.

Mayo, Katherine. *The Isles of Fear: The Truth about the Philippines*. New York: Harcourt Brace, 1924.

McLaughlin, Allan J. "The Suppression of a Cholera Epidemic in Manila." *PJS* 4B (1909): 43–58.

McLaughlin, Allan J., assisted by James A. Tobey. *Personal Hygiene: The Rules of Right Living*. New York: Funk and Wagnalls, 1924.

Meacham, Franklin A. "Report of Major Franklin A. Meacham, Chief Surgeon 3rd Military District of the Department of Northern Luzon, to Chief Surgeon Department of Northern Luzon, May 31, 1900." In George M. Sternberg, *Report of the Surgeon-General of the Army to the Secretary of War*, 137–42. Washington, D.C.: Government Printing Office, 1900.

Mearns, Lilian Hathaway. *A Philippine Romance*. New York: Aberdeen, 1910.

Miller, George Amos. *Interesting Manila*. Manila: E. C. McCullough, 1912.

Morris, Charles. *Our Island Empire: A Handbook of Cuba, Porto Rico, Hawaii and the Philippine Islands*. Philadelphia: Lippincott, 1899.

Moses, Bernard. "Control of Dependencies Inhabited by Less Developed Races." *University of California Chronicle* 7 (1905): 83–99.

Moses, Edith. *Unofficial Letters of an Official's Wife*. New York: D. Appleton, 1908.

Munson, Edward L. *The Theory and Practice of Military Hygiene*. London: Ballière, Tindall and Cox, 1902.

———. *The Principles of Sanitary Tactics: A Handbook on the Use of Medical Department Detachments and Organizations in Campaign*. Menasha, Wis.: Banta Publishing, 1911.

———. *The Management of Men: A Handbook on the Systematic Development of Morale and the Control of Human Behavior*. New York: Henry Holt, 1921.

———. "The Ideal Ration for an Army in the Tropics," *JAMS* 9 (1900): 298–333.

——. "The Civil Sanitary Function of the Army Medical Department in Territory under Military Control." *Military Surgeon* 25 (1909): 273–304.

——. "Cholera Carriers in Relation to Cholera Control." *PJS* 10B (1915): 1–9.

Musgrave, W. E. "Progress of Medicine in the Philippines." *Bulletin of the Manila Medical Society* 8 (1911): 122–26, 138–44.

——. "Tropical Neurasthenia, Tropical Hysteria and Some Special Tropical Hysteria-like Neuropsychoses." *Archives of Neurology and Psychiatry* 5 (1921): 398–407.

Musgrave, W. E., and A. G. Sison. "Blood Pressure in the Tropics: A Preliminary Report." *PJS* 5 (1910): 325–29.

——. "Mali-mali, a Mimic Psychosis in the Philippine Islands: A Preliminary Report." *PJS* 5 (1910): 335–39.

Notter, J. Lane. "On the Sanitary Methods of Dealing with Epidemics." *JMSI* 35 (1899): 111–24.

O'Reilly, G. A. "Manila's Grand Annual Carnival: The Great Unexpected Success of 1908 and the Splendid Spectacle Assured for 1909." *Colonial and Philippines Monthly Review* 2 (1908): 55–59.

Osler, William. "The Nation and the Tropics." *The Lancet* ii (Nov. 13, 1909): 1401–06.

Page, Henry. "Malaria and Mosquitoes at Lucena Barracks, Philippine Islands." *JMSI* 19 (1906): 65–76.

Palmer, G. G. "Notes on Luzon." *JMSI* 33 (1903): 223–30.

Pardo de Tavera, T. H. *El Legado del ignorantismo*. Manila: Bureau of Printing, 1921.

——. "Filipino Views of American rule." *North American Review* 174 (January 1902): 73–84.

Parker, James. "Some Random Notes on the Fighting in the Philippines." *JMSI* 27 (1900): 317–40.

Parsons, A. L. "Malaria Control at Camp Stotsenberg, P.I." *Military Surgeon* 63 (1928): 816–29.

Phalen, James M. "An Experiment with Orange-red Underwear." *PJS* 5 (1910): 525–46.

Phalen, James M., and H. J. Nichols. "Notes on the Distribution of *Filaria nocturna* in the Philippine Islands." *PJS* 3B (1908): 305–10.

Phelan, Henry du Rest. "Sanitary Service in Surigao, a Filipino Town on the Island of Mindanao." *JAMS* 14 (1904): 1–18.

Quezon, Manuel L. *The Good Fight*. New York: D. Appleton-Century, 1946.

Rattray, Alexander. "On Some of the More Important Physiological Changes Induced in the Human Economy by Change of Climate, as from Temperate to Tropical, and the Reverse." *Proceedings of the Royal Society of London* 18 (1869–70): 513–29; 19 (1870–71): 295–316.

Recto, Claro M. "Most Ignominious Surrender." In *Vintage Recto: Memorable Speeches and Writing*, edited by Renato Constantino, 13–24. Quezon City: Nationalist Studies, 1986 [1933].

——. "Our Mendicant Foreign Policy." In *Vintage Recto: Memorable Speeches and Writing*, edited by Renato Constantino, 63–83. Quezon City: Nationalist Studies, 1986 [1951].

——. "Our Lingering Colonial Complex." In *Vintage Recto: Memorable Speeches and*

Writing, edited by Renato Constantino, 84–94. Quezon City: Nationalist Studies, 1986 [1951].

Reed, Walter, Victor C. Vaughan, and E. O. Shakespeare. *Abstract of the Report of the Origin and Spread of Typhoid Fever in United States' Military Camps During the Spanish War of 1898*. Washington D.C.: War Department, 1900.

Rhodes, Charles D. "The Utilization of Foreign Troops in Our Foreign Possessions." *JMSI* 30 (1902): 1–26.

Rizal, José. *Noli Me Tangere*. Translated by Priscilla G. Valencia. Manila: National Book Store, 1967 [1887].

——. *El Filibusterismo*. Translated by Jovita Ventura Cruz. Manila: Asean Committee on Culture and Information, 1991 [1891].

Roosevelt, Nicholas. *The Philippines: A Treasure and a Problem*. New York: J. H. Sears, 1926.

Roosevelt, Theodore. *The Strenuous Life*. New York: Century, 1901.

——. *A Book Lover's Holidays in the Open*. New York: Scribner's, 1919.

——. "At Arlington, Memorial Day, May 30, 1902." In *Presidential Addresses and State Papers*, 1:56–67. New York: Review of Reviews, 1904 .

——. "At the Banquet Tendered for Gen. Luke E. Wright, at Memphis, Tennessee, Nov. 19, 1902." In *Presidential Addresses and State Papers*, 1:202–08. New York: Review of Reviews, 1904 .

——. "Message of the President of the U.S., Communicated to the Two Houses of Congress at the Beginning of the First Session of the 57th Congress." In *Presidential Addresses and State Papers*, 1:529–606. New York: Review of Reviews, 1904 [1901].

——. "At the Coliseum, Hartford, Conn., Aug. 22, 1902." In *Presidential Addresses and State Papers*, 2:85–98. New York: Review of Reviews, 1904.

——. "Message of the President of the US, Communicated to the Two Houses of Congress at the Beginning of the Second Session of the 57th Congress." In *Presidential Addresses and State Papers*, 2:606–45. New York: Review of Reviews, 1904 [1902].

Root, Elihu. "Report for 1902." In *Annual Reports of the Secretary of War to the President of the United States, 1898–1903*, 245–323. Washington, D.C.: Government Printing Office, 1904.

Rose, Wickliffe. "Field Experiments in Malaria Control." *JAMA* 73 (1919): 1414–20.

Ross, Ronald. *The Prevention of Malaria*. New York: Dutton, 1910.

——. *Memoirs, with a Full Account of the Great Malaria Problem and Its Solution*. London: John Murray, 1923.

——. *Studies on Malaria*. London: John Murray, 1928.

Russell, Frederick F. *The Results of Anti-Typhoid Vaccination in the Army in 1911, and Its Suitability for Use in Civil Communities*. Chicago: American Medical Association, 1912.

——. "War on Disease, Particularly Yellow Fever and Malaria." *Sigma Xi Quarterly* 13 (1925): 11–32.

Russell, Paul F. *Malaria and Culicidae in the Philippine Islands: History and Critical Bibliography*. Manila: Bureau of Printing, 1934.

——. *Man's Mastery of Malaria*. London: Oxford University Press, 1955.

——. "Malaria in the Philippine Islands." *American J. Tropical Medicine* 12 (1933): 167–78.

——. "Malaria in India: Impressions from a Tour." *American J. Tropical Medicine* 16 (1936): 653–64.

Russell, Paul F., and Fred W Knipe. "Malaria Control by Spray-killing Adult Mosquitoes." *J. of the Malaria Institute of India* 2 (1939): 229–37.

Russell, Paul F., L. S. West, and R. D. Manwell. *Practical Malariology*. Philadelphia: W. B. Saunders, 1946.

Sambon, Luigi W. "Remarks on Acclimatisation in Tropical Regions." *British Medical J.* 1 (1897): 61–66.

Scarborough, W. S. "The Negro and Our New Possessions." *Forum* 34 (1901): 341–49.

Schöbl, Otto. "Observations Concerning Cholera Carriers." *PJS* 10B (1915): 11–17.

Schurz, Carl. *For American Principles and American Honor*. New York: Anti-Imperialist League, 1900.

Seale, A. "The Mosquito Fish, *Gambusia affinus* in the Philippine Islands." *PJS* 12 (1917): 177–89.

Seaman, Louis L. "Observations in China and the Tropics" *JAMS* 10 (1901–02): 149–50.

——. "Native Troops for Our Colonial Possessions." *JAMS* 10 (1901–02): 240.

Sellards, Andrew Watson. "Bonds of Union between Tropical Medicine and General Medicine." *Science* 66ns (1927): 93–100.

Shaklee, Alfred O. "Experimental Acclimatization to the Tropical Sun." *PJS* 12 (1917): 1–22.

Shaler, Nathaniel S. "The Transplantation of a Race." *Popular Science Monthly* 56 (March 1900): 513–24.

——. "The Future of the Negro in the Southern States." *Popular Science Monthly* 57 (June 1900): 145–54.

Simmons, J. S., J. H. St. John, and F. H. K Reynolds. "Malaria Survey at Camp Stotsenberg, P.I." *Military Surgeon* 67 (1930): 1–13.

Sison, Agerico B. M. "Educating Our Educators." *Bulletin of the San Juan de Dios Hospital* 1 (1927): 123–24.

Smart, Charles. "Medical Department of the Army." *TAMS* 3 (1893): 193–203.

——. "Transport of the Wounded in War." *TAMS* 4 (1894): 22–45.

Smith, Goldwin. *Commonwealth or Empire: A Bystander's View of the Question*. London: Macmillan, 1902.

Snodgrass, John E. *Leprosy in the Philippine Islands*. Manila: Bureau of Printing, 1915.

Soper, Fred L., and D. B. Wilson. *Anopheles gambiae in Brazil, 1930–1940*. New York: Rockefeller Foundation, 1943.

Stein, Stanley, with Lawrence Blochman. *Alone No Longer*. New York: Funk and Wagnalls, 1963.

Stelle, Matthew F. "Some Notes on the Clothing and Equipment of the Soldier for Service in the Tropics." *JMSI* 29 (1901): 14–23.

Sternberg, George M. *Report of the Surgeon-General of the Army to the Secretary of*

War, *For the Fiscal Year Ended June 30, 1898.* Washington D.C.: Government Printing Office, 1898.

Sternberg, George M. *Report of the Surgeon-General of the Army to the Secretary of War, For the Fiscal Year Ended June 30, 1900.* Washington D.C.: Government Printing Office, 1900.

——. *Infection and Immunity, with Special Reference to the Prevention of Infectious Disease.* New York: G. P. Putnam's Sons, 1903.

——. "A Fatal Form of Septacemia in the Rabbit Produced by Subcutaneous Injection of Human Saliva." *National Board of Health Bulletin* 2 (1881): 781–83.

——. "Presidential Address." *TAMS* 5 (1895): 8–22.

Sterne, Albert E. "Neurasthenia and Its Treatment by Actinic Rays." *JAMA* 42 (1904): 500–507.

Stillman, James W. *Republic or Empire? An Argument in Opposition to the Establishment of an American Colonial System.* Boston: George H. Ellis, 1900.

Stitt, E. R. *The Diagnostics and Treatment of Tropical Diseases.* Philadelphia: Blakiston, 1914.

——. *The Diagnostics and Treatment of Tropical Diseases.* 5th ed. Philadelphia: Blakiston, 1922.

——. "A Study of the Intestinal Parasites Found in Cavite Province." *PJS* 6B (1911): 211–14.

Stone, Hamilton. "Our Troops in the Tropics — From the Surgeon's Standpoint." *JMSI* 26 (1900): 358–69.

Strong, Richard P. "Leprosy." In *Forchheimer's Therapeusis of Internal Diseases,* edited by Frank Billings and Ernest E. Irons, 387–400. New York and London: D. Appleton, 1914.

——. "The Importance of Ecology in Relation to Disease." *Science* 82ns (1935): 307–17.

Strong, Richard P., et al. "Medical Survey of the Town of Taytay." *PJS* 4B (1909): 247–52.

Suarez Caopalleja, Victor. *Le salud del europeo en América y Filipinas y del repatriado y criollo en Europa.* Madrid: Gabriel Pedraza, 1897.

Taft, Helen. *Recollections of Full Years.* New York: Dodd, Mead, 1914.

Taft, William H. *Special Report of W. H. Taft to the President on the Philippine Islands.* Washington, D.C.: Government Publications Office, 1908.

——. "The Work of the United States in the Philippines." In *William Howard Taft, the Man of the Hour: His Biography and His Views on the Great Questions of the Day,* edited by Oscar King Davis, 229–65. Philadelphia: P. W. Ziegler, 1908 [1907].

——. "Progress of the Negro." In *William Howard Taft, the Man of the Hour: His Biography and His Views on the Great Questions of the Day,* edited by Oscar King Davis, 319–28. Philadelphia: P. W. Ziegler, 1908.

——. "Address of President Taft at the 15th International Congress on Hygiene and Demography." *Science* 36ns (October 18, 1912): 504–08.

Taylor, Frederick Winslow. *Principles of Scientific Management.* New York: Harper, 1911.

Terry, C. E. "The Negro, a Public Health Problem." *Southern Medical J.* 7 (1915): 458–67.

Thompson, Joseph C. " 'Tropical Neurasthenia': A Deprivation Psychoneurosis." *Military Surgeon* 54 (1924): 319–24.

Tianco, Mamero, under direction of J. D. Long. *Philippine Health Service Sanitary Almanac for 1919 and Calendars for 1920 and 1921.* Health Bulletin No. 19. Manila: Bureau of Printing, 1918.

Tiedemann, W. D. "Malaria in the Philippines." *J. Preventive Medicine* 1 (1927): 205–54.

Traub, P. E. "Military Hygiene: How Best to Enforce Its Study." *JMSI* 36 (1905): 1–38.

Tucker, E. F. Gordon. "Neurasthenia in Anglo-Indians." *Indian Medical Gazette* 38 (1903): 43–49.

Turner, Frederick Jackson. "The Significance of the Frontier in American History." In *The Frontier in American History*, 1–38. Huntington N.Y.: Robert E. Krieger, 1976 [1893]).

Twain, Mark [Samuel Clemens]. "To the Person Sitting in Darkness." *North American Review* 172 (February 1901): 161–76.

Vaughan, Victor C. *Infection and Immunity.* Chicago: AMA, 1915.

——. "Typhoid Fever among the American Soldiers in the Recent War with Spain." *JMSI* 35 (1899): 85–88.

Vedder, Edward B. *Beriberi.* New York: W. Wood, 1913.

——. "Report on the Seventh Congress of the Far Eastern Association of Tropical Medicine." *Military Surgeon* 62 (1928): 275–82.

Wade, H. W., and José Avellana Basa. "The Culion Leper Colony." *American J. of Tropical Medicine* 3 (1923): 395–417.

Walker, E. L., and A. W. Sellards. "Experimental Entamoebic Dysentery." *PJS* 8B (1913): 253–329.

Walker E. L., and M. A. Barber "Malaria in the Philippine Islands I." *PJS* 9 (1914): 381–439.

Washburn, W. S. "The Relation between Climate and Health, with Special Reference to American Occupation of the Philippine Islands." *American J. of the Medical Sciences* 130 (1905): 497–517.

——. "Health Conditions in the Philippines." *PJS* 3B (1908): 269–84.

Watkins, V. E. "Neurasthenia among Blondes in the Southwest." *New York Medical J.* 82 (1905): 1373–74.

Watson, Malcolm. *The Prevention of Malaria in the Federated Malay States.* 2nd ed. London: John Murray, 1921.

Willets, D. G. "A Statistical Study of Intestinal Parasites in Tobacco Haciendas of the Cagayan Valley." *PJS* 6B (1911): 77–92.

Williams, Daniel R. *The United States and the Philippines.* New York: Doubleday, 1924.

Wilson, R. M. "Industrial Therapy in Leprosy." *Southern Medical J.* 23 (March 1930): 218–22.

Wilson, Woodrow. *Constitutional Government in the United States*. New York: Columbia University Press, 1921.

Winslow, Charles-Edward Amory. "Man and the Microbe." *Popular Science Monthly* 85 (1914): 5–20.

Wood, Leonard. *Report of the Governor-General of the Philippines, 1925*. Washington D.C.: Government Printing Office, 1926.

——. "Progress Fighting Leprosy at Culion: Better Facilities Might Open the Way to Complete Victory." *The World's Work* (Dec. 1925): 144–47.

Woodhull, Alfred A. *Notes on Military Hygiene for Officers of the Line: A Syllabus of Lectures at the United States Infantry and Cavalry School*. New York: Wiley, 1904 [1890].

Woodruff, Charles E. *The Effects of Tropical Sunlight Upon the White Man*. New York: Rebman, 1905.

——. *Expansion of Races*. New York: Rebman, 1909.

——. "Military Medical Problems." *TAMS* 3 (1893): 220–38.

——. "The Military Uses of Bacteriology." *JMSI* 35 (1899): 178–202.

——. "Hygiene in the Tropics." *JMSI* 35 (1899): 296–99.

——. "The Neurasthenic States Caused by Excessive Light." *Medical Record* 68 (Dec. 23, 1905): 1005–09.

Woodward, C. M. "The Sanitation of Camps." *TAMS* 2 (1892): 138–46.

Woodward, Joseph Janvier. *Outlines of the Chief Camp Diseases of the United States' Armies as Observed During the Present War*. Philadelphia: J. B. Lippincott, 1863.

Worcester, Dean C. *History of Asiatic Cholera in the Philippine Islands*. Manila: Bureau of Printing, 1908.

——. *The Philippines, Past and Present*. 2 vols. New York: Macmillan, 1930 [1914].

Wu, T. C. "Fighting Leprosy in the Philippines." *Leper Quarterly* 4 (1930): 3–14.

Zinsser, Hans. *Infection and Resistance: An Exposition of the Biological Phenomena Underlying the Occurrence of Infection and the Recovery of the Animal Body from Infectious Disease*. 2nd ed. New York: Macmillan, 1922.

SECONDARY SOURCES

Abel, Emily K. " 'Only the Best Class of Immigration': Public Health Policy toward Mexicans and Filipinos in Los Angeles, 1910–1940." *American J. Public Health*. 94 (2004): 932–39.

——. "From Exclusion to Expulsion: Mexicans and Tuberculosis Control in Los Angeles, 1914–1940." *Bulletin of the History of Medicine* 77 (2003): 823–49.

Ackerknecht, Erwin. *History and Geography of the Most Important Diseases*. New York: Hafner, 1965.

Adas, Michael. *Machines as the Measure of Men: Science, Technology, and Ideologies of Western Dominance*. Ithaca: Cornell University Press, 1989.

——. "Improving on the Civilizing Mission? Assumptions of U.S. Exceptionalism in the Colonization of the Philippines." *Itinerario* 22 (1998): 44–66.

Adelman, Jeremy, and Stephen Aron. "From Borderlands to Borders: Empires, Nation-states and Peoples in between in North American History." *American Historical Review* 104 (1999): 814–41.

Agamben, Giorgio. *Homo Sacer: Sovereign Power and Bare Life.* Translated by Daniel Heller-Roazen. Stanford: Stanford University Press, 1998.

Agoncillo, Teodoro A. *The Revolt of the Masses: The Story of Bonifacio and the Katipunan.* Manila: University of the Philippines Press, 1956.

Agoncillo, Teodoro A., and O. M. Alfonso. *Short History of the Philippine People.* Manila: University of the Philippines Press, 1963.

Alatas, Syed Hussein. *The Myth of the Lazy Native: A Study of the Image of Malays, Filipinos and Javanese from the 16th to the 20th Century and Its Function in the Ideology of Colonial Capitalism.* London: F. Cass, 1977.

Alfonso, Oscar M. *Theodore Roosevelt and the Philippines, 1897–1909.* Quezon City: University of the Philippines Press, 1970.

Allen, Charles E. "World Health and World Politics." *International Organization* 4 (1950): 27–43.

Anderson, Benedict. *Imagined Communities: Reflections on the Origins and Spread of Nationalism.* Revised ed. London: Verso, 1991.

——. *The Spectre of Comparisons: Nationalism, Southeast Asia and the World.* London: Verso, 1998.

Anderson, Warwick. "Colonial Pathologies: American Medicine in the Philippines, 1898–1921." Ph.D. diss., University of Pennsylvania, 1992.

——. "Excremental Colonialism: Public Health and the Poetics of Pollution." *Critical Inquiry* 21 (1995): 640–69.

——. "Immunities of Empire: Race, Disease, and the New Tropical Medicine." *Bulletin of the History of Medicine* 70 (1996): 94–118.

——. "The Trespass Speaks: White Masculinity and Colonial Breakdown." *American Historical Review* 102 (1997): 1343–70.

——. "Leprosy and Citizenship." *Positions: East Asia Cultures Critique* 6 (1998): 707–30.

——. "Victor G. Heiser." In *American National Biography*, edited by John A. Garraty and Mark C. Carnes, 10:522–24. New York: Oxford University Press, 1999.

——. "Richard Pearson Strong." In *American National Biography*, edited by John A. Garraty and Mark C. Carnes, 21:46–48. New York: Oxford University Press, 1999.

——. "The 'Third-World' Body." In *Medicine in the Twentieth Century*, edited by Roger Cooter and John Pickstone, 235–46. Amsterdam: Harwood Academic, 2000.

——. "Going through the Motions: American Hygiene and Colonial 'Mimicry.'" *American Literary History* 14 (2002): 686–719.

——. *The Cultivation of Whiteness: Science, Health and Racial Destiny in Australia.* New York: Basic Books, 2003.

——. "The Natures of Culture: Environment and Race in the Colonial Tropics." In *Nature in the Global South: Environmental Projects in South and Southeast Asia*, edited by Paul Greenough and Anna L. Tsing, 29–46. Durham, N.C.: Duke University Press, 2003.

Anderson, Warwick. "Natural Histories of Infectious Disease: Ecological Vision in Twentieth-century Biomedical Science." *Osiris* 19 (2004): 39–61.

——. "Postcolonial Histories of Medicine." In *Locating Medical History: The Stories and Their Meanings*, edited by Frank Huisman and John Harley Warner, 285–307. Baltimore: Johns Hopkins University Press, 2004.

——. "States of Hygiene: Race 'Improvement' and Biomedical Citizenship in Australia and the Colonial Philippines." In *Haunted by Empire: Geographies of Intimacy in North American History*, edited by Ann Laura Stoler. Durham, N.C.: Duke University Press, 2006.

——. "Science in the Philippines." In *Cambridge History of Science*, edited by Ronald L. Numbers and David Lindberg, vol. 8: *National Sciences*, edited by Ronald Numbers and David Livingstone. Cambridge: Cambridge University Press, forthcoming.

Appleby, Joyce. *Liberalism and Republicanism in the Historical Imagination*. Cambridge: Harvard University Press, 1992.

Aretxaga, Begoña. "Dirty Protest: Symbolic Overdetermination and Gender in Northern Ireland Ethnic Violence." *Ethnos* 23 (1995): 123–48.

Arnold, David. *Colonizing the Body: State Medicine and Epidemic Disease in Nineteenth-Century India*. Berkeley: University of California Press, 1993.

——. "Introduction: Disease, Medicine and Empire." In *Imperial Medicine and Indigenous Society*, edited by David Arnold, 1–26. Manchester: Manchester University Press, 1989.

——. " 'An Ancient Race Outworn': Malaria and Race in Colonial India, 1860–1930." In *Race, Science and Medicine, 1700–1960*, edited by Waltraud Ernst and Bernard Harris, 123–43. London: Routledge, 1999.

Ashburn, Percy M. *A History of the Medical Department of the United States Army*. Boston: Houghton Mifflin, 1929.

[Ashburn, Percy M.] "A Synopsis of the Work of the Army Medical Research Boards in the Philippines." *Army Medical Bulletin* (1929): 2–179.

Azicate, Enrico. "Medicine in the Philippines: An Historical Perspective." M.A. thesis, University of the Philippines, 1989.

Bakhtin, Mikhail M. *Rabelais and His World*. Translated by Helène Iswolsky. Bloomington: Indiana University Press, 1984 [1964].

Bankoff, Greg. "A Question of Breeding: Zootechny and Colonial Attitudes toward the Tropical Environment in the Late Nineteenth-century Philippines." *J. of Asian Studies* 60 (2001): 413–37.

Bantug, J. P. *A Short History of Medicine in the Philippines under the Spanish Regime, 1565–1898*. Manila: Colegio Médico-farmacéutico de Filipinas, 1953.

——. "Rizal and the Progress of the Natural Sciences." *Philippine Studies* 9 (1961): 3–16.

Barrett, Frank A. *Disease and Geography: The History of an Idea*. Toronto: Geography Department, York University, 2000.

Bauman, Zygmunt. *Modernity and Ambivalence*. Cambridge: Polity Press, 1991.

Bederman, Gail. *Manliness and Civilization: A Cultural History of Gender and Race in the United States, 1880–1917*. Chicago: University of Chicago Press, 1995.

Beisner, Robert L. *Twelve Against Empire: The Anti-Imperialists, 1898–1900*. New York: McGraw Hill, 1968.

Benjamin, Walter. "On the Mimetic Faculty." In *Reflections*, edited by Peter Demetz, translated by E. Jephcott, 333–36. New York: Harcourt Brace Jovanovich, 1979.

Berkhofer, Robert F., Jr. *The White Man's Indian: Images of the American Indian from Columbus to the Present*. New York: Alfred A. Knopf, 1978.

Bhabha, Homi. *The Location of Culture*. London: Routledge, 1994.

——. "Of Mimicry and Man: The Ambivalence of Colonial Discourse." *October* 28 (1984): 125–33.

——. "Remembering Fanon." Foreword to Frantz Fanon, *Black Skin, White Masks*, vii–xxvi. London: Pluto Press, 1986.

Bickel, Keith B. *Mars Learning: The Marine Corps Development of Small Wars Doctrine, 1915–1940*. New York: Westview Press, 2001.

Biehl, João. "Other Life: AIDS, Brazil, and Subjectivity in Brazil's Zones of Social Abandonment." PH.D. diss., University of California-Berkeley, 1999.

Birn, Anne-Emanuelle. "A Revolution in Rural Health? The Struggle over Local Health Units in Mexico, 1928–1940." *J. of History of Medicine and Allied Sciences* 53 (1998): 43–76.

——. "Revolution, the Scatological Way: The Rockefeller Foundation's Hookworm Campaign in 1920s Mexico." In *Disease in the History of Modern Latin America: From Malaria to AIDS*, edited by Diego Armus, 158–82. Durham, N.C.: Duke University Press, 2003.

Birn, Anne-Emanuelle, and Armando Solorzano. "Public Health Policy Paradoxes: Science and Politics in the Rockefeller Foundation's Hookworm Campaign in Mexico in the 1920s." *Social Science and Medicine* 49 (1999): 1197–1213.

Birtle, Andrew J. "The U.S. Army's Pacification of Marinduque, Philippine Islands, April 1900–April 1901." *J. of Military History* 61 (1997): 255–82.

Bourdieu, Pierre. *Outline of a Theory of Practice*. Translated by Richard Nice. Cambridge: Cambridge University Press, 1977.

Bradley, D. J. "The Particular and the General: Issues of Specificity and Verticality in the History of Malaria Control." *Parassitologia* 40 (1998): 5–10.

Braeman, John. *Albert J. Beveridge, American Nationalist*. Chicago: University of Chicago Press, 1971.

Brieger, Gert H. "Fielding H. Garrison: The Man and His Book." *Trans. and Studies of the College of Physicians of Philadelphia* 3 (1981): 1–21.

Briggs, Charles L., and Clara Mantini-Briggs. *Stories in a Time of Cholera: Racial Profiling During a Medical Nightmare*. Berkeley: University of California Press, 2003.

Briggs, Laura. *Reproducing Empire: Race, Sex, Science, and U.S. Imperialism in Puerto Rico*. Berkeley: University of California Press, 2002.

Brown, Jo Anne. "Purity and Danger in Color: Notes on Germ Theory, and the Semantics of Segregation." In *Heredity and Infection: The History of Disease Transmission*, edited by J. P. Gaudillière and Ilana Löwy, 101–31. London: Routledge, 2001.

Brown, Norman O. "The Excremental Vision." In *Life Against Death: The*

Psychoanalytic Meaning of History. 2nd ed., 179–201. Middletown, Conn.: Wesleyan University Press, 1985 [1959].

Brugger, Bill. *Republican Theory in Political Thought: Virtuous or Virtual?* New York: St. Martin's Press, 1999.

Buckingham, Jane. *Leprosy in Colonial South India*. Basingstoke: Palgrave, 2002.

Burkitt, Ian. "Civilization and Ambivalence." *British J. of Sociology* 47 (1996): 135–50.

Burnet, F. Macfarlane. *Biological Aspects of Infectious Disease*. Cambridge: Cambridge University Press, 1940.

Bynum, W. F. "An Experiment that Failed: Malaria Control at Mian Mir." *Parassitologia* 36 (1994): 107–20.

———. "Malaria in Inter-war British India." *Parassitologia* 42 (2000): 25–31.

Bynum, W. F., and Caroline Overy, eds. *The Beast in the Mosquito: The Correspondence of Ronald Ross and Patrick Manson*. Amsterdam: Rodopi, 1998.

Callaway, Helen. *Gender, Culture and Empire: European Women in Colonial Nigeria*. Urbana: University of Illinois Press, 1987.

Cannell, Fenella. *Power and Intimacy in the Christian Philippines*. Cambridge: Cambridge University Press, 1999.

Carter, Richard, and Kamini N. Mendis. "Evolutionary and Historical Aspects of the Burden of Malaria." *Clinical Microbiology Reviews* 15 (2002): 564–94.

Cassedy, James H. *Charles V. Chapin and the Public Health Movement*. Cambridge: Harvard University Press, 1962.

———. "The 'Germ of Laziness' in the South, 1901–1915: Charles Wardell Stiles and the Progressive Paradox." *Bulletin of the History of Medicine* 45 (1971): 161.

Cell, John W. "Anglo-Indian Medical Theory and the Origins of Segregation in West Africa." *American Historical Review* 91 (1986): 307–35.

Chakrabarty, Dipesh. *Provincializing Europe: Postcolonial Thought and Historical Difference*. Princeton: Princeton University Press, 2000.

———. "Of Garbage, Modernity and the Citizen's Gaze." *Economic and Political Weekly* (March 7–14, 1992): 541–47.

Chapman, Carleton B. *Order Out of Chaos: John Shaw Billings and America's Coming of Age*. Boston: Boston Medical Library, 1994.

Chapman, Ronald Fettes. *Leonard Wood and Leprosy in the Philippines: The Culion Leper Colony 1921–27*. N.p.: University Press of America, 1982.

Chatterjee, Partha. *The Nation and Its Fragments: Colonial and Postcolonial Histories*. Princeton: Princeton University Press, 1993.

Chaudhuri, Nupur, and Margaret Strobel, eds. *Western Women and Imperialism: Complicity and Resistance*. Bloomington: Indiana University Press, 1992.

Chernin, Eli. "Richard Pearson Strong and the Iatrogenic Plague Disaster in Bilibid Prison, Manila, 1906." *Reviews of Infectious Diseases* 11 (1989): 996–1004.

———. "Richard Pearson Strong and Manchurian Epidemic of Bubonic Plague, 1910–11." *J. of History of Medicine and Allied Sciences* 44 (1989): 296–319.

Choy, Catherine Ceniza. *Empire of Care: Nursing and Migration in Filipino-American History*. Durham, N.C.: Duke University Press, 2003.

Cirillo, Vincent J. *Bullets and Bacilli: The Spanish-American War and Military Medicine*. New Brunswick, N.J.: Rutgers University Press, 2004.

Cohen, Nancy. *The Reconstruction of American Liberalism, 1865–1914*. Chapel Hill: University of North Carolina Press, 2002.

Cohen, Nathaniel A. "Public Health in the Philippines." *Far Eastern Survey* 15 (1946): 87–90.

Coleman, William. "Science and Symbol in the Turner Frontier Hypothesis." *American Historical Review* 72 (1966): 22–49.

Collini, Stefan. "The Idea of 'Character' in Victorian Political Thought." *Trans. of the Royal Historical Society* 35 (1985): 29–50.

Comaroff, John, and Jean Comaroff. *Ethnography and the Historical Imagination*. Boulder: Westview, 1992.

Conklin, Alice L. *A Mission to Civilize: The Republican Idea of Empire in France and West Africa, 1895–1930*. Stanford: Stanford University Press, 1997.

Cooper, Frederick. "Modernizing Bureaucrats, Backward Africans, and the Development Concept." In *International Development and the Social Sciences: Essays on the History and Politics of Knowledge*, edited by Frederick Cooper and Randall Packard, 64–92. Berkeley: University of California Press, 1997.

———. "Modernizing Colonialism and the Limits of Empire." *Items* 4 (2003): 1–9.

Cooper, Frederick, and Randall Packard, ed. *International Development and the Social Sciences: Essays on the History and Politics of Knowledge*. Berkeley: University of California Press, 1997.

Cooter, Roger. *Surgery and Society in Peace and War: Orthopaedics and the Organization of Modern Medicine, 1880–1948*. Manchester: Manchester University Press, 1993.

Corbellini, G. "Acquired Immunity against Malaria as a Tool for the Control of the Disease: The Strategy Proposed by the Malaria Commission of the League of Nations Health Organization in 1933." *Parassitologia* 40 (1998): 109–16.

Corbin, Alain. *The Foul and the Fragrant: Odor and the French Social Imagination*. Translated by Miriam L. Kochan, Roy Porter, and Christopher Prendergast. Cambridge: Harvard University Press, 1986.

Cosmas, Graham A. *An Army for Empire: The United States Army in the Spanish-American War*. St. Louis: University of Missouri Press, 1971.

Craddock, Susan. *City of Plagues: Disease, Poverty and Deviance in San Francisco*. Minneapolis: University of Minnesota Press, 2000.

Craig, Charles F. "The Army Medical Service." *Yale Medical J.* 16 (1910): 415–27.

Cruz, Romeo Victorino. *America's Colonial Desk and the Philippines 1898–1934*. Quezon City: University of the Philippines Press, 1974.

Cueto, Marcos, ed. *Missionaries of Science: The Rockefeller Foundation and Latin America*. Bloomington: Indiana University Press, 1994.

———. "Tropical Medicine and Bacteriology in Boston and Peru: Studies of Carrión's Disease in the Early Twentieth Century." *Medical History* 40 (1996): 344–64.

———. "The Origins of Primary Health Care and Selective Primary Health Care." *American J. Public Health* 94 (2004): 1864–74.

Cullinane, Michael. "Ilustrado Politics: The Response of the Filipino Educated Elite to American Colonial Rule, 1898–1907." ph.d. diss., University of Michigan, 1989.

Cunningham, Andrew, and Perry Williams, eds. *The Laboratory Revolution in Medicine*. Cambridge: Cambridge University Press, 1992.

Curtin, Philip D. *Death by Migration: Europe's Encounter with the Tropical World in the Nineteenth Century*. Cambridge: Cambridge University Press, 1989.

———. "Medical Knowledge and Urban Planning in Tropical Africa." *American Historical Review* 90 (1985): 594–613.

Cushner, Nicolas. *Spain in the Philippines*. Quezon City: Ateneo de Manila University Press, 1974.

Darwin, John. "What Was the Late-Colonial State?" *Itinerario* 23 (1999): 73–82.

Dayrit, Conrado S., Perla Dizon Santos Ocampo, and Eduardo R. de la Cruz. *History of Philippine Medicine, 1899–1999*. Pasig City: Anvil, 2002.

Deacon, Harriet Jane. "A History of the Medical Institutions on Robben Island, Cape Colony, 1846–1910." PH.D. diss., University of Cambridge, 1994.

Dean, Mitchell, *Governmentality: Power and Rule in Modern Society*. London: Sage, 1999.

De Bevoise, Ken. "The Compromised Host: The Epidemiological Context of the Philippine-American War." PH.D. diss., University of Oregon, 1986.

———. *Agents of Apocalypse: Epidemic Disease in the Colonial Philippines*. Princeton: Princeton University Press, 1995.

De Certeau, Michel. *Heterologies: Discourse on the Other*. Translated by Brian Massumi. Minneapolis: University of Minnesota Press, 1986.

De la Cruz, Eduardo R. *History of Philippine Medicine and the* PMA. Manila: PMA, 1983.

Delaporte, François. *The History of Yellow Fever: An Essay on the Birth of Tropical Medicine*. Cambridge: MIT Press, 1991.

Dery, Luis. "Prostitution in Colonial Manila." *Philippine Studies* 39 (1991): 475–89.

Desmond, Jane C., and Virginia R. Domínguez. "Resituating American Studies in a Critical Internationalism." *American Quarterly* 48 (1996): 475–90.

Deutschman, Zygmunt. "Public Health and Medical Services in the Philippines." *Far Eastern Q*. 4 (1945): 148–57.

Deverell, William. "Plague in Los Angeles, 1924: Ethnicity and Typicality." In *Over the Edge: Remapping the American West*, edited by Valerie J. Matsumoto and Blake Allmendinger, 172–200. Berkeley: University of California Press, 1999.

Dirks, Nicholas B., ed., *Colonialism and Culture*. Ann Arbor: University of Michigan Press, 1992.

Dobson, M. J., M. Malowany, and R. W. Snow. "Malaria Control in East Africa: The Kampala Conference and the Pare-Taveta Scheme: A Meeting of Common and High Ground." *Parassitologia* 42 (2000): 149–66.

Doeppers, Daniel F. *Manila, 1900–1941: Social Change in a Late-Colonial Metropolis*. New Haven: Yale University Southeast Asian Studies, 1984.

Douglas, Mary. *Purity and Danger: An Analysis of the Concepts of Pollution and Taboo*. London: Routledge and K. Paul, 1966.

———. "Witchcraft and Leprosy: Two Strategies of Exclusion." *Man* 264 (1991): 723–36.

Drinnan, Richard. *Facing West: The Metaphysics of Indian-Hating and Empire-Building*. Minneapolis: University of Minnesota Press, 1980.

Duffy, John. *A History of Public Health in New York City*. 2 vols. New York: Russell Sage, Foundation, 1968.

———. *The Sanitarians: A History of American Public Health*. Urbana: University of Illinois Press, 1990.

Dumett, Raymond E. "The Campaign against Malaria and the Expansion of Scientific Medical and Sanitary Services in British West Africa, 1898–1910." *African Historical Studies* 1 (1968): 153–97.

Dyer, Thomas. *Theodore Roosevelt and the Idea of Race*. Baton Rouge: Louisiana State University Press, 1980.

Edmond, Rod. "Abject Bodies/Abject Sites: Leper Islands in the High Imperial Era." In *Islands in History and Representation*, edited by Rod Edmond and Vanessa Smith, 133–45. London: Routledge, 2003.

Ee, Heok Kua. "Amok in Nineteenth-century British Malaya History." *History of Psychiatry* 3 (1991): 429–36.

Elias, Norbert. *The Civilizing Process*. Translated by E. Jephcott. New York: Pantheon, 1978 [1939].

Ernst, Waltraud. *Mad Tales from the Raj: The European Insane in British India, 1800–1858*. London: Routledge, 1991.

———. "European Madness and Gender in Nineteenth-century British India." *Social History of Medicine* 9 (1996): 357–82.

Eschscholtzia, L. Lucia, and Laura S. Haymond. *An Analysis of Certain Causes of Mortality in the Philippine Islands with Reference to Changes in Administrative Policy*. University of California Publications in Public Health No. 1. Glendale, Calif.: Arthur H. Clark, 1928.

Escobar, Arturo. *Encountering Development: The Making and Unmaking of the Third World*. Princeton: Princeton University Press, 1995.

Esty, Joshua D. "Excremental Postcolonialism." *Contemporary Literature* 40 (1999): 22–59.

Etherington, Norman. *Theories of Imperialism: War, Conquest and Capital*. London: Croom Helm, 1984.

Ettling, John. *The Germ of Laziness: Rockefeller Philanthropy and Public Health in the New South*. Cambridge: Harvard University Press, 1981.

Evans, Hughes. "European Malaria Policy in the 1920s and 1930s: The Epidemiology of Minutiae." *Isis* 80 (1989): 40–59.

Fairchild, Amy L. *Science at the Borders: Immigrant Medical Inspection and the Shaping of the Modern Industrial Labor Force*. Baltimore: Johns Hopkins University Press, 2003.

Fanon, Frantz. *Black Skin, White Masks*. Translated by Charles Lam Markmann. New York: Grove Press, 1967.

Farley, John. *Bilharzia: A History of Imperial Tropical Medicine*. Cambridge: Cambridge University Press, 1991.

———. *To Cast Out Disease: A History of the International Health Division of the Rockefeller Foundation, 1913–1951*. Oxford: Oxford University Press, 2004.

———. "The International Health Division of the Rockefeller Foundation: The Russell Years, 1920–1934." In *International Health Organizations and Movements, 1918–*

1939, edited by Paul Weindling, 203–21. Cambridge: Cambridge University Press, 1995.

Feierman, Steven. "Struggles for Control: The Social Roots of Health and Healing in Modern Africa." *African Studies Review* 28 (1985): 73–128.

Feinstein, Howard. "The Use and Abuse of Illness in the James Family Circle." In *Our Selves/Our Past: Psychological Approaches to American History*, edited by Robert J. Brugger, 228–43. Baltimore: Johns Hopkins University Press, 1981.

Feldman, Allen. *Formations of Violence: The Narrative of the Body and Political Terror in Northern Ireland*. Chicago: University of Chicago Press, 1991.

Ferguson, James. *The Anti-Politics Machine: Development, Depoliticization, and Bureaucratic Power in Lesotho*. Cambridge: Cambridge University Press, 1990.

Fieldhouse, D. K. *The Colonial Empires: A Comparative Survey from the Eighteenth Century*. London: Weidenfeld and Nicolson, 1966.

Filiberti, Edward J. "The Roots of U.S. Counterinsurgency Doctrine." *Military Review* 58 (1988): 50–61.

Foreman, Carolyn T. "General Eli Lundy Huggins." *Chronicles of Oklahoma* 13 (1935): 255–65.

Fosdick, Raymond B. *The Story of the Rockefeller Foundation*. New Brunswick, N. J.: Transaction Publishers, 1989 [1952].

Foucault, Michel. *Discipline and Punish: The Birth of the Prison*. Translated by Alan Sheridan. New York: Pantheon Books, 1977.

——. *Power/Knowledge: Selected Interviews and Other Writings, 1972–77*. Edited by Colin Gordon, translated by Colin Gordon, Leo Marshall, John Mephan, Kate Soper. Brighton: Harvester Press, 1980.

——. *The History of Sexuality. Volume 1: An Introduction*. Translated by Robert Hurley. New York: Vintage, 1980.

——. *Technologies of the Self: A Seminar with Michel Foucault*. Edited by Luther H. Martin, Huck Gutman, and Patrick H. Hutton. Amherst: University of Massachusetts Press, 1988.

——. *Abnormal: Lectures at the Collège de France, 1974–75*. Translated by Graham Burchell. New York: Picador, 2003.

——. *"Society Must be Defended": Lectures at the Collège de France, 1975–76*. Translated by David Macey. New York: Picador, 2003.

——. "Governmentality." In *The Foucault Effect: Studies in Governmentality*, edited by Graham Burchell et al., 87–104. Chicago: University of Chicago Press, 1991.

Fredrickson, George M. *The Black Image in the White Mind: The Debate on Afro-American Character and Destiny, 1817–1914*. Hanover N.H.: Wesleyan University Press, 1987 [1971].

Freud, Sigmund. *Civilization and Its Discontents*. Translated by Joan Riviere. London: Hogarth Press, 1973 [1929].

——. "The Uncanny." In *The Standard Edition of the Complete Psychological Works of Sigmund Freud*, translated by James Strachey, vol. 17 (1917–19), 219–52. London: Hogarth Press, 1955 [1919].

Friend, Theodore. *Between Two Empires: Philippine Ordeal and Development from the*

Great Depression through the Pacific War, 1929–46. New Haven: Yale University Press, 1965.

Furner, Mary O. "The Republican Tradition and the New Liberalism: Social Investigation, State Building, and Social Learning in the Gilded Age." In *The State and Social Investigation in Britain and the United States,* edited by Michael J. Lacey and Mary O. Furner, 171–241. Cambridge: Woodrow Wilson Center Press and Cambridge University Press, 1993.

Gaerlan, Barbara S. "The Pursuit of Modernity: Trinidad H. Pardo de Tavera and the Educational Legacy of the Philippine Revolution," *amerasia j.* 24 (1998): 87–108.

Galambos, Louis. "The Emerging Organizational Synthesis in American History." *Business History Review* 44 (1970): 279–90.

———. "Technology, Political Economy and Professionalization: Central Themes of the Organizational Synthesis." *Business History Review* 57 (1983): 471–93.

Galishoff, Stuart. "Germs Know No Color Line: Black Health and Public Policy in Atlanta, 1900–1918." *J. of History of Medicine and Allied Sciences* 40 (1985): 22–41.

Gamble, Vanessa Northington, ed. *Germs Have No Color Line: Blacks and American Medicine, 1900–1940.* New York: Garland, 1989.

Garrison, Fielding H. *John Shaw Billings: A Memoir.* New York: G. P. Putman's Sons, 1915.

Gates, Henry Louis, Jr., "Critical Fanonism." *Critical Inquiry* 17 (1991): 457–70.

Gates, John Morgan. *Schoolbooks and Krags: The United States Army in the Philippines, 1898–1902.* Westport, Conn.: Greenwood Press, 1973.

Gatewood, Willard B. Jr. *Black Americans and the White Man's Burden, 1898–1903.* Urbana: University of Illinois Press, 1975.

Gerstle, Gary. *American Crucible: Race and Nation in the Twentieth Century.* Princeton: Princeton University Press, 2001.

Gibson, John. *Soldier in White: The Life of General George Miller Sternberg.* Durham, N.C.: Duke University Press, 1958.

Gijswijt-Hofstra, Marijke, and Roy Porter, ed. *Cultures of Neurasthenia from Beard to the First World War.* Amsterdam: Rodopi, 2001.

Gillett, Mary. *The Army Medical Department, 1865–1917.* Washington, D.C.: Center of Medical History, 1995.

———. "Medical Care and Evacuation during the Philippine Insurrection, 1899–1901." *J. of History of Medicine and Allied Sciences* 42 (1987): 169–85.

———. "U.S. Army Medical Officers and Public Health in the Philippines in the Wake of the Spanish-American War, 1898–1905." *Bulletin of the History of Medicine* 64 (1990): 567–87.

Gilman, Sander L. *Difference and Pathology: Stereotypes of Sexuality, Race and Madness.* Ithaca: Cornell University Press, 1985.

Glenn, Susan A. "'Give Me an Imitation of Me': Vaudeville Mimics and the Play of the Self." *American Quarterly* 50 (1998): 47–76.

Go, Julian. "Colonial Reception and Cultural Reproduction: Filipino Elites and United States Tutelary Rule." *J. of Historical Sociology* 12 (1999): 337–68.

Go, Julian. "Introduction: Global Perspectives on the U.S. Colonial State in the Philippines." In *The American Colonial State in the Philippines: Global Perspectives*, edited by Julian Go and Anne L. Foster, 1–42. Durham, N.C.: Duke University Press, 2003.

Goffman, Erving. *Asylums: Essays on the Social Situation of Mental Patients and Other Inmates*. New York: Anchor Books, 1961.

Gonzalez Flores, Luis Felipe. *Historia de la influencia extranjera en el desenvolvimiento educacional y científico de Costa Rica*. San José: Editorial Costa Rica, 1976.

Gorgas, William C., and Burton J. Hendrick. *William Crawford Gorgas, His Life and Work*. London: Heinemann, 1924.

Gosling, F. G. *Before Freud: Neurasthenia and the American Medical Community, 1867–1910*. Urbana: University of Illinois Press, 1987.

Gottman, Jean. "Bugeaud, Galliéni, Lyautey: The Development of French Colonial Warfare." In *Makers of Modern Strategy: Military Thought from Machiavelli to Hitler*, edited by Edward Mead Earle, 234–59. Princeton: Princeton University Press, 1952.

Goubert, Jean-Peirre. *The Conquest of Water: The Advent of Health in the Industrial Age*. Translated by Andrew Wilson. Cambridge: Polity Press, 1989.

Gouda, Frances. *Dutch Culture Overseas: Colonial Practice in the Netherlands Indies, 1900–1942*. Amsterdam: Amsterdam University Press, 1995.

Griffen, Clyde. "Reconstructing Masculinity from the Evangelical Revival to the Waning of Progressivism: A Speculative Synthesis." In *Meanings for Manhood: Constructions of Masculinity in Victorian America*, edited by Mark C. Carnes and Griffen, 183–204. Chicago: University of Chicago Press, 1990.

Grmek, Mirko. "Géographie médicale et histoire des civilisations." *Annales: Economies, Sociétés, Civilisations* 18 (1963): 1071–87.

Guerra, Francisco. *El Médico político: Estudios biográficos sobre la influencia del médico en la historia política de Hispanoamérica y Filipinas*. Madrid: Afrodisio Aguado, 1975.

Gupta, Akhil. *Postcolonial Developments: Agriculture in the Making of Modern India*. Durham, N.C.: Duke University Press, 1998.

Gussow, Zachary. *Leprosy, Racism, and Public Health: Social Policy in Chronic Disease*. Boulder, Colo.: Westview Press, 1989.

Gussow, Zachary, and George S. Tracy. "Stigma and the Leprosy Phenomenon: The Social History of a Disease in the Nineteenth and Twentieth Centuries." *Bulletin of the History of Medicine* 44 (1970): 425–49.

Haber, Samuel. *Efficiency and Uplift: Scientific Management in the Progressive Era, 1890–1920*. Chicago: University of Chicago Press, 1964.

Hagedorn, Hermann. *Leonard Wood: A Biography*. 2 vols. New York: Harper and Bros., 1931.

Hale, Nathan G., Jr. *Freud and the Americans: The Beginnings of Psychoanalysis in the United States, 1876–1917*. New York: Oxford University Press, 1987.

——. *The Rise and Crisis of Psychoanalysis in the United States: Freud and the Americans, 1917–85*. New York: Oxford University Press, 1995.

Hansen, Karen Tranberg, ed. *African Encounters with Domesticity*. New Brunswick, N.J.: Rutgers University Press, 1992.

Haraway, Donna. *Primate Visions: Gender, Race and Nature in the World of Modern Science*. New York: Routledge, 1989.

Harrison, Gordon. *Mosquitoes, Malaria and Man: A History of the Hostilities Since 1880*. New York: E. P. Dutton, 1978.

Harrison, Mark. *Climates and Constitutions: Health, Race Environment and British Imperialism in India, 1600–1850*. New Delhi: Oxford University Press, 1999.

——. "The Medicalization of War—The Militarization of Medicine." *Social History of Medicine* 9 (1996): 267–76.

Hartnack, Christiane. "British Psychoanalysts in Colonial India." In *Psychology in Twentieth-Century Thought and Society*, edited by Mitchell G. Ash and William R. Woodward, 233–52. New York: Cambridge University Press, 1987.

——. "Vishnu on Freud's Desk: Psychoanalysis in Colonial India." *Social Research* 57 (1990): 921–49.

Hattori, Anne Perez. *Colonial Dis-Ease: U.S. Navy Health Policies and the Chamorros of Guam, 1898–1941*. Honolulu: University of Hawaii Press, 2004.

Hayden, Joseph R. *The Philippines: A Study in National Development*. New York: Macmillan, 1942.

Haynes, Douglas M. *Imperial Medicine: Patrick Manson and the Conquest of Tropical Disease*. Philadelphia: University of Pennsylvania Press, 2001.

Heidegger, Martin. *The Question Concerning Technology, and Other Essays*. Translated by William Lovitt. New York: Harper Torchbooks, 1977.

Hewa, Soma. *Colonialism, Tropical Disease and Imperial Medicine: Rockefeller Philanthropy in Sri Lanka*. Lanham, Md.: University Press of America, 1995.

Higham, John. *Strangers in the Land: Patterns of American Nativism, 1860–1925*. New Brunswick, N.J.: Rutgers University Press, 1955.

Hobsbawm, Eric. *The Age of Empire 1875–1914*. New York: Vintage, 1989.

Hofstadter, Douglas. "Manifest Destiny and the Philippines." In *American Imperialism in 1898: Problems in American Civilization*, edited by Theodore P. Greene, 54–70. Boston: D. C. Heath, 1955.

——. "Cuba, the Philippines and Manifest Destiny." In *The Paranoid Style in American Politics and Other Essays*, 145–87. New York: Knopf, 1965.

Hoganson, Kristin. *Fighting for American Manhood: How Gender Politics Provoked the Spanish-American and the Philippine-American Wars*. New Haven: Yale University Press, 1998.

Holborn, Hojo. "Moltke and Schlieffen: The Prussian-German School." In *Makers of Modern Strategy: Military Thought from Machiavelli to Hitler*, edited by Edward Mead Earle, 172–205. Princeton: Princeton University Press, 1952.

Horsman, Reginald. *Race and Manifest Destiny: The Origins of American Anglo-Saxonism*. Cambridge: Harvard University Press, 1989.

Howard-Jones, Norman. *International Health Between the Two World Wars—The Organizational Problems*. Geneva: W.H.O., 1978.

Hoxie, Frederick E. *A Final Promise: The Campaign to Assimilate the Indians, 1880–1920*. Lincoln, Neb.: University of Nebraska Press, 1984.

Hoy, Suellen M. *Chasing Dirt: The American Pursuit of Cleanliness*. New York: Oxford University Press, 1995.

Humphreys, Margaret. *Malaria: Poverty, Race and Public Health in the United States.* Baltimore: Johns Hopkins University Press, 2001.

Hutchcroft, Paul D. "Colonial Masters, National Politicos, and Provincial Lords: Central Authority and Local Autonomy in the American Philippines, 1900–1913." *J. of Asian Studies* 59 (2000): 277–306.

Hyam, Ronald. *Empire and Sexuality: The British Experience.* Manchester: Manchester University Press, 1990.

Ileto, Reynaldo C. *Pasyon and Revolution: Popular Movements in the Philippines, 1840–1910.* Quezon City: Ateneo de Manila University Press, 1979.

———. "Cholera and the Origins of the American Sanitary Order in the Philippines." In *Imperial Medicine and Indigenous Society*, edited by David Arnold, 125–48. Manchester: Manchester University Press, 1989.

———. "Outlines of a Non-linear Emplotment of Philippines History." In *The Politics of Culture in the Shadow of Capital*, edited by Lisa Lowe and David Lloyd, 98–131. Durham, N.C.: Duke University Press, 1997.

Jacobson, Matthew Frye. *Whiteness of a Different Color: European Immigrants and the Alchemy of Race.* Cambridge: Harvard University Press, 1998.

Jamison, Perry D. *Crossing the Deadly Ground: United States Army Tactics, 1865–1899.* Tuscaloosa: University of Alabama Press, 1994.

Jardine, Alice. *Gynesis: Configurations of Women and Modernity.* Ithaca: Cornell University Press, 1985.

Johnson, Terence. "Imperialism and the Professions." In *Professionalisation and Social Change*, edited by Paul Halmos, 281–309. Keele: University of Keele Press, 1973.

Jones, David Shumway. "Rationalizing Epidemics: Meanings and Uses of American Indian Mortality since 1600." ph.d. diss., Harvard University, 2001.

———. *Rationalizing Epidemics: Meanings and Uses of American Indian Mortality since 1600.* Cambridge: Harvard University Press, 2004.

Kagan, Solomon R. *Life and Letters of Fielding H. Garrison.* Boston: Medico-Historical Press, 1938.

Kakar, Sanjiv "Leprosy in British India, 1860–1940: Colonial Politics and Missionary Medicine." *Medical History* 40 (1996): 215–30.

———. "Medical Developments and Patient Unrest in the Leprosy Asylum, 1860–1940." *Social Scientist* 24 (1996): 62–81.

Kakar, Sudhir. "Encounters of a Psychological Kind: Freud, Jung, and India." In *Culture and Psyche: Selected Essays*, 20–32. Delhi: Oxford University Press, 1997.

Kaplan, Amy. "Romancing the Empire: The Embodiment of American Masculinity in the Popular Historical Novel of the 1890s." *American Literary History* 2 (1990): 659–70.

———. " 'Left Alone with America': The Absence of Empire in the Study of American Culture." In *Cultures of United States Imperialism*, edited by Amy Kaplan and Donald E. Pease, 3–21. Durham, N.C.: Duke University Press, 1993.

Katz, J. *Experimentation with Human Beings.* New York: Russell Sage Foundation, 1972.

Keller, Richard. "Madness and Colonization: Psychiatry in the British and French Empire, 1800–1962." *J. of Social History* 35 (2001): 295–326.

Kennedy, Dane. *The Magic Mountains: Hill Stations and the British Raj*. Berkeley: University of California Press, 1996.

———. "The Perils of the Midday Sun: Climatic Anxieties in the Colonial Tropics." In *Imperialism and the Natural World*, edited by John M. McKenzie, 118–40. Manchester: Manchester University Press, 1990.

Kimmel, Michael S. "The Contemporary 'Crisis' in Masculinity in Historical Perspective." In *The Making of Masculinities: The New Men's Studies*, edited by Harry Brod, 121–54. Boston: Allen and Unwin, 1987.

Kipp, Rita Smith. "The Evangelical Uses of Leprosy." *Social Science and Medicine* 39 (1994): 165–78.

Kleinman, Arthur, and Joan Kleinman. "How Bodies Remember: Social Memory and the Bodily Experience of Criticism, Resistance, and Delegitimation Following China's Cultural Revolution." *New Literary History* 25 (1994): 707–23.

Kramer, Paul A. "The Pragmatic Empire: U.S. Anthropology and Colonial Politics in the Occupied Philippines, 1898–1916." ph.d. diss., Princeton University, 1998.

———. "Making Concessions: Race and Empire Revisited at the Philippine Exposition, St. Louis, 1901–05." *Radical History Review* 73 (1999): 74–114.

———. "Empires, Exceptions, and Anglo-Saxons: Race and Rule between the British and United States Empires, 1880–1910." *J. American History* 88 (2002): 1315–53.

Kraut, Alan M. *Silent Travelers: Germs, Genes, and the "Immigrant Menace."* Baltimore: Johns Hopkins University Press, 1994.

Kristeva, Julia. *Powers of Horror: An Essay in Abjection*, Translated by Leon S. Roudiez. New York: Columbia University Press, 1982.

Kunitz, Stephen J. "Efficiency and Reform in the Financing and Organization of American Medicine in the Progressive Era." *Bulletin of the History of Medicine* 55 (1981): 497–515.

———. "The History and Politics of U.S. Health Care Policy for American Indians and Alaskan Natives." *American J. Public Health* 86 (1996): 1464–73.

Lacey, Michael J. "The World of the Bureaus: Government and the Positivist Project in the Late Nineteenth Century." In *The State and Social Investigation in Britain and the United States*, edited by Lacey and Furner, 127–70. Washington, D.C., Woodrow Wilson Center Press; Cambridge: Cambridge University Press, 1993.

Laporte, Dominique. *Histoire de la Merde*. Paris: Christian Bourgois Editeur, 1979.

Lasch, Christopher. "The Anti-imperialists, the Philippines and the Rights of Man." *J. of Southern History* 24 (1958): 319–31.

Latour, Bruno. *Pandora's Hope: Essays on the Reality of Science Studies*. Cambridge: Harvard University Press, 1999.

———. "Give Me a Laboratory and I Will Raise the World." In *Science Observed: Perspectives on the Social Study of Science*, edited by Karin Knorr-Cetina and Michael Mulkay, 141–70. London: Sage, 1983.

Lawrence, Christopher. "Disciplining Disease: Scurvy, the Navy and Imperial

Expansion." In *Visions of Empire*, edited by D. Miller and P. Reill, 80–106. Cambridge: Cambridge University Press, 1994.

Lears, T. J. Jackson. "The Destructive Element: Modern Commercial Society and the Martial Ideal." In *No Place of Grace: Antimodernism and the Transformation of American Culture 1880–1920*, 97–140. New York: Pantheon, 1981.

Leavitt, Judith Walzer. *Healthiest City: Milwaukee and the Politics of Health Reform*. Princeton: Princeton University Press, 1982.

———. *Typhoid Mary: Captive to the Public's Health*. Boston: Beacon Press, 1996.

Lee, Chistopher. "Toilet Training the Settler Subject: An Exercise in Civic Regulation." *Southern Review* 29 (1996): 50–63.

Lefebvre, Henri. *The Production of Space*. Translated by Donald Nicholson-Smith. Oxford: Blackwell, 1991 [1971].

Levine, Philippa. "Venereal Disease, Prostitution and the Politics of Empire: The Case of British India." *J. History of Sexuality* 4 (1994): 579–602.

Levinson, Julie. "Beyond Quarantine: A History of Leprosy in Puerto Rico, 1898–1930s." *História, Ciéncias, Saúde—Manguinhos* 10, Suppl. 1 (2003): 225–45.

Linn, Brian McA. *The United States Army and Counter-Insurgency in the Philippine War, 1899–1902*. Chapel Hill: University of North Carolina Press, 1989.

———. *Guardians of Empire: The U.S. Army and the Pacific, 1902–1940*. Chapel Hill: University of North Carolina Press, 1997.

———. *The Philippines War, 1899–1902*. Lawrence: University of Kansas Press, 2000.

Litsios, Socrates. "René Dubos and Fred L. Soper: Their Contrasting Views on Vector and Disease Eradication." *Perspectives in Biology and Medicine* 41 (1997): 138–49.

———. "The Christian Medical Commission and the Development of the World Health Organization's Primary Health Care Approach." *American J. Public Health* 94 (2004): 1884–93.

Liu, Shiyung. "Building a Strong and Healthy Empire: The Critical Period of Building Colonial Medicine in Taiwan." *Japanese Studies* 24 (2004): 301–14.

Livingstone, David N. "Science and Society: Nathaniel S. Shaler and Racial Ideology." *Trans. Institute of British Geography* 9 (1984): 181–210.

———. "Human Acclimatisation: Perspectives on a Contested Field of Inquiry in Science, Medicine and Geography." *History of Science* 25 (1987): 359–94.

———. "Climate's Moral Economy: Science, Race and Place in Post-Darwinian British and American Geography." In *Geography and Empire*, edited by Anna Godlewska and Neil Smith, 132–54. Oxford: Blackwell, 1994.

———. "Tropical Climate and Moral Hygiene: The Anatomy of a Victorian Debate." *British J. of the History of Science* 32 (1999): 93–110.

Lo, Ming-Cheng M. *Doctors Within Borders: Profession, Ethnicity, and Modernity in Colonial Taiwan*. Berkeley: University of California Press, 2002.

Lull, G. "The Days Gone By: A Brief History of the Army Medical School, 1893–1933." *Military Surgeon* 74 (1934): 78–86.

Lutz, Tom. *American Nervousness 1903: An Anecdotal History*. Ithaca: Cornell University Press, 1991.

MacKinnon, Aran S. "Of Oxford Bags and Twirling Canes: The State, Popular Responses and Zulu Antimalaria Assistants in the Early-twentieth-century Zululand Malaria Campaigns." *Radical History Review* 80 (2001): 76–100.

Madison, Donald L. "Preserving Individualism in the Organizational Society: 'Cooperation' and American Medical Practice, 1900–1920." *Bulletin of the History of Medicine* 70 (1996): 442–83.

Manderson, Lenore. *Sickness and the State: Health and Illness in Colonial Malaya, 1870–1940*. Cambridge: Cambridge University Press, 1996.

Markel, Howard. *Quarantine! East European Jewish Immigrants and the New York City Epidemics of 1892*. Baltimore: Johns Hopkins University Press, 1997.

Martellone, Anna Maria. "In the Name of Anglo-Saxondom, for Empire and Democracy: The Anglo-American Discourse, 1880–1920." In *Reflections on American Exceptionalism*, edited by David K. Adams and Cornelis A. van Minnen, 83–96. Keele: Keele University Press, 1994.

Mauss, Marcel. "Techniques of the Body." *Economy and Society* 2 (1973): 70–88.

May, Glenn A. *Social Engineering in the Philippines: The Aims, Execution, and Impact of American Social Policy, 1900–13*. Westport, Conn.: Greenwood Press, 1980.

———. *Battle for Batangas: A Philippine Province at War*. New Haven: Yale University Press, 1991.

———. "Filipino Resistance to American Occupation: Batangas, 1899–1902." *Pacific Historical Review* 4 (1979): 531–56.

Mbembe, Achille. "The Banality of Power and the Aesthetics of Vulgarity in the Postcolony." Translated by Janet Roitman. *Public Culture* 4 (1992): 1–30.

McClain, Charles. "Of Medicine, Race and American Law: The Bubonic Plague Outbreak of 1900." *Law and Social Inquiry* 13 (1988): 447–513.

McClintock, Anne. *Imperial Leather: Race, Gender and Sexuality in the Colonial Contest*. London: Routledge, 1995.

McCoy, Alfred W. "The Colonial Origins of Philippine Military Traditions." In *The Philippine Revolution of 1896: Ordinary Lives in Extraordinary Times*, edited by Florentino Rodao and Felice Noelle Rodriguez, 83–124. Quezon City: Ateneo de Manila University Press, 2001.

McCoy, Alfred, and Ed J. de Jesus, eds. *Philippine Social History: Global Trade and Local Transformations*. Quezon City: Ateneo de Manila University Press, 1982.

McCulloch, Jock. *Colonial Psychiatry and "the African Mind."* Cambridge: Cambridge University Press, 1995.

McFerson, Hazel M., ed. *Mixed Blessing: The Impact of the American Colonial Experience on Politics and Society in the Philippines*. Westport, Conn.: Greenwood Press, 2002.

Mehta, Uday S. "Liberal Strategies of Exclusion." In *Tensions of Empire: Colonial Cultures in a Bourgeois World*, edited by Frederick Cooper and Ann L. Stoler, 59–86. Berkeley: University of California Press, 1997.

Memmi, Albert. *The Colonizer and the Colonized*. Translated by Howard Greenfeld. New York: Orion Press, 1965.

Mendelsohn, J. Andrew. "Medicine and the Making of Bodily Inequality in Twentieth-century Europe." In *Heredity and Infection: The History of Disease Transmission*, edited by J. P. Gaudillière and Ilana Löwy, 21–79. London: Routledge, 2001.

Miller, Stuart C. *"Benevolent Assimilation": The American Conquest of the Philippines, 1899–1903*. New Haven: Yale University Press, 1982.

Mills, James H. *Madness, Cannabis, and Colonialism: The "Native Only" Lunatic Asylums of British India, 1857–1900*. New York: St. Martin's Press, 2000.

Mitchell, Timothy. *Colonizing Egypt*. Berkeley: University of California Press, 1991.

Mohanty, Chandra Talpade. "Under Western Eyes: Feminist Scholarship and Colonial Discourse." *boundary* 2 12 (1984): 333–58.

Monnais-Rousselot, Laurence. *Médecine et Colonisation: L'Aventure Indochinoise, 1860–1939*. Paris: CNRS Editions, 1999.

Moore, John H. "Senator John Tyler Morgan and Negro Colonization in the Philippines, 1901–2." *Phylon* 24 (1968): 65–67.

Mrozek, Donal D. J. "The Habit of Victory: The American Military and the Cult of Manliness." In *Manliness and Morality: Middle-Class Masculinity in Britain and America, 1800–1940*, edited by J. A. Mangan and James Walvin, 220–41. Manchester: Manchester University Press, 1987.

Mullan, Fitzhugh. *Plagues and Politics: The Story of the U.S. Public Health Service*. New York: Basic Books, 1989.

Najera, J. A. "Malaria Control: Present Situation and Need for Historical Research." *Parassitologia* 32 (1990): 215–29.

Nandy, Ashis. *The Intimate Enemy: Loss and Recovery of Self under Colonialism*. Delhi: Oxford University Press, 1983.

———. "The Psychology of Colonialism." *Psychiatry* 45 (1982): 197–218.

———. "The Savage Freud: The First Non-Western Psychoanalyst and the Politics of Secret Selves in Colonial India." In *The Savage Freud, and Other Essays on Possible and Retrievable Selves*, 81–144. Princeton: Princeton University Press, 1995.

Nichols, H. "Notes on the History of the Laboratories of the Army Medical School." *Military Surgeon* 60 (1927): 52–58.

Nussbaum, Felicity A. *Torrid Zones: Maternity, Sexuality and Empire in Eighteenth-Century English Narratives*. Baltimore: Johns Hopkins University Press, 1995.

Obregón, Diana. *Batallas contra la lepra: Estado, medicina y ciencia en Colombia*. Bogotá: Banco de la República, 2002.

———. "The Anti-leprosy Campaign in Colombia: The Rhetoric of Hygiene and Science, 1920–1940." *História, Ciéncias, Saúde—Manguinhos* 10, Suppl. 1 (2003): 179–207.

O'Connor, Erin. *Raw Material: Producing Pathology in Victorian Culture*. Durham, N.C.: Duke University Press, 2000.

Olch, Peter D. "Medicine in the Indian-fighting Army, 1866–1890." *J. of the West* 21 (1982): 32–41.

Ong, Aihwa. "Making the Biopolitical Subject: Cambodian Immigrants, Refugee Medicine, and Cultural Citizenship in California." *Social Science and Medicine* 40 (1995): 1243–57.

Oppenheim, Janet. *"Shattered Nerves": Doctors, Patients and Depression in Victorian England*. Oxford: Oxford University Press, 1991.

Owen, Norman G., ed. *Compadre Colonialism: Studies on the Philippines under American Rule*. Ann Arbor: University of Michigan Papers on South and Southeast Asia No. 3, 1971.

———, ed. *Death and Disease in Southeast Asia: Explorations in Social, Medical and Demographic History*. Singapore: Oxford University Press, 1987.

Packard, Randall M. *White Plague, Black Labor: Tuberculosis and the Political Economy of Health and Disease in South Africa*. Berkeley: University of California Press, 1989.

———. "Malaria Dreams: Visions of Health and Development in the Third World." *Medical Anthropology* 17 (1997): 279–96.

———. "Visions of Postwar Health and Development and Their Impact on Public Health Interventions in the Developing World." In *International Development and the Social Sciences: Essays on the History and Politics of Knowledge*, edited by Frederick Cooper and Randall M. Packard, 93–115. Berkeley: University of California Press, 1997.

———. " 'No Other Logical Choice': Global Malaria Eradication and the Politics of International Health in the Post-war Era." *Parassitologia* 40 (1998): 217–29.

Packard, Randall M., and P. Gadelha. "A Land Filled with Mosquitoes: Fred L. Soper, the Rockefeller Foundation, and the *Anopheles gambiae* Invasion of Brazil." *Parassitologia* 36 (1994): 197–213.

Palmer, Steven. "Central American Encounters with Rockefeller Public Health, 1914–21." In *Close Encounters of Empire: Writing the Cultural History of U.S.-Latin American Relations*, edited by Gilbert Joseph, Catherine C. LeGrand, Ricardo Salvator, 311–32. Durham, N.C.: Duke University Press, 1998.

Pandya, S. S. "The First International Leprosy Conference, Berlin, 1897: The Politics of Segregation." *História, Ciências, Saúde—Manguinhos* 10, Suppl. 1 (2003): 161–77.

Paredes, Ruby R. "The Ilustrado Legacy: The Pardo de Taveras of Manila." In *An Anarchy of Families: State and Family in the Philippines*, edited by Alfred W. McCoy. Quezon City: Ateneo de Manila University Press, 1994.

Parekh, Bhiku. "Liberalism and Colonialism: A Critique of Locke and Mill." In *The Decolonization of Imagination*, edited by Jan Nederveen Pieterse and Bhiku Parekh, 81–98. London: Zed Books, 1995.

Parreñas, Rhacel Salazar. "Transgressing the Nation State: The Partial Citizenship and 'Imagined Community' of Migrant Filipina Domestic Workers." *Signs* 26 (2001): 1129–54.

Pateman, Carole. *The Sexual Contract*. Cambridge: Polity Press, 1988.

Pegg, M. G. "Le corps et l'authorité: La lèpre de Badouin IV." *Annales: Economies, Sociétés, Civilisations* 45 (1990): 265–87.

Petryna, Adriana. *Life Exposed: Biological Citizens After Chernobyl*. Princeton: Princeton University Press, 2002.

Pick, Daniel. *Faces of Degeneration: A European Disorder, c. 1848–c. 1918*. Cambridge: Cambridge University Press, 1989.

Pickens, Donald K. "The Turner Thesis and Republicanism: A Historiographic Commentary." *Pacific Historical Review* 61 (1992): 319–40.

Pigg, Stacy Leigh. " 'Found in Most Traditional Societies': Traditional Medical

Practitioners between Culture and Development." In *International Development and the Social Sciences: Essays on the History and Politics of Knowledge*, edited by Frederick Cooper and Randall Packard, 259–90. Berkeley: University of California Press, 1997.

Poovey, Mary. *Making a Social Body: British Cultural Formation, 1830–1864*. Chicago: University of Chicago Press, 1995.

Porter, Dorothy. *Health, Civilization and the State: A History of Public Health from Ancient to Modern Times*. New York: Routledge, 1999.

Prakash, Gyan. *Another Reason: Science and the Imagination of Modern India*. Princeton: Princeton University Press, 1999.

Pringle, Henry F. *The Life and Times of William H. Taft*. 2 vols. New York: Farrer and Rinehart, 1939.

Quisumbing, Eduardo. "Development of Science in the Philippines." *J. of East Asiatic Studies* 6 (1957): 127–53.

Rabinbach, Anson. *The Human Motor: Energy, Fatigue and the Origins of Modernity*. New York: Basic Books, 1990.

Rabinow, Paul. *French Modern: Norms and Forms of the Social Environment*. Cambridge: MIT Press, 1989.

Rafael, Vicente L. *White Love, and Other Events in Filipino History*. Durham, N.C.: Duke University Press, 2000.

———. "White Love: Surveillance and Nationalist Resistance in the United States' Colonization of the Philippines." In *Cultures of United States Imperialism*, edited by Amy Kaplan and Donald E. Pease, 185–218. Durham, N.C.: Duke University Press, 1993.

———. "Colonial Domesticity: White Women and United States Rule in the Philippines," *American Literature* 67 (1995): 639–65.

———. "Mimetic Subjects: Engendering Race at the Edge of Empire." *differences: A Journal of Feminist Cultural Studies* 7 (1995): 127–49.

———, ed. *Discrepant Histories: Translocal Essays on Filipino Cultures*. Philadelphia: Temple University Press, 1995.

Ramos, Paz G. "Historical Background of Health Education in the Philippines." *Education Quarterly* 14 (1966): 4–13.

Reed, Robert R. *City of Pines: The Origins of Baguio as a Colonial Hill Station and Regional Capital*. 2nd ed. Baguio City: A-Seven Publishing, 1999 [1976].

Renan, Ernest. *Qu'est-ce qu'une nation? Et autres essais politiques*. Paris: Presses-Pochet, 1992.

Renbourn, E. T. "The Spine Pad: A Discarded Item of Tropical Clothing." *J. of the Royal Army Medical Corps* 102 (1956): 217–33.

———. "Life and Death of the Solar Topi." *J. of Tropical Medicine and Hygiene* 65 (1962): 203–18.

Robertson, Jo. "Leprosy and the Elusive *M. leprae*: Colonial and Imperial Medical Exchanges in the Nineteenth Century." *História, Ciéncias, Saúde — Manguinhos* 10, Suppl. 1 (2003): 13–40.

Robinson, Ronald. "Non-European Foundations of European Imperialism: Sketch for a

Theory of Collaboration." In *Studies in the Theory of Imperialism*, edited by Roger Owen and Bob Sutcliffe, 117–42. London: Longman, 1972.

Rodgers, Daniel T. "In Search of Progressivism." *Reviews in American History* 10 (1982): 113–32.

Rogaski, Ruth. *Hygienic Modernity: The Meanings of Health in Treaty-Port China*. Berkeley: University of California Press, 2004.

Rogers, Naomi. "Germs with Legs: Flies, Disease and the New Public Health." *Bulletin of the History of Medicine* 63 (1989): 599–617.

Rose, Nikolas. *Powers of Freedom: Reframing Political Thought*. Cambridge: Cambridge University Press, 1999.

Rosen, George. *A History of Public Health*. New York: MD Publications, 1958.

———. *From Medical Police to Social Medicine: Essays on the History of Health Care*. New York: Science History Publications, 1974.

———. *Preventive Medicine in the United States, 1900–75: Trends and Interpretations*. New York: Prodist, 1977.

———. "Nostalgia: A 'Forgotten' Psychological Disorder." *Psychological Medicine* 5 (1975): 340–54.

———. "The Efficiency Criterion in Medical Care, 1900–1920: An Early Approach to the Evaluation of Health Service." *Bulletin of the History of Medicine* 50 (1976): 28–44.

Rosenberg, Charles E. "George M. Beard and American Nervousness." In *No Other Gods: On Science and American Social Thought*, 98–108. Baltimore: Johns Hopkins University Press, 1976.

———. "Sexuality, Class and Role in Nineteenth-century America." In *The American Man*, edited by Elizabeth H. Pleck and Joseph H. Pleck, 219–54. Englewood Cliffs, N.J.: Prentice-Hall, 1980.

———. "Framing Disease: Illness, Society and History." In *Framing Disease: Studies in Cultural History*, edited by Charles E. Rosenberg and Janet Golden, xii–xxvi. New Brunswick, N.J.: Rutgers University Press, 1992.

Rosenkrantz, Barbara Gutmann. *Public Health and the State: Changing Views in Massachusetts, 1842–1936*. Cambridge: Harvard University Press, 1972.

Rotundo, E. Anthony. *American Manhood: Transformations in Masculinity from the Revolution to the Modern Era*. New York: Basic Books, 1993.

Russell, Edmund. *War and Nature: Fighting Humans and Insects with Chemicals from World War I to Silent Spring*. Cambridge: Cambridge University Press, 2001.

Russell, Paul F. "The United States and Malaria: Debits and Credits." *Bulletin of the New York Academy of Medicine* 44 (1968): 623–53.

Sadowsky, Jonathan. *Imperial Bedlam: Institutions of Madness in Colonial Southwest Nigeria*. Berkeley: University of California Press, 1999.

Said, Edward W. *Orientalism*. London: Routledge and Kegan Paul, 1978.

Saldivar, José David. "Looking Awry at 1898: Roosevelt, Montejo, Paredes, and Mariscal." *American Literary History* 12 (2000): 386–406.

Salman, Michael. "The United States and the End of Slavery in the Philippines, 1898–

1914: A Study of Imperialism, Ideology and Nationalism." ph.d. diss., Stanford
University, 1993.

Sangari, Kumkum, and Sudesh Vaid. *Recasting Women: Essays in Colonial History*.
New Delhi: Kali for Women, 1989.

Santiago, Luciano P. R. "The First Filipino Doctors of Medicine and Surgery (1878–
97)." *Philippine Quarterly of Culture and Society* 22 (1997): 103–40.

Scheper-Hughes, Nancy. "Rotten Trade." *J. of Human Rights* 2 (2003): 197–226.

Schneider, William H., ed. *Rockefeller Philanthropy and Modern Biomedicine:
International Initiatives from World War I to the Cold War*. Bloomington: Indiana
University Press, 2002.

Schumacher, John N. *The Propaganda Movement 1880–1895*. Manila: Solidaridad,
1973.

———. "Rizal and Blumentritt." *Philippine Studies* 2 (1954): 85–101.

———. "Philippine Higher Education and the Origins of Nationalism." *Philippine
Studies* 23 (1975): 53–65.

Scott, David. "Colonial Governmentality." *Social Text* 43 (1995): 191–220.

Scott, Joan W. *Only Paradoxes to Offer: French Feminists and the Rights of Man*.
Cambridge: Harvard University Press, 1996.

———. "Gender: A Useful Category of Historical Analysis." *American Historical
Review* 91 (1986): 1053–75.

Shah, Nayan. *Contagious Divides: Epidemics and Race in San Francisco's Chinatown*.
Berkeley: University of California Press, 2001.

Shirmer, Daniel B. *Republic or Empire: American Resistance to the Philippine War*.
Cambridge: Schenkman, 1972.

Showalter, Elaine. *The Female Malady: Woman, Madness and English Culture 1830–
1980*. Harmondsworth: Penguin, 1985.

Sicherman, Barbara. "The Uses of a Diagnosis: Doctors, Patients and Neurasthenia."
J. of the History of Medicine and Allied Sciences 32 (1977): 33–54.

Sinha, Mrinalini. *Colonial Masculinities: The "Manly Englishman" and the "Effeminate
Bengali" in the Late Nineteenth Century*. Manchester: Manchester University Press,
1995.

Skowronek, Stephen. *Building a New American State: The Expansion of National
Administrative Capacities, 1877–1920*. Cambridge: Cambridge University Press,
1982.

Smallman-Raynor, Matthew, and Andrew D. Cliff. "The Epidemiological Legacy of
War: The Philippine-American War and the Diffusion of Cholera in Batangas and La
Laguna, South-West Luzón, 1902–4." *War in History* 7 (2000): 29–64.

Smith, Dale. "Edward L. Munson, m.d.: A Biographical Study in Military Medicine."
Military Medicine 164 (1999): 1–5.

Smith-Rosenberg, Carroll, and Charles E. Rosenberg. "The Female Animal: Medical
and Biological Views of Woman and Her Role in Nineteenth-century America." *J. of
American History* 60 (1973): 332–56.

Sobredo, James D. "From American 'Nationals' to the 'Third Asiatic Invasion': Racial

Transformation and Filipino Exclusion (1898–1934)." ph.d. dissertation, University of California-Berkeley, 1998.

Spivak, Gayatri Chakravorty. *In Other Worlds: Essays in Cultural Politics*. New York: Methuen, 1987.

Stallybrass, Peter, and Allon White. *The Politics and Poetics of Transgression*. Ithaca: Cornell University Press, 1986.

Stanley, Peter W. *A Nation in the Making: The Philippines and the United States 1899–1921*. Cambridge: Harvard University Press, 1974.

——. "William Cameron Forbes: Proconsul in the Philippines." *Pacific Historical Review* 35 (1966): 285–301.

——. " 'The Voice of Worcester Is the Voice of God': How One American Found Fulfillment in the Philippines." In *Reappraising an Empire: New Perspectives on Philippine-American History*, edited by Peter W. Stanley, 117–42. Cambridge: Committee on American–East Asian Relations, Harvard University, 1984.

Stapleton, Darwin H. "Technology and Malaria Control, 1930–1960: The Career of Rockefeller Foundation Engineer Frederick W. Knipe." *Parassitologia* 42 (2000): 59–68.

——. "Internationalism and Nationalism: The Rockefeller Foundation, Public Health, and Malaria in India, 1923–51." *Parassitologia* 42 (2000): 127–34.

Stauffer, Robert B. *The Development of an Interest Group: The Philippine Medical Association*. Quezon City: University of the Philippines Press, 1966.

Stepan, Nancy Leys. "Race, Gender, Science and Citizenship." In *Cultures of Empire: Colonizers in Britain and the Empire in the Nineteenth and Twentieth Centuries*, edited by Catherine Hall, 61–86. New York: Routledge, 2000.

Stern, Alexandra Minna. *Eugenic Nation: Faults and Frontiers of Better Breeding in America*. Berkeley: University of California Press, 2005.

Sternberg, Martha L. *George Miller Sternberg: A Biography*. Chicago: AMA, 1920.

Stewart, Susan. *On Longing: Narratives of the Miniature, the Gigantic, the Souvenir, the Collection*. Durham, N.C.: Duke University Press, 1993.

Stoler, Ann Laura. *Race and the Education of Desire: Foucault's History of Sexuality and the Colonial Order of Things*. Durham, N.C.: Duke University Press, 1995.

——. "Rethinking Colonial Categories: European Communities and the Boundaries of Rule." *Comparative Studies in Society and History* 31 (1989): 134–61.

——. "Carnal Knowledge and Imperial Power: Gender, Race, and Morality in Colonial Asia." In *Gender at the Crossroads of Knowledge: Feminist Anthropology in the Postmodern Era*, edited by Micaela di Leonardo, 51–101. Berkeley: University of California Press, 1991.

——. "Sexual Affronts and Racial Frontiers: European Identities and the Cultural Politics of Exclusion in Colonial Southeast Asia." *Comparative Studies in Society and History* 34 (1992): 514–51.

——. "Tense and Tender Ties: The Politics of Comparison in North American History and (Post) Colonial Studies." *J. of American History* 88 (2001): 829–96.

——. *Carnal Knowledge and Imperial Power: Race and the Intimate in Colonial Rule*. Berkeley: University of California Press, 2002.

Stoler, Ann Laura, and Frederick Cooper. "Tensions of Empire: Rethinking a Research Agenda." In *Tensions of Empire: Colonial Cultures in a Bourgeois World*, edited by Frederick Cooper and Ann L. Stoler, 1–56. Berkeley: University of California Press, 1997.

Stone, Martin. "Shellshock and the Psychologists." In *The Anatomy of Madness: Essays in the History of Psychiatry*. Vol. 2: *Institutions and Society*, edited W. F. Bynum, Roy Porter, and M. Shepherd, 242–71. New York: Tavistock, 1985.

Sturdy, Steve. "From the Trenches to the Hospitals at Home: Physiologists, Clinicians and Oxygen Therapy, 1914–30." In *Medical Innovations in Historical Perspective*, edited by J. V. Pickstone, 104–23. New York: St. Martin's Press, 1992.

Sturdy, Steve, and Roger Cooter. "Science, Scientific Management, and the Transformation of Medicine in Britain, c. 1870–1950." *History of Science* 36 (1998): 421–66.

Sullivan, Rodney J. " 'Exemplar of Americanism': The Philippine Career of Dean C. Worcester." ph.d. diss., James Cook University of North Queensland, 1986.

———. *Exemplar of Americanism: The Philippines Career of Dean C. Worcester*. Ann Arbor, Mich.: Center for South and Southeast Asian Studies, University of Michigan, 1991.

———. "Cholera and Colonialism in the Philippines." In *Disease, Medicine and Empire: Perspectives on Western Medicine and the Experience of European Expansion*, edited by Roy MacLeod and Milton Lewis, 284–300. London: Routledge, 1988.

Tadiar, Neferti X. "Filipina Domestic Bodies." *Sojourn: A Journal of Social Issues in Southeast Asia* 12 (1997): 153–91.

Taussig, Michael. *Mimesis and Alterity: A Particular History of the Senses*. London: Routledge, 1993.

Temkin, Owsei. "The Scientific Approach to Disease: Specific Entity and Individual Sickness." In *The Double Face of Janus and Other Essays in the History of Medicine*, 441–55. Baltimore: Johns Hopkins University Press, 1977.

Thomas, Howard Elsworth. *A Study of Leprosy Colony Policies*. N.p.: American Mission to Lepers, 1947.

Thomas, Nicholas. *Colonialism's Culture: Anthropology, Travel and Government*. Princeton: Princeton University Press, 1994.

Tomes, Nancy. *The Gospel of Germs: Men, Women and the Microbe in American Life*. Cambridge: Harvard University Press, 1998.

Trask, David F. *The War with Spain in 1898*. New York: Macmillan, 1981.

Trauner, Joan B. "The Chinese as Medical Scapegoats in San Francisco, 1870–1905." *California History* 57 (1978): 70–87.

Trennert, Robert A. *White Man's Medicine: Government Doctors and the Navajo, 1863–1955*. Albuquerque: University of New Mexico Press, 1998.

Trigo, Benigno. "Anemia and Vampires: Figures to Govern the Colony, Puerto Rico, 1880–1904." *Comparative Studies in Society and History* 41 (1999): 104–23.

Ugarte, Eduardo F. "Muslims and Madness in the Southern Philippines," *Pilipinas* 19 (1992): 1–24.

———. " 'Like a Mad Dog': The Perceived Savageness of 'the Malay' in Euro-British and Euro-American Colonial Writing," *Pilipinas* 29 (1999): 97–118.

Utley, Robert M. *Frontier Regulars: The United States Army and the Indian, 1866–1891*. New York: Macmillan, 1973.

Valenčius, Conevery Bolton. "Histories of Medical Geography." In *Medical Geography in Historical Perspective*, edited by Nicolaas Rupke, 3–29. London: Wellcome Trust Centre for the History of Medicine, 2000.

Van Hise, Joseph B. "American Contributions to Philippine Science and Technology, 1898–1916." ph.d. diss., University of Wisconsin-Madison, 1957.

Vaughan, Christopher A. "Ogling Igorots: The Politics and Commerce of Exhibiting Otherness, 1898–1913," In *Freakery: The Cultural Spectacle of the Extraordinary Body*, edited by Rosemary Garland Thompson, 219–33. New York: New York University Press, 1996.

Vaughan, Megan. *Curing Their Ills: Colonial Power and African Illness*. Stanford: Stanford University Press, 1991.

Velasco, José R., and Luz Baens-Arcega. *The National Institute of Science and Technology, 1901–1982: A Facet of Science Development in the Philippines*. Manila: Philippine Association for the Advancement of Science, 1984.

Vergara, Benito M., Jr. *Displaying Filipinos: Photography and Colonialism in Early-Twentieth-Century Philippines*. Quezon City: University of the Philippines Press, 1995.

Vergès, Françoise. "Chains of Madness, Chains of Colonialism: Fanon and Freedom." In *The Fact of Blackness: Frantz Fanon and Visual Representation*, edited by Alan Read, 47–75. Seattle: Bay Press, 1996.

Vigarello, Georges. *Concepts of Cleanliness: Changing Attitudes in France since the Middle Ages*. Translated by Jean Birrell. Cambridge and Paris: Cambridge University Press and Editions de la maison des sciences de l'homme, 1988.

Visvanathan, Shiv. "On the Annals of the Laboratory State." In *Science, Hegemony and Violence: A Requiem for Modernity*, edited by Ashis Nandy, 257–88. New Delhi: Oxford University Press, 1988.

Vogel, Morris J. "Managing Medicine: Creating a Profession of Hospital Administration in the United States, 1895–1915." In *The Hospital in History*, edited by Lindsay Granshaw and Roy Porter, 243–60. New York: Routledge, 1989.

[Wade, H. W., ed.]. *Culion: A Record of Fifty Years Work with the Victims of Leprosy at the Culion Sanitarium*. Manila: Bureau of Printing, 1956.

Walker, David. *A Selected Bibliography of Malaria in the Philippines*. Manila: Bureau of Printing, 1953.

Warner, John Harley. *The Therapeutic Perspective: Medical Practice, Knowledge and Identity in America, 1820–1885*. Cambridge: Harvard University Press, 1986.

———. "The Idea of Southern Medical Distinctiveness: Medical Knowledge and Practice in the Old South." In *Sickness and Health in America: Readings in the History of Medicine and Public Health*. 2nd ed. Edited by Judith Walzer Leavitt and Ronald L. Numbers, 53–70. Madison: University of Wisconsin Press, 1985.

Weigley, Russell F. *History of the United States Army*. Bloomington: Indiana University Press, 1984.

Weindling, Paul, ed. *International Health Organizations and Movements, 1918–1939*. Cambridge: Cambridge University Press, 1995.

Welch, Richard E., Jr. *Response to Imperialism: The United States and the Philippine-American War, 1899–1902*. Chapel Hill: University of North Carolina Press, 1979.

Whorton, James C. "Insecticide Spray Residues and Public Health, 1865–1938." *Bulletin of the History of Medicine* 45 (1971): 219–41.

Wiebe, Robert H. *The Search for Order, 1877–1920*. New York: Hill and Wang, 1967.

Williams, Ralph Chester. *The United States Public Health Service, 1798–1950*. Washington, D.C.: Commissioned Officers Association of the USPHS, 1951.

Williams, Walter L. "United States Indian Policy and the Debate over Philippine Annexation: Implications for the Origins of American Imperialism." *J. of American History* 66 (1980): 810–31.

Williams, William Appleman. *Empire as a Way of Life: An Essay on the Causes and Consequences of America's Present Predicament*. New York: Oxford University Press, 1980.

———. "The Frontier Thesis and American Foreign Policy." *Pacific Historical Review* 24 (1955): 379–95.

Wilson, Rob. *American Sublime: The Genealogy of a Poetic Genre*. Madison: University of Wisconsin Press, 1991.

———. "Techno-euphoria and the Discourse of the American Sublime." *boundary 2* 19 (1992): 205–29.

Winichakul, Thongchai. *Siam Mapped: A History of the Geo-Body of the Nation*. Honolulu: University of Hawaii Press, 1993.

Winslow, Charles-Edward Amory. *The Life of Hermann M. Biggs, Physician and Statesman of Public Health*. Philadelphia: Lea and Febiger, 1929.

———. *The Conquest of Epidemic Disease: A Chapter in the History of Ideas*. Madison: University of Wisconsin Press, 1980 [1943].

Winzeler, R. "Amok: Historical, Psychological, and Cultural Perspectives." In *Emotions of Culture: A Malay Perspective*, edited by Wazir Jahan Karim, 96–122. Singapore: Oxford University Press, 1990.

Worboys, Michael. *Spreading Germs: Disease Theories and Medical Practice in Britain, 1865–1900*. Cambridge: Cambridge University Press, 2000.

———. "Manson, Ross and Colonial Medical Policy: Tropical Medicine in London and Liverpool, 1899–1914." In *Disease, Medicine and Empire: Perspectives on Western Medicine and the Experience of European Expansion*, edited by Roy MacLeod and Milton Lewis, 21–33. London: Routledge, 1988.

Wright, Gwendolyn. *The Politics of Design in French Colonial Urbanism*. Chicago: Chicago University Press, 1991.

Wright, Lawrence. *Clean and Decent: The Fascinating History of the Bathroom and the Water Closet*. London: Routledge Kegan Paul, 1960.

Young, Iris Marion. "Polity and Group Difference: A Critique of the Ideal of Universal Citizenship." *Ethics* 99 (1989): 250–74.

Young, Kenneth Ray. *The General's General: The Life and Times of Arthur MacArthur*. Boulder: Westview Press, 1994.

Young, Robert J. C. *Colonial Desire: Hybridity in Theory, Culture and Race*. London: Routledge, 1995.

Zaide, Gregorio F. *Philippine Political and Cultural History*. 2 vols. Manila: Philippine Educational Co., 1957.

———. *The Philippine Revolution*. Manila: Modern Book Co., 1968.

Zinoman, Peter. *The Colonial Bastille: A History of Imprisonment in Vietnam, 1862–1940*. Berkeley: University of California Press, 2001.

Index

de Witt, Wallace, 81, 104, 261n.28
dichloro-diphenyl-trichloroethane (DDT), 224–25
dietary needs, 43
discipline: in leper colonies, 162, 171, 177–79; in military medicine, 26–30; in tropical neurasthenia prevention, 144–47
disease control: American military programs for, 15–17; in colonial Philippines, 2–3; Filipinization of, 181–82, 189–93; scientific approach to, 137–42
Dutch East Indies, 4, 99
dysentery, 61, 129, 143–44, 272n.107

ecological intervention, 208–26
economic conditions, 207–8
Edger, Benjamin J., 108–9
educational programs: changes in focus of, 208; for hookworm eradication, 199, 202; for malaria control, 211–12, 221; on sanitation and hygiene, 116–20, 202–3, 289nn.100–101. See also medical education
Egan, Eleanor Franklin, 167–68
Eighth Army Corps, 241n.10
El Ideal, 125, 147
elite Filipinos: Americans viewed by, 204; at Baguio, 145–47, 277n.61; colonial collaborative compromise with, 187, 286n.32; Filipinization resisted by, 183, 286n.29; public health policies and, 51–52; response to cholera epidemic among, 67–68
Elliot, Charles Burke, 146, 277n.61
Emerson, Haven, 229, 297n.7
environmental conditions: malarial control programs and, 208–26; military medical research on, 24–30; racial economy in tropics and, 37–43
epidemic disease: colonial politics and, 61–69; military medical control procedures for, 28–30, 244n.55. See also specific epidemics
Escobar, Arturo, 285n.16
ethnic identity of Filipinos: American

homogenization and, 3, 238n.8, 239n.24; carnival and, 124–28; nationalism movement and, 20–22; Spanish classification, 19–22, 241n.16. See also racial typologies
evangelism, 162–63
excrement: as colonial racial obsession, 8–11, 104–29; military medical policies on, 27–30; parasite research and, 194–205. See also toilets

Fabella, José, 227
Fajardo, Jacobo, 202, 227, 289n.100
Fales, Louis, 138–40, 275nn.31–32
Fanon, Franz, 278n.79
Fauntleroy, P. C., 37, 231
Federal Party, 186, 258n.101
Federated Malay states, 281n.31
Fee, Mary H., 89
feminist theory, 3
fiesta, 120–28
Filaria nocturna, 194
Filipino culture: carnival and, 123–28, 271n.86; civic virtue rhetoric and, 54–58; Filipinization campaign and racialization of, 186–93; human waste habits in, 104–29; immunity mechanisms assumed in, 92–95; leprosy policy in, 175–77; "mimicry" aspects of, 180–205; psychoanalysis in, 132; racialization of, 3–11, 59–61, 69–73, 128–29, 238n.8; response to cholera epidemic in, 66–68; sanitary immunity and supposed resistance, 95–101; tropical disease concepts rejected in, 147
Filipino physiology: immunity and, 88–95, 102–3; leprosy research and, 166–68; tropical medicine research and, 74–76, 85–87; tropical neurasthenia and, 141–42, 157, 278n.79
Finlay, Carlos, 215
Fleming, Kenneth, 35, 246n.84
Flexner, Simon, 32, 79, 255n.74, 260n.19
Forbes, W. Cameron, 1, 89, 123–25, 130–31, 253n.45, 266n.8; Baguio sanitarium and, 142, 146–47, 276n.49,

Hospital de San José, 18

Hospital de San Juan de Dios, 18

hospitals in Philippines: American military construction of, 33–35, 245n.77, 246n.83; Filipinization of, 184–93; for lepers, 162–63; military oversight of, 50; Spanish construction of, 18

Hoyt, Henry F., 31–33, 35, 194, 245nn.64, 68

Huggins, Eli, 141, 275n.41

humidity hypothesis of neurasthenia, 152

Hunt, William H., 195

Huntington, Ellsworth, 139–40, 275n.33

Hyam, Ronald, 132–33

hygiene policies: among American Indians, 58, 254n.59; in bubonic plague outbreak, 62–69; cholera epidemic and Filipino practices of, 63–64; at Culion leper colony, 158–61, 168–75; economic factors in, 207–9; Filipinization and, 3, 181–93; in hookworm eradication programs, 195–205; human waste disposal policies and, 105–29; immunity and, 89–95, 101–3; leprosy and, 162–68; in military medical infrastructure, 1–11, 23–30, 45–73, 237n.1, 244n.59, 249n.5; in postwar Philippines, 69–73; racialization of, 3–4, 8–11, 37–43; sanitary immunity concept and, 96–101; state-run Filipino health program and, 227–33; as surveillance apparatus, 128–29; in tropical conditions, 30–37, 42–43; in tropical neurasthenia prevention, 144–47; in United States, 229–33; white male dominance of, 6; white physiology in tropics and, 82–87

Ide, Henry C., 253n.45

identity formation, 4–11

Igorots: classification of, 242n.16; in Philippine-American war, 33; physiological studies of, 86–87, 92; racialized exhibitions of, 124–25

Ileto, Reynaldo C., 2–3, 5, 249n.2, 251n.23

ilustrados, 191–93

immigration: by Filipinos to United States, 232–33; by white Americans to Philippines, 79–81, 260n.22

immunity: Filipinization of programs and, 189–93; imperialist concepts of, 87–95; to malaria, 211, 213, 291n.14; sanitary immunity concept, 95–101

imperialism: civic virtue rhetoric and, 52–58; immunity concepts and, 87–95; masculinity and, 132–34; race and, 2

India: British health policies in, 99; leprosy in, 169, 281n.31; malaria control in, 214, 223–24, 292n.28, 295n.75

Indian Psychoanalytic Society, 152, 277n.71

indios, 19–20, 241n.16

industrial hygiene, 231–32, 298n.17

Instituto di Sanità Pubblica (Italy), 217

international health and development programs, 10–11, 232–33

International Health Commission (Board), 196–99, 203–4, 215–16, 223, 232–33, 293n.42

International Journal of Leprosy, 283n.75

International Leprosy Association, 283n.75

interracial sex, 5, 239n.20

intimacy: in colonial hygiene policies, 4–5, 239n.19; in leper colonies, 160–61

Iwahig Prison Colony, 221–22, 295n.68

Jackson, Thomas W., 101

Jagor, Fedor, 77

James, William, 187, 266n.8

Jansen, Paul F., 283n.73

Japan: Culion quarantined by, 284n.88; leprosy, 281n.31; Philippines invaded by, 228; public health programs, 99

Jenks, Albert E., 284n.86

Joaquin, Nick, 127–28

Johnson, Richard, 65, 166, 257n.90

Jones Act, 188

Jordan, David Starr, 260n.25

Katipunan, 20

Kemp, Franklin M., 32–33

masculinity (*continued*)
    sexual identity and, 148–50, 152–54;
    tropical disease among white males and,
    74–76; tropical neurasthenia as threat
    to, 132–34, 154–57, 182, 273n.9,
    278n.75. *See also* gender; women
Mason, Charles F., 39–40, 42, 248n.109
Maus, Anna Page Russell, 66, 257n.98
Maus, L. Mervin, 251n.25, 275n.41;
    Baguio sanitarium and, 276n.47; chol-
    era epidemic and, 66–68; on colonial
    sanitation, 48, 51–52; Heiser and, 70;
    on immunity, 88; leprosy research and,
    164; on prostitution and venereal dis-
    ease, 251n.27; racialization of hygiene
    and, 59; Worcester and, 252n.29,
    256n.84
Mayo, Katherine, 115, 167–68, 269n.49
McDill, John, 82, 231
McDonnell, P. G., 147, 277n.63
McIntyre, Frank, 190
McKinley, E. B., 199, 220
McKinley, William, 17
McLaughlin, Allan J., 101, 119, 171, 230–
    31
Meacham, Franklin A., 48–49, 251n.25
Mearns, Lilian Hathaway, 110
medical education: of Filipino physicians,
    184–87, 198; hygiene principles in, 29–
    30; international developments in,
    244n.59; lack of training in tropical
    medicine in, 30–37; military training
    programs for, 29–30, 244n.59;
    nationalist politics and, 191–93; racial-
    ization in Philippines of, 20–21
Medical Field Service School, 49, 231
medical geography: military medical pol-
    icies and, 24–25, 243nn.35–36; racial
    and ethnic characteristics and, 41–42
Mencken, H. L., 134–36, 149–51
mental deterioration: climate and, 87; colo-
    nial concepts of, 9; in leper colonies,
    172–73; military medical research on,
    40–43, 248nn.109–10; as moral
    failure, 154–57; psychic burden of
    whiteness and, 130–57; psychoanalytic

theories of, 150–54; tropical neuras-
    thenia concept and, 132–42, 147–50
Mercado, Eliodoro, 281n.42
Merritt, Wesley, 14
Mestizos, 19–20, 241n.16; racial stereo-
    typing of, 56, 259n.11
microbiological research: on leprosy, 163,
    280nn.17–18; military medical policies
    and, 24–25, 28–30; Philippine sanita-
    tion policies and, 58–61; in postwar
    Philippines, 71–73; racial concepts of
    immunity and, 90–95, 102–3; wartime
    limitations on, 47
Mieldazis, J. J., 198, 218–19
military medicine: Army Medical Depart-
    ment transformations of, 22–30; ascen-
    dancy of, 29–30, 245n.61; characteris-
    tics of, in Philippines, 17–22; codifica-
    tion of, during Philippine-American
    war, 15; colonial public health in Phil-
    ippines and, 45–73; history of, in Phil-
    ippines, 8–11; limitations of, in tropics,
    30–37; malaria control models of,
    210–11, 224–25, 295n.79; race-based
    health policies of, in Philippines, 2;
    racial economy of tropics and, 37–43;
    research legacy of, 231; tropical neuras-
    thenia research and, 141–42, 275n.40
mimesis: in Filipinization of bureaucracy,
    183–84, 205–6, 290n.114; in hook-
    worm eradication programs, 199–205
Minier, John F., 142–43
missionaries, 162
Molokai, Hawaii, 175, 282n.71
Monnais-Rousselot, Laurence, 98
morality: human waste disposal policies
    and, 106–7; racialized colonial con-
    cepts of, 9, 47, 89–90; in military medi-
    cal policies, 26–30, 40; tropical neuras-
    thenia and, 139–42, 154–57
morbidity and mortality statistics: in chol-
    era epidemic, 65–66, 68, 257n.89; Fil-
    ipinization of health service and, 189–
    90, 287n.44; on malaria, 210–12; dur-
    ing Philippine-American war, 14–17,
    38, 240n.4, 247n.95; tropical climate

and, 79–81; white physiology in tropics and, 81–87; for whites in Philippines, 74–76

Morel, Bénédict Augustin, 138

Moriarty, C. F., 199–200, 204–5, 219

Moros: American colonial policies and, 5, 58, 239n.24; classification of, 242n.16; racialized stereotypes of, 142

Morris, Charles, 79, 260n.16

Moses, Bernard, 56, 253nn.45, 49, 275n.40

Moses, Edith, 93, 110, 121

mosquito control programs, 211–26

mosquito netting, 209–11, 221–22

Munson, Edward L., 243n.33; 250n.16; cholera epidemic and, 65–66, 68, 108, 190; on diet in tropics, 43; Heiser and, 70; hookworm eradication program and, 199; on human waste disposal, 105; hygiene policies and, 27–28, 49, 231; on medical geography, 24–25; on mental and moral health, 40–41; on sanitation, 58; on tuberculosis prevalence, 291n.3; on venereal disease, 243n.44

Musgrave, W. E., 85, 100, 157, 229, 261n.43, 278n.79

Muslim Filipinos, 141–42

Musset, Alfred de, 141

Mycobacterium leprae, 163, 167

Najera, J. A., 295nn.77–78

Nandy, Ashis, 132–33, 271n.71, 278n.77

nastin, 170, 281n.46

National Association of Manufacturers, 231–32

National Guard, 30

nationalism: Filipino ethnic identity and, 20–21; leprosy management policies and, 160–62, 175–77, 283n.74; in medicine and science, 191–93, 206; opposition to carnival and, 124–28, 272n.105

National Library of Medicine, 242n.24

Necator americanus, 194–95

Nesbitt, Charles T., 195–96

New York City Public Health Department, 229–30, 297n.13

New York Herald, 189

Nichols, H. J., 85, 194

Nietzsche, Friedrich, 135

non-Christian Filipinos, 3, 238n.8

Notes on Military Hygiene, 49

Notter, J. Lane, 24–25, 39

nursing, 201–5, 233

O'Reilly, G. A., 123

Osgood, H. D., 251n.25

Osler, William, 142, 276n.46

Osmeña, Sergio, 283n.73

Panama Canal Zone, 214–15, 229, 292n.31, 297n.6

Pan-American Sanitary Bureau, 233

parasitology research, in Philippines, 194–205

Pardo de Tavera, T. H., 67–68, 186–87, 258n.101, 286n.27

Paris Green, 218–19, 221–24, 293n.44, 295n.71

Parke, Glenn V., 13–15

Pasteur, Louis, 87

pathology, 8–11, 25

peninsulares, 19–20, 241n.16

Phalen, James M., 84–85, 194

Phelan, Henry du Rest, 107

Philippine-American War: American military medicine and, 8, 13–17, 30–37; civil morbidity and mortality during, 14–15, 21–22, 240n.4; military strategy in, 46–47

Philippine Civil Affairs Unit, 228

Philippine Commission, 43, 54–56, 67–68, 111, 186

Philippine Expeditionary Force, 241n.10

Philippine General Hospital, 190

Philippine Health Service, 197, 220–21, 227–33, 251n.24, 294n.64

Philippine Islands Medical Association, 82, 176, 231

Philippine Journal of Science, 185

Philippine Republic, 20

regional health programs in Asia of, 175, 265n.102, 289n.84

Rodgers, James B., 282n.63

Rogaski, Ruth, 10

Roosevelt, Nicholas, 114, 131

Roosevelt, Theodore: immigration policies of, 254n.57; imperialism and, 52–55, 57, 190, 237n.2

Roosevelt, Theodore, Jr., 208, 221

Root, Elihu, 52–53

Rose, Wickliffe, 195–97, 216, 293n.37

Ross, Ronald, 76, 209–10, 214–15, 243n.36, 291n.6

Roxas, Manuel, 283n.74

rural health programs, in Philippines, 199–205

Russell, F. F., 203, 205, 290n.105, 295n.70

Russell, Paul F., 198, 201, 204, 215, 217, 220–27, 233, 294n.64, 296n.81

St. Louis Exhibition, 125

Saldivar, José David, 8

Salman, Michael, 5, 279n.3

San Francisco, 230, 297n.10

San Francisco Corporation, 18

Sanitary Commission for the Eradication of Hookworm Disease, 195, 197–98

sanitary commissions, 116–20

sanitary engineering, 108, 267n.18

sanitary immunity, 87–88, 95–101

Sanitary Model House exhibit, 126–27

sanitation infrastructure: bubonic plague outbreak and, 62–69; at Carnival celebrations, 121–28; cholera epidemic and, 65–68, 249n.2; Clean-Up Week campaign for, 127–28; colonial policies on, 1–3, 18–19, 69–73, 237n.1, 241n.13; at Culion leper colony, 169–75; Filipinization of, 181, 189–93, 200–205; in Filipino culture, 92–95; hookworm eradication programs and, 195–205; in marketplace, 114–16, 259nn.53–54; military medical policies on, 15–17, 23–30, 48–53, 58–60, 244n.59, 245n.74; racialized concepts

of, 8–11, 107–29; Rockefeller Foundation programs for, 199–200; in tropical conditions, 30–37; in United States, 241n.13

San Lazaro Hospital, 18, 64, 162–63, 165, 190, 256n.86

Sardinia, 217–18, 225, 293n.42

Schapiro, Louis , 229

School of Sanitation and Public Health (Manila), 217

self-government: at Culion leper colony, 175–77, 179; education linked to, 207; Filipinization and, 186–93, 286n.29; racialized colonial policy and, 4–11, 54–58, 182–84, 203–5, 285n.12

Sellards, Andrew W., 129, 231, 272n.107

sexuality, 149–54. *See also* gender; masculinity

Shakespeare, E. O., 244n.55

Shaklee, Alfred O., 83

Shaler, Nathaniel Southgate, 101–2, 265n.111

Sibul Springs, 276n.47

Sinha, Mrinalini, 132–33

Sison, Agerico B. G., 85, 202

Sloper, Mary E., 35

smallpox: Filipinization of vaccination program, 189–90; immunity to, 88; in San Francisco, 98; vaccination programs for, 38–39

Smart, Charles, 29

Smith, James F., 115, 253n.45, 269n.50

Snodgrass, John, 170–71, 233, 281n.42

social gospel, 2–3, 237n.2

Soper, Fred L., 225

Southall, E. A., 256n.86

Spanish occupation of Philippines, 17–22; leper colonies during, 162–63; medical geographies and, 76–78, 259nn.10–11; response to cholera and, 64, 256n.85

Stanley, Peter, 253n.45, 286n.32

Stapleton, Darwin H., 217, 293n.42

Stelle, Matthew F., 42

Stepan, Nancy, 3

Stephens, J. W. W., 213–14

vertical disease control techniques, 225–26, 295n.79

Von Ezdorf, R. H., 215–16

Wade, H. W., 283n.75

Walker, E. L., 129, 213, 272n.107

Washburn, William S., 81–82, 261n.29

Watson, Malcolm, 214

Welch, William, 246n.77

Welfareville Institution, 159

Wherry, W. B., 298n.15

"White Man's Burden," 4, 132–34, 273n.16

whiteness: American military concepts of, 15–17, 43–44, 241n.8; climatic burden of, 76–81; fragility and ambivalence of, 134, 273n.18; immunity and, 87–95; physiology in tropics and, 81–87, 262n.51; psychic burden of, 130–57; in public health programs, 6–11, 239n.28; racialization of human waste disposal and, 106–7; sexuality and, 152–54; tropical disease morbidity and mortality analysis and, 74–76; tropical neurasthenia and, 38–43, 137–42, 156–57, 278n.77

Who Walk Alone, 173–74

Wickline, W. A., 262n.57

Widal typhoid test, 28, 94

Wilkinson, H. B., 165

Willets, David, 119, 270n.70

Williams, Daniel R., 114–15, 189, 287n.40

Wilson, Woodrow, 182–84, 187

Winslow, Charles-Edward Amory, 97

Wolley, Paul G., 298n.15

women: tropical climate effects on, 79; in Filipino hygiene programs, 6; as health-care workers, 200, 233; in leper colonies, 160, 171–75,

282n.49; tropical neurasthenia research and, 140, 275n.37. *See also* gender

Wood, Leonard, 82, 122, 175–77, 191, 217, 272n.104, 283n.75, 287n.52

Wood, W. T., 83–84

Woodhull, Alfred A., 34–37, 49, 245n.77

Woodruff, Charles E., 15, 43, 249n.124; malaria advice of, 91, 208; military medical authority and, 245n.61, 248n.120; tropical neurasthenia research by, 80–81, 83, 87, 137–40, 156, 260nn.23–25, 274n.27

Woodward, C. M., 25

Worcester, Dean C., 124–25, 250n.20, 253n.45, 275n.41; Baguio sanitarium and, 143, 146, 276n.47; on cholera epidemic, 63, 257n.97; colonial hygiene policies and, 52, 72–73; Filipinization resisted by, 185–86, 188, 284n.38; on leper colonies, 164, 176–77; Maus and, 68, 252n.29, 256n.84; Philippine hospital construction and, 50

World Health Organization, 295n.77

Wright, George "Skypilot," 283n.73

Wright, Luke, 66, 253n.45, 258n.113, 276n.47

Wu, T. C., 282n.61

Wyman, Walter, 70

x-ray treatment, for leprosy, 281n.42

Yaeger, C. H., 181, 200–204, 219

Yeater, Charles H., 189

yellow fever, 215, 225

Yellow Fever Commission, 244n.55

Yersin, Alexandre, 61

Zinoman, Peter, 279n.3

Warwick Anderson is Robert Turell Professor of Medical History and Population Health and professor of the history of science, as well as a faculty associate of the Center for Southeast Asian Studies, at the University of Wisconsin, Madison. He is the author of *The Cultivation of Whiteness: Science, Health, and Racial Destiny in Australia* (Melbourne University Press, 2002; Basic Books, 2003; paperback, Duke, 2006).

Library of Congress Cataloging-in-Publication Data
Anderson, Warwick
Colonial pathologies : American tropical medicine, race, and hygiene in the Philippines / Warwick Anderson.
p. cm.
Includes bibliographical references and index.
ISBN-13: 978-0-8223-3804-8 (cloth : alk. paper)
ISBN-10: 0-8223-3804-1 (cloth : alk. paper)
ISBN-13: 978-0-8223-3843-7 (pbk. : alk. paper)
ISBN-10: 0-8223-3843-2 (pbk. : alk. paper)
1. Tropical medicine — Philippines — History. 2. Military hygiene — Philippines — History.
3. Philippines — Colonization — History. I. Title.
RC962.P6A53 2006
616.9′883009599 — dc22   2006004594